# Bioethics, Healthcare and the Soul

This thought-provoking book explores the connections between health, ethics, and soul. It analyzes how and why the soul has been lost from scientific discourses, healthcare practices, and ethical discussions, presenting suggestions for change.

Arguing that the dominant scientific worldview has eradicated talk abou the soul and presents an objective and technical approach to human life and it vulnerabilities, Ten Have and Pegoraro look to rediscover identity, humanity, an meaning in healthcare and bioethics. Taking a multidisciplinary approach, the investigate philosophical, scientific, historical, cultural, social, religious, economi and environmental perspectives as they journey toward a new, global bioethi emphasizing the role of the moral imagination.

*Bioethics, Healthcare and the Soul* is an important read for students, research and practitioners interested in bioethics and person-centered healthcare.

**Henk ten Have** is Professor Emeritus at the Center for Healthcare Ethic Duquesne University, Pittsburgh, USA, and Research Professor at Anal University in Mexico.

**Renzo Pegoraro** is Chancellor of the Pontifical Academy for Life in Rom Professor of Bioethics at the Faculty of Theology of North-East of Italy.

# Bioethics, Healthcare and the Soul

Henk ten Have and Renzo Pegoraro

Routledge
Taylor & Francis Group
LONDON AND NEW YORK

First published 2022
by Routledge
2 Park Square, Milton Park, Abingdon, Oxon OX14 4RN

and by Routledge
52 Vanderbilt Avenue, New York, NY 10017

*Routledge is an imprint of the Taylor & Francis Group, an informa business*



*British Library Cataloguing-in-Publication Data*
A catalogue record for this book is available from the British Library

*Library of Congress Cataloging-in-Publication Data*
A catalog record for this book has been requested

ISBN: 978-1-032-07156-5 (hbk)
ISBN: 978-1-032-07603-4 (pbk)
ISBN: 978-1-003-20565-4 (ebk)

Typeset in Goudy
by Apex CoVantage, LLC

# Contents

# 1 Introduction

## The soul in healthcare and ethics

Surgeon and writer Sherwin Nuland published a collection of stories, first-person narratives of various medical specialists, titled *The Soul of Medicine*. [1] Nuland does not explain the title, but the stories illustrate his point. Physicians cannot be technicians. They play a diversity of roles: pastor, counselor, advocate, guide but also friend and confidant. Only at the closing page of the book, Nuland concludes that while diagnosis has much improved, and is faster and more accurate today than ever before, something has been lost in healthcare. More data, information, and, perhaps, knowledge will enable us to categorize patients but what is more important is clinical judgment: the particular understanding of the treating physician about what is best for this individual patient. Another medical writer, internist Jerome Groopman, points out how medicine desperately tries to combine two different dimensions, an objective, disease-centered one and a subjective, patient-centered one. Healing requires a mixture of science and soul. [2] A third medical writer, Atul Gawande, also a surgeon, explains that contemporary medicine has a narrow focus; it concentrates on repair of health, "not sustenance of the soul." [3] This is especially important now that many people live longer and have chronic diseases and disabilities. They do not want treatment but care. First of all, they want an existence that is worthwhile and meaningful and has a purpose, rather than the continuation of treatment, or the safety and protection in a nursing home when they become dependent and vulnerable.

The above-mentioned authors of bestselling books continue a long tradition of physicians who are also writers and involved in literary activities. It is often assumed that doctors are good storytellers because they are, perhaps more than other people, able to observe intense and dramatic human experiences. They see, meet, and talk to people in the most vulnerable circumstances. In their writings, they may not directly focus on medical issues but they frequently highlight the travails of daily life and the precariousness of the human predicament. An example is Anton Chekhov (1860–1904). He practiced as a medical doctor and wrote many stories and plays to earn money to support his family and his education. He is regarded as the master of the short story, portraying human misery, tragic dimensions of life, and what is below the surface of everyday existence. Mikhail Bulgakov (1891–1940) is another example. He worked as a provincial physician but abandoned medical practice after a serious illness. He wrote feuilletons for newspapers, plays, and novels. Well known is his collection of short stories (*A Country Doctor's Notebook*) about his experiences as a young doctor in a small village in Smolensk province. Louis-Ferdinand Céline (1894–1961) first worked in Paris at a maternity hospital and later started a private practice as obstetrician. His two most famous novels, *Journey to the End of the Night* (1932) and *Death on the Installment Plan* (1936), present a shocking vision of suffering and despair as well as the banality and absurdity of human life. All human weaknesses are exploited but at the same time there is compassion with suffering fellow beings. The Dutch writer Simon Vestdijk (1989–1971) worked as general practitioner and ship's doctor. After 1932, he no longer practiced medicine but focused on writing literature and poems. He was one of the most productive Dutch authors, publishing approximately 200 books. Many doctors figure in his work, but usually not in a positive way. In his view, physicians as human beings are less interesting than their professional activities would suggest. An important Portuguese writer today is psychiatrist António Lobo Antunes (1942). He uses his experiences in the psychiatric hospital as well as in the colonial war in Angola as material for his novels, especially the early ones. Medicine and travel are frequent topics in his work.

Faced with the realities of human suffering, physician-writers show in different ways what they regard as essential for medicine. In his stories, Anton Chekhov outlines the details of suffering in order to emphasize that it is not acceptable. Human beings have the capacity of empathy so that they can share suffering. This capacity is fundamental for medicine. Chekhov as a materialist did not believe in the existence of the human soul. In his view, mental and physical phenomena are similar. Human life is characterized by stagnation, stupidity, degradation, and mediocrity. Nonetheless, the "soul" of medicine for him is not accepting indifference and detachment in regard to suffering. The medical perspective entails the conviction that life can and should be changed. Being a physician implies a sense of dignity that cannot accept these miserable conditions of human life. [4] The work of Louis-Ferdinand Céline is frequently regarded as dark and nihilistic. It celebrates the death of compassion. At the same time, it is paradoxical in that it struggles to reconnect with basic humanity. Bardamu, the main character in *Journey to the End of the Night*, and alter ego of Céline, is a dehumanized physician beyond compassion but he attempts to recover his lost humanity. [5] The soul is associated with darkness, exile, death, and weakness but is also the source of meaningfulness. Bardamu's experiences as a physician, his lack of empathy, and his cynical interactions with patients can serve as a negative role model for medical students, while Céline himself apparently was a caring doctor for the poor. [6]

Physician-writers often have their own burden of disease. Chekhov suffered and eventually died from tuberculosis. Bulgakov was badly injured in the first World War; to deal with the chronic pain, he became addicted to morphine. Céline was also wounded in this war, making him disabled for the rest of his life. Vestdijk was plagued by depressions since his adolescence. As doctors, they see their patients at the most vulnerable moments of their life, but they likewise become aware of their own vulnerability. Writing and reading stories expand the worldview of physicians, making them aware of ethical dilemmas but first of all teach them the importance of subjectivity and the primacy of care. This is why, these stories refer to the notion of soul; they are concerned with what is the core, the essence of medicine and healthcare.

Talk of the soul is paradoxical. In contemporary culture and society, the soul is no longer regarded as an existing entity or substance. In the age of scientific materialism, the soul is dead. [7] According to the dominating worldview of science, it is a myth, an illusion. It should be erased since it is not a necessary or useful concept to explain the world. It can be reduced to something else, to brains or genes. There is only matter. Every mental phenomenon can be explained in terms of physical principles and laws. The soul or the mind therefore is the brain. The concept of soul is perhaps useful as a metaphor, a figure of speech. Nonetheless, despite these negative assessments, the soul is often addressed in a wide range of human activities: in philosophy, in religion, in poetry and art, in literature, and in music. Many people believe in soulmates. In some countries, there is soul music and soul food. The soul is connected to many positive images: a vital force, the core of individuality, the stream of consciousness, the persistence of things, the depth dimension of human experiences, the heart of things, breath, the live-giving principle. [8] If the soul is lost, something essential will be missing. Erasure of the soul generates alienation, rootlessness, apathy, inauthenticity, meaninglessness, and inhumanity. Even if we do not understand what soul is, it will be important to cultivate it, to contemplate what it means, and to sustain it with care. [9]

Soul is a fuzzy concept. It is associated with a wide range of ideas and themes. Its field of application is also very broad. Questions can be asked about the soul of medicine or the soul of a nation. [10] These questions are taken seriously because suggestions that the soul is missing signal that something crucial that used to be determinative has now vanished. The term "soul" is frequently connected to and exchanged with other words such as mind, spirit, psyche, and pneuma. It is not clear to what the soul refers. However, its basic function is that it identifies what is characteristic for an entity, substance, practice, or activity. The soul of medicine refers to what is the essence of medicine. It is what inspires, drives, gives life to medical activities. In this sense, soul is used as a metaphor. The purpose is to criticize and denounce the prevailing materialism of science, showing that more is at stake than simple physical interactions. The metaphor refers to another, more fundamental use of the notion of soul. This use applies to human beings. Soul is considered as the realm of unique human capacities and experiences. It identifies and explains what is typically human in human beings. The soul is the personal, individual essence of every human. Specific human capacities such as self-awareness, rationality, morality, language, memory, free agency, responsibility, future orientation, spirituality, and relations with other human beings and God are all attributed to the soul. The term soul is therefore used to refer not only to distinctive aspects of human beings as a special category of beings but also to characteristics of individual persons. The basic idea conveyed by the concept is that human nature transcends the physical and biological world. Human nature cannot be reduced to DNA or brain activities. How the soul is specifically conceptualized is a matter of long-standing debates, especially in philosophy and religion.

Is it a real entity or force? How is it connected or interacting with the body? Is it a part of the self that continues beyond death?

This book will explore the connections between healthcare, ethics, and soul. It will examine the complaints that the soul has been lost in healthcare as well as in bioethics. These charges express the uneasiness, dissatisfaction, and disquiet that many people today experience with healthcare and also with the ethical queries that emerge in the medical setting. That such uneasiness is expressed in terms of loss of soul has something to do with the dominant scientific worldview that has completely eradicated any soul-talk and that presents an objective and technical approach to human life and its vulnerabilities.

The aim of this book is to use the notion of soul and its loss to review a wide range of familiar criticisms of contemporary medicine and bioethics in order to arrive at a broader understanding of bioethics. We do not intend to provide a rigorous philosophical or theological analysis of the concept of the soul, nor to scrutinize the philosophical foundations of medicine and healthcare, but our aim is to propose a moral vision for medicine and bioethics that goes beyond the narrow and technical forms of ethical thinking that dominate current practices, using a variety of sources and disciplines. Although we are attracted to the Aristotelian-Thomist concept of the soul, we do not develop a theoretical formulation of this concept, but use "soul" as container term and as a metaphor to essential aspects of human existence that are not accounted for in the practice of medicine and discourse of ethics, in the hope to recover these aspects.

## The erasure of the soul

This book will first analyze how and why the soul has been lost from scientific discourses, healthcare practices, and ethical discussions.

The notion of soul has almost disappeared from theological and philosophical discourse. Theologians have substituted the word "spirit" for soul so that they can distinguish between secular and spiritual aspects of human life. For many philosophers, soul is the ghost in the machine, and no longer a serious object of reflection. Psychology has discarded the soul as a relic from ancient times, and is studying the mind and consciousness. Science is most radical: the idea that people have souls is superstition. Nonetheless, the term "soul" is widely used in ordinary life as well as in cultural and popular literature. In almost every culture, belief in the soul is persistent since ancient times. Nowadays, more than half of secondary school pupils in Britain (54%) believe that people have souls (with 23% disagreeing), with 45% professing to believe in God. [11] A survey in 2009 found that 70% of people in the United Kingdom believe in the human soul, while 53% believe in life after death. [12] In Western Europe, 76% of religious people say they have a soul, while 43% of people who are neither religious nor spiritual also affirm they have a soul. [13] While fewer Americans believe in God, belief in life after death in the United States is stable since decades and increasing recently (80% in 2014). [14] A similar majority of Americans believe that every person has an immortal soul (79%).

This divergence between the scientific discourse of eradication of the soul and the active experiences of soul in everyday life explains why there is a continuous argumentation, and frequently dissatisfaction and unhappiness concerning the loss of soul.

## Medicine lost its soul

Modern medicine has become "sick care," and does not create health. [15] It does not recognize the power of emotions in care and healing. The ideal is detachment, making the physician neglect his or her own emotions. As we will discuss later, the role of empathy is often downplayed so that patients do not have the feeling that the doctor is concerned about their suffering. Spiritual needs of patients, particularly at the end of life, are disregarded. Medicine also lost its soul because it does no longer provide holistic care, focused on the whole person. It is guided by a materialistic and mechanistic ideology that reduces the patient to a complex body machinery. Many patients are therefore disappointed and appeal to alternative approaches for a broader vision of health. [16] The focus of medicine is also primarily on treatment and cure, neglecting the wider context of the life story in which illness has emerged and developed. [17] Furthermore, the context of healthcare itself is disregarded: economic pressures, lack of time for interpersonal communication, and fragmentation of care lead to dehumanizing experiences for patients. For example, increasing attention for prevention without a population perspective will only reinforce the individualistic orientation of healthcare, overemphasizing personal responsibility for health and individual choice, thus violating the soul of public health. [18]

However, losing the soul of medicine has further implications for healthcare providers. More attention is currently given to their vulnerability and limitations. Dissatisfaction with medical practice is widespread among healthcare professionals. [19] Physician burnout, suicide, and moral distress are relatively common and are higher than in the general population. Among medical students, anxiety and depression are prevalent. Many clinicians are clinically depressed and consider dropping out of the profession. [20] The ideal of compassionate and empathic care with which they started medical school has not been achieved in daily practice. On the contrary, medical training has made them cynical, nihilistic, and numb. [21] It has encouraged professional distance and detachment. Like their patients, healthcare providers feel depersonalized. Current medicine offers no room for physicians as persons; in the words of some commentators, they have been reduced to automatons. [22] In this perspective, practicing medicine requires intellectual development, training of competencies, and skills but it is not considered a work of the heart and the soul.

## Bioethics lost its soul

Bioethics started as a social movement to balance medical power and to articulate the human dimensions of medicine but it became institutionalized and professionalized within relatively short time. It has lost its soul, according to Gilbert Meilaender, because it developed in a particular direction that made it impossible to address background beliefs about human nature and destiny. It has become a specific technology to resolve moral dilemmas, while fundamental questions about who we are and should be cannot be examined. Nonetheless, such basic queries of meaning and humanity were the initial inspiration for bioethical discourse. Nowadays, such discourse is primarily concerned with regulation and public policy with the goal of forging a social consensus. [23]

Soul defines what is essential to human beings. It is the reason why we have intrinsic moral status and dignity. It determines what makes the human organism into a person. It also defines life and death. If the soul is what makes us more than a biological organism, it is essential for ethics. [24] This fundamental idea is underlined by Thomas Moore in his bestselling book on *Care of the Soul*: "If we neglect our souls, we lose both our humanity and our individuality and risk becoming more like our machines and more absorbed into a crowd mentality." [25]

Neglect or loss of soul leads to loss of core values. That depersonalized and distanced conduct without compassion or empathy is quite remarkable, and is illustrated by the upsetting example of a physician who used a robot to tell a seriously ill patient in intensive care that nothing could be done to treat him and that he is going to die. [26] We will argue that complaints about lack of empathy and compassion are often associated with dissatisfaction with the dominant scientific worldview of naturalism. This is the philosophy that only those things are real that are within the scope of a purely scientific description of the world. Everything that exists is part of nature; there is no reality beyond or outside of nature. And only scientific beliefs are justified. Morality, values, and normativity are not part of the natural world. [27] Interpreting medicine as a natural science implies that there is no soul; thus, ethics, values, moral responsibility, and freedom of will are illusions. It also implies that first-person perspectives are eliminated. Focusing on biological mechanisms will be sufficient for diagnosis and treatment. The third-person perspective of the detached expert will provide a complete understanding of what the patient is experiencing. This naturalistic worldview is not frequently criticized in bioethical debate. It is often taken for granted as an implicit metaphysical background.

Eradicating the soul furthermore frames the bioethical debate in a specific direction. It is common to reject soul–body dualism. The philosopher Descartes is usually praised for defining the body as a mechanism that can be explored and improved by medical science, but at the same time, he is blamed for separating the soul (or preferably conceptualized as the mind) from the body. Bioethics has introduced the notion of respect for personal autonomy as a basic ethical principle, assuming that there is a subject owning and governing the human body. However, in this perspective, the idea is lost that the soul does not merely refers to the individual. It is also a dimension of human experience that arises out of relatedness. The soul cannot be confined within the individual. The soul is a "form of communion." [28] The individual soul is connected to a community; individuals are related to self, others, and creation. This interconnectedness has two ethical consequences. One is that the individualism of present-day ideologies is located in a broader framework in which other values than competition, self-interest, and rationality may emerge. The other is that human existence is located within creation, within a partnership of humans and earth. Soul-centric societies are eco-centric, based on cooperation, compassion, and sustainability. The notion of soul refers to the entanglements of human existence with social and natural contexts. Erosion of soul means loss of connection with others, society, and creation.

## What is lost when the soul is dead?

Contemporary sciences have pronounced the death of the soul. For the natural sciences and psychology, the soul is irrelevant and even an illusion. For theology and philosophy, it is no longer a useful concept. Chapter 2 will examine how the soul has been banned from scientific discourse. It will also analyze how its role in medicine, healthcare, and bioethics has been eradicated. The chapter will explain this erasure of the soul. It is argued that the specific scientific worldview of naturalism is responsible for the soul's demise. This is the view that the universe consists of matter and energy. The implication is that mental events are in fact physical events. Human persons are bodies that can be objectively observed, examined, analyzed, and dissected. Everything in the world can be clarified in terms of scientific explanations. There is no need for first-person perspectives. [29]

Naturalism, and its specific form of physicalism, is a powerful ideology in contemporary medicine and healthcare. It assumes that diseases, suffering, disabilities, and bodily dysfunction can be explained in terms of physical processes and laws. The machine metaphor is used to explain living organisms. For medical diagnosis and treatment, there is no need to separate the physical body and the person since focusing on the body will suffice for understanding the person.

However, this ideology has been criticized for a long time. Human beings are not merely entities within nature. Their being-in-the-world cannot be understood on the model of physical systems. Furthermore, it is argued that human persons are not the same as material substances. As beings in the world, they are connected to other beings, and at the same time they transcend the natural order. [30]

The final part of this chapter relates what has happened to the soul to the long-standing discourse of dualism, which is still influential in medicine. It is often argued that the philosopher Descartes has removed the soul from the domain of medicine. He has advanced the body as the proper object for medical science. However, this common view that soul and body are different substances needs to be critically examined since Descartes has developed a more nuanced argument.

It is clear that most contemporary scientific views reject substance dualism. Generally, scientists defend reductive materialism: material objects are the only substances; persons are bodies; there are no mental events, only physical events. Even when they believe that there are mental events, they are convinced that they can be explained solely in terms of physical events. [31] Nonetheless, ordinary experiences have not discredited dualism. Talking about persons is not the same as talking about bodies and their connected mental life. Persons are not the same as their bodies. This is a common experience in healthcare, as voiced by the physician-writers in the beginning of this chapter. More knowledge about the body and detailed information about body parts and organs does not provide sufficient knowledge about the patient.

## The disenchantment of the world

The disappearance of the soul in modern times is not an isolated phenomenon. It is the manifestation of a process, explored in Chapter 3, that sociologist Max Weber has called the "disenchantment of the world." The world, especially in Western cultures, is understood as less mysterious and magical; it has become knowable, predictable, and manipulable by humans. Rationalization and intellectualization are typical of our times: we can, in principle at least, master all things by calculation. [32] The thesis of Weber has two aspects: declining magic and increasing rationalization. The first aspect is related to the process of secularization, and the second to the dominance of science and rational government in modern societies. The disenchantment thesis implies that modernity is ruled by instrumental rationality but also by formal rationality that has emerged through bureaucracy and industrialization. This last type of rationality uses means–end calculations referring to abstract and universally applied rules, laws, or regulations. It creates a form of domination that is completely impersonal. The consequence is that we live in what Weber calls the Iron Cage. Modern people are trapped in a rationalistic, bureaucratized organization that restricts their freedom and creativity – an order of things that cannot be altered. [33]

The next section of Chapter 3 examines disenchantment in medicine and healthcare. Much of the dissatisfaction with medicine mentioned earlier is the result of disenchantment. Modern medicine focuses on the ideal of systematic observation. Physicians learn how to see the body in a specific way, distinguishing between objectivity and subjectivity. This "clinical gaze" is the first step toward mastering the human body and human life. Present-day medicine also uses the rational and bureaucratic language of the market as technological production of goods and services. The effect is a disenchanted world: the personal and the professional are separated.

Disenchantment has furthermore affected the discipline of bioethics. Weber's thesis implies that the supposed moral unity of the premodern world is lost and fragmented. Moral values have moved from the public realm into the private sphere of personal relationships. The role of bioethics is therefore limited. Moral values have become the subject of empirical observation, mathematical measurement, and testing.

The final part of Chapter 3 focuses on re-enchantment. Many scholars question whether disenchantment is the universal phenomenon that Weber assumes. It seems that nowadays mystery and ambiguity are commonly accepted, scientific theories and approaches are rejected, and values, religion, and spirituality have not become irrelevant for many people. Scholars also doubt whether there ever was a unified and homogenous world that has increasingly fragmented in modern times. [34]

Weber's thesis of disenchantment explains why and how the soul has disappeared from the contemporary worldview. We live in a fully rationalized world without mystery or magic. Science and technology are the driving forces of rationalization and bureaucratization. They are characterized by fragmentation and specialization. However, science is not as neutral and value-free as Weber suggests. With its ideology of naturalism is assumed that physics alone can explain what the world is like. According to science, questions about values, meaning, love, and morality are simple to answer. They are illusions. Scientists therefore often take a normative stance. They promote a particular way of interpreting life, assuming that this is a superior view. They assume that they have the authority to determine how life should be manipulated and improved. Scientists, as Sheila Jasanoff argues, are "myth-makers." [35] They advance the idea that science is pure, disinterested, and not embedded in society and industry, asserting that it should be free of external controls and regulate itself. This current role of science and technology does not reflect what Weber intended with his thesis. On the contrary, it seems that science and technology have themselves transformed into a magical, mysterious, and transcendent worldview that claims superiority and dominance as the overriding rational framework to attribute meaning to contemporary life. Eradicating the soul or dividing it in manageable parts and pieces, it promulgates a view of humanity as controllable and perfectible.

## Images without soul

The scientific worldview of naturalism and the thesis of the disenchanted world disseminate specific images and metaphors that predetermine the normative debate of bioethical issues. Chapter 4 will critically analyze the images that dominate the current ethical debates in healthcare and medicine: the ideas of *homo economicus*, body machine, lone ranger, detached concern, and consumer/client.

In contemporary scientific and market thinking, the human person is considered as a rational individual, first of all concerned with material self-interest. The organization of social life is dominated by the metaphor of the "market." As a self-regulating force, the market will give room to self-actualizing individuals whose productivity and creativity will work for the benefit of all. There is only a limited role for the state and the community. Areas of social life such as education, care, and security should be transformed into commodities and transacted in a trading market. Competition is the core value. The image of the market has engendered a specific discourse and set of practices that dominate processes of globalization since the 1980s. These are often summarized under the label "neoliberalism." This refers to a set of particular economic and political views, as well as policy practices, that have a pervasive influence in politics, social relations, and everyday life.

Daniel Cohen has called the image of *homo economicus* an "anthropological monster." It promotes a kind of Darwinian logic according to which the weak are losing and the stronger prosper. Shared communal life is disintegrating. Vulnerability is primarily an individual affair. [36] The image presents an erroneous and fictitious model. Research in behavioral economics has shown that the standard assumptions of economic theory do not work. Human actions are often flawed and irrational because human beings lack complete information and self-control. They are frequently motivated by other things than material self-interest. [37]

Another dominating image is that of the body machine. Persons are reduced to bodies without soul. This view of the body promotes a mechanistic approach in healthcare. Diseases are defects of the biological machinery. Medical knowledge is derived from empirical experience; data is collected by observation, tested in experiments, and verified or falsified by others. Medical problems therefore require rational and objective biological approaches. [38] As a result of the market ideology, the body (and its parts) has furthermore become a commodity. The body is the private property of the individual person. Regarding the body as a commodity has effects on altruistic practices; the meaning of a gift is changing, and the motivation to give is impacted. The assumption of this image of the body as mechanism is that everything we value can be subject of market exchange. However, as this chapter will argue, this is not the way how people value things. Between different groups of people and between different historical times, values are often radically different and incommensurable.

Another powerful image is individualism. Through our bodies, we are situated in the world as independent selves and we can act on our surroundings. Individual capacities determine what people make of their lives. This is the image of the autonomous subject that is dominant in mainstream bioethics. Almost from its beginning, bioethics has been criticized for its limited moral vocabulary, centered on the value complex of individual rights, self-determination, and privacy, at the expense of social responsibility and social justice. [39] One consequence of this image of the lone ranger is that human vulnerability is denied or translated into impairment or deficiency of the person's capacity to make autonomous decisions. [40] Another consequence is that the interconnectedness of human life is lost. What has disappeared is the significance of dependency, networking, and cooperation.

Declarations that the soul has been expelled from medicine and healthcare are often associated with the idea that the belief in technology and medication has eliminated subjective experiences from the realm of medicine. While medical professionals would not deny that emotions and feelings such as empathy and compassion play a role in the proceedings of medical practice, many adhere to the image of detached concern. However, this image is contested. Traditionally, sympathy and compassion have always been regarded as contributing to healing. In medical practice, it is impossible to ignore the needs of patients for emotional interactions with physicians and other care providers. Attending to the subjective experiences of patients will not only provide important information but also engage physicians in more effective communication. It will build trust with patients and will improve the effectiveness of medical treatment. The image of detached concern therefore is unsatisfactory. Empathy should supplement objective knowledge. [41]

Another image that dominates bioethical discourse is that of the consumer/client. The modern citizen is a choosing self, a responsible subject. Consumer language has been introduced in healthcare since the 1960s and 1970s. [42] Nowadays, healthcare is regarded as a business. Consumerism promises to liberate patients from the paternalism of medicine. Policies suppose that citizens will be active consumers who not only search and check the available information relevant for their health, but also are interested in a healthy lifestyle and will demonstrate responsible conduct in the decisions they make.

It is clear that in the domain of healthcare this consumer image is deficient. Adequate information as basis for choices and decisions is often lacking or does not exist or is kept private. If information is available, it is less reliable and harder to evaluate than elsewhere. The major flaw of the consumer model, however, is that it is based on misconceptions about human nature. People do not make decisions all the time in search of control, seeking the best combination of cost and quality. Also, human beings do not want to be reduced to "aggregates of data," self-tracking and moving around continuously gathering detailed health data about themselves. Furthermore, the human context changes when people are ill, disabled, or suffering. While consumers are driven by desires and preferences, patients are in need of care, assistance, or treatment. Patients, in distinction to consumers, are vulnerable. It is precisely this aspect of vulnerability that is omitted in consumer discourse. [43]

## Moral imagination

More and more bioethicists nowadays argue that bioethical discourse needs to change. Solomon Benatar has suggested that what is necessary for remedies and alternatives is a greater moral imagination, enabling us to alter our outlook and actions. [44] Chapter 5 will discuss the role of moral imagination as a faculty of the soul in bioethics. Imaginary visions are not just rhetorical devices. They provide ways of thinking and give structure to ideas. In her final book, philosopher Mary Midgley discusses patterns, world pictures, and frameworks, ways of thinking to explore the constantly changing world. She argues that there are always different perspectives available for interpreting the world. In her view, imaginative visions of how the world is "are the necessary background of all our living. They are likely to be much more important to us, much more influential than our factual knowledge." [45] Philosophy suggests new ways of thinking which call for different ways of living.

The chapter will point out that it is important to emphasize that bioethics is not a homogeneous discourse. It comprises various discursive practices. Moral deliberation moves from cases and specific situations to more elaborate and abstract arguments. This can be done in multiple ways. Imaginary processes play a role in this movement so that a richer and broader conceptual and analytical apparatus may emerge, giving voice to discourses that are easily silenced. The chapter will argue that imagination is important to facilitate interpretation; it generates and produces worldviews, ideals, and values to guide moral perception. Imagination is reshaping and reconstructing our experiences. We all have the capacity to imagine. [46] It is the creative ability to make the absent become present. Imagination projects ideals and values, offers possibilities for thinking and acting, helps us to bring new realities into existence, and conceives alternatives to problematic situations. It also makes use of past experiences as they suggest alternative possibilities. Imagination is therefore a crucial activity for ethics.

The capabilities of imagination will be further elaborated in the chapter. Moral imagination is not merely an inventive power that gives us different ways of seeing the world. It is especially important for global bioethics. First of all, it provides the capability to empathize with others. It helps us to experience the situation of other human beings, to recognize situations like ours, and to notice the moral demands that others make upon us. Second, moral imagination identifies various possibilities for acting. It encourages us to envision how action might help or hurt, to anticipate possible consequences of action, and to project possibilities into the future. [47]

## Recovering the soul: inspiring images

How can moral imagination activate, produce, or instigate images that rehabilitate and reinsert the soul in bioethical discourse? Chapter 6 will examine images and metaphors that are providing potential answers, particularly the ideas of the warm doctor, holistic care, stories and narratives, sacred values, and the blue marbles.

Research indicates that having a doctor who is warm and reassuring improves the patient's health. For example, symptoms are relieved faster when the doctor is nice and encouraging. [48] Also, placebo treatment has a more powerful effect if the physician is projecting warmth and competency. [49] In practice, there is no opposition between an objective, rational, and distanced health professional and a warm doctor with empathy and communicative skills. Such opposition assumes that medical competence is a technical ability based on biological knowledge and specific expertise in procedures. It disregards that there is also interpersonal competence, reflecting skills in social interaction and communication. At the same time, this view implies a restricted vision of empathy as a relational ability. This is not only the ability to share emotions of others, and thus an affective ability. Empathy is also a cognitive ability, that is to understand the emotions of other people. In good healthcare, both competence and empathy are necessary for patient-centered care. [50]

In an influential publication, George Engel has argued that medicine is in need for a new medical model. [51] The dominating biomedical model focuses medical attention on the underlying processes in the patient's body, not on the patient's experiences, social context, or healthcare system. Engel advocates a broader biopsychosocial model of holistic care. However, this model has not significantly changed medical practice. This chapter discusses several reasons for this lack of impact. One is that the biopsychosocial model itself does not escape the mind–body dualism that it criticizes in the biomedical model. It still assumes that the physical body is a necessary condition for the existence of the mind. The holistic model simply seems to add some additional dimensions to the mainstream approach of medicine without producing a new or alternative approach. Another reason might be the processes of rationalization described by Weber, and his concept of the Iron Cage. Nurses, for example, complain that their profession – while from its inception orientated toward humanitarian concerns for patients, treating them as total human beings – is increasingly caught in a system of technological medicine and mechanized care. They have become subordinated to the mechanistic and technical approaches of medical science. [52] A third reason might be that the delivery of healthcare has become more and more bureaucratic and commercial. There is hardly any time for communication. Most people want quick solutions and "magic bullets." At the same time, many patients use alternative and complementary healing approaches. Recent studies show the healing effects of the mind: hypnosis, biofeedback, and conditioning. They also show the harmful effects of loneliness, poverty, lack of social support, and deficient social relations on health. There is increasing interest for the health benefits of religion. [53]

Another image that suggests different approaches in bioethics is the metaphor of life as a story. The basic idea is that our lives are narratable; they can be presented as stories. Human beings are storytellers; they specifically express their values through their stories. Narratives play a central role in the medical context as is reflected traditionally in the importance of the anamnesis. Stories restore the voice of patients that is usually privatized and silenced.

Narratives and stories are frequently used in bioethics as instruments in the teaching of ethics, illustrating how abstract and general principles can be applied in specific contexts. Furthermore, stories have a critical function for bioethics. They exemplify what is a good life but also what is good medical practice, as many physician-writers are arguing in their books. They instigate moral reflection and motivate ethical action. The emphasis on stories therefore presents a different view of ethics and therefore challenges biomedical principles. [54]

Finally, the image of stories sheds a particular light on Weber's thesis of disenchantment. In Weber's view, the stories peculiar for Western civilization and religion are disappearing from the public realm. However, the increasing interest in narrative ethics shows that this diagnosis is only partially true. On the one hand, it illustrates the move from public to private realm. Stories give priority to particular people and situations, rather than abstract principles. They focus the ethical attention to desires, wants, and values rather than rules, norms, and principles. Because of these characteristics, stories are influencing the mind of listeners and readers; they transform their imagination. This is why they are regarded as agents of ethical empathy. They make it possible to imagining ourselves in the place of the other. The world is narratable, and therefore a place that we can make sense of by means of stories. On the other hand, narratives are intersubjective. Stories are shared. Many of our stories originate with others. They are produced by relationships. Telling a story means responding to it. Stories are assumed to express the soul because they make clear what really matters to people. Our basic experience of the world is gained directly from our own particular perspective. Science provides a second-order expression. This is why first-person perspectives as expressed in narratives are important. Contrary to the disenchantment thesis, they make the world personal. At the same time, while human beings are unique in having first-person perspectives, they have them because they are social beings. [55]

Another class of images that is associated with the soul concerns values. They determine what is worthwhile and what might provide meaning. However, in the process of disenchantment, they have been relocated from the public to the private domain. Weber does not deny that there are values, and that there are different values, but his point is that the "ultimate" values have been removed from public life. As all spheres of life are dominated by the rationalization of scientific progress, values cannot play a public role. Due to the process of disenchantment, the universe is no longer understood as a sacred order.

Nonetheless, especially in healthcare, values cannot be ignored. Patients' stories demonstrate what is valued in life. Concepts of health and disease are defined in connection to values. Goals of medicine embody values such as quality of life and prolongation of life. Health policies impose particular values such as competition and efficiency. Commodification as a basic component of market discourse presupposes that all commodities are fungible, that is interchangeable without loss in value. But this presupposition is a form of reductionism. It does not reflect the way how people, in fact, value things. In reality, there is significant incommensurability and pluralism. It may be very difficult to translate values between different groups of people and between distinct historical times. [56] Certain activities such as child abuse and dwarf-tossing elicit strong moral outrage and repugnance. They are regarded as inappropriate activities; even if they express individual values, these should be rejected because they are an affront to human dignity as a fundamental value. Repugnance indicates that not all values are the same. Some values are sacred; they cannot be balanced with other values. In this perspective, it is necessary to limit the scope of commodification and to protect some realms of social life against market forces.

The retreat of values in the private sphere has also raised critical questions. Weber's point of view is ambiguous. He argues that the modern world is characterized by impersonal structures of domination, while, at the same time, the self is described as autonomous. Weber proposes the concept of "inner distance" to protect the inner core of the persons against the depersonalizing forces of the world and to maintain individuality and power of self-expression. As a personality, the self affirms constantly some values. Weber therefore advocates "adaptation" to the possible. The modern individual adheres self-consciously to certain values and refuses to yield to circumstances in his surroundings and life world. Apparently, there are only two choices: submission to the demands of the modern world, or preservation of a sense of individuality by maintaining "inner distance." [57] This view has been criticized from two perspectives. One is that values are not simply individual desires or preferences. They are associated with a wide range of emotions such as respect, honor, affection, and love. What people value is often plural and different in quality. They also differ over time depending on the context, conditions, and challenges of life. [58] Another critique is that not only the world but also the self, and particularly its intimate relations, has been rationalized. Intimate life and emotions have been made into measurable and calculable objects. The modern subject is regarded as a self-manager. He or she has to do introspection and to clarify his or her self-image in a continuous process of communication. This has implications for values; the subject has to take values as the guides to his or her life. But the process is ambivalent. It is intensifying subjective life as the expression of personal values and authenticity but simultaneously it objectifies the means to express and exchange emotions so that others will recognize the values as components of a rational lifestyle. The self needs to show self-restraint and moral autonomy in order to maintain interpersonal relationships. This requires the ability to combine two sets of values: care, cooperation, and social concern, and autonomy and self-reliance. [59]

A final set of images is related to processes of globalization, referring to a series of pictures of the planet Earth taken from spacecrafts Apollo 11 and 17, the so-called "blue marbles." They became the iconic symbols for environmental concern. [60] These images express the growth of global consciousness. People are aware that they live on the same planet, that they share the same future, and that they all have responsibility for their destiny. This sense of common home triggers the imagination. People, especially in developing countries, are redefining themselves as "citizens of the world." This notion is part of the long-standing philosophy of cosmopolitanism. Basically, this is the idea that there is a global moral community. All human beings are members of that community since they share common values and responsibilities. [61] In many cultures, it has been acknowledged that human beings are born, and therefore rooted, in a specific place; they are localized in a native community and state. They have a common origin, language, and culture with fellow citizens. At the same time, they are inhabitants of the same planet; they are situated in a similar space. They share the same dignity and equality as members of humanity. As citizens of the world, they can go beyond their localization and boundedness of culture, tradition, community, and history. Being born in a specific place and within a particular culture with its often restrictive and traditional customs, laws, and morals can be overcome in a cosmopolitan perspective. Cosmopolitanism is the aspiration to live beyond bounded horizons. Human beings are not defined, and should not be defined, by a particular location, community, culture, or religion. From this philosophical perspective, much older than the modern processes of globalization, boundaries have no moral significance; the focus should be on what human beings have in common. Cosmopolitanism therefore expresses the moral ideal of the unity of humanity. There is a universal community that includes the whole of humanity.

## Another bioethics

The final chapter will address the question how bioethics can rehabilitate or reinfuse the soul into medicine and healthcare. Previous chapters discussed the reasons why the soul has disappeared or has been erased from medical science, healthcare, and bioethics. The chapters analyzed what has been lost with the eclipse of the soul. It is pointed out that medical writers, health practitioners, and patients regret that medicine has lost its soul. The chapters explained that the removal of the soul is part of a wider cultural and historical process in which rationalization and bureaucratization came to determine social life, and in which the sense of mystery and wonder but also emotions and meaning have been displaced from the public to the private sphere.

Given this context, and given the argument that the eradication of the soul from healthcare is a loss and impoverishment for medical and healthcare practices, what kind of bioethics or what bioethical approach will be needed? First of all, it is important to stress that "soul" has different meanings. As illustrated earlier, the notion refers to the principle of life, an immaterial substance, and to the core or essence of human beings. There are many different theories and interpretations of soul in religion, theology, and philosophy. We have been using the notion of soul mostly in the last sense of the term. Soul refers to the deep structure of beings. It is connected to what fundamentally characterizes a being: its value, depth, heart, personality. The soul of human beings thus refers to what is specifically human. Whether or not one prefers to imagine the soul as a substance or entity, it is first of all, as formulated by Moore, "a quality or a dimension of experiencing life and ourselves." [62] This view also articulates that the soul is not confined to the individual. As "activity of self-transcendence," it refers to community, other people, and the social context. It brings individuals in relation to self, but also others. The soul therefore is a "form of communion" – it "inhabits a collective home." [63] The departure of the soul implies loss of connections with others, society, and creation.

In his argument that bioethics has lost the soul, Gilbert Meilaender regards the soul as "attention to the meaning of being human." [64] Losing the soul means that fundamental issues about human nature and destiny cannot be addressed. It is futile to ask questions about who we are and who we should be. However, in his view, that will be an impoverishment of bioethics. Retrieving its soul requires alternative imaginations. A significant implication of this view is that the role of bioethics will change. It will resemble a prophetic activity, proposing what is worthwhile and valuable. This is not how bioethics is perceived today. Mainstream bioethics addresses the query: what can be done and what should be allowed? How can particular interventions be justified from a moral point of view? How can different ethical principles be balanced and how can arguments be provided for a specific decision? Ethics is regarded as an abstract system that can provide rules for conduct and decision-making. It is furthermore regarded as a series of momentary decisions that follow discrete events. Thus, it is attractive to view ethics as a human technology that facilitates the application of medical science and technology. New approaches can be added to make it even more attractive, for example narrative ethics or the biopsychosocial model. However, in our view, these additions will not change the basic nature of bioethics if they do not reach out to the soul. In order to focus on subjective patient experiences and a new ideal of empathic care, several considerations should be taken into account. First, ethics is a lifelong project, a way of life. It is not a succession of discrete events but the result of a continuous nurturing of emotions and moral sensibilities. Second, ethical life is shared with other people. It arises in the realm of interpersonal interactions, within the tension between interpersonal demands and individual inclinations. Ethics emerges in a succession of perspectives: from first-person individual concerns, to the second-person stance of mutual engagement, to the third-person perspective of detached onlooker. A complete understanding of ethical life cannot be provided by the third-person point of view. A crucial feature of ethics is the capacity to move back and forth between perspectives. [65] Such orientation is fundamentally what has been suggested in the ethical tradition as the moral point of view. Ethics exists because our sympathies are limited; we are therefore encouraged to take the point of view of other persons. It relates to what is called the expanding circle of moral concern. The scope of ethics is widening, and more beings are taken into account as morally relevant. A third consideration is that ethics is a social enterprise. Social interactions are not simply communications between autonomous individuals. They are intersubjective and reciprocal. They involve the sharing and exchanging of perspectives. Ethics as social ethics designates not only a distinct field but also a distinctive frame. The main purpose is to widen the usual scope of bioethics from individual to social, cultural, and economic concerns. [66] This means that another field of concerns will be addressed. Bioethical analysis will have a different starting point. Instead of focusing on individual clinical encounters, it will focus attention to social dynamics. Injustices hurt individual people but they usually take place in specific social contexts. Bioethics should therefore start in communities of marginalized and vulnerable people where social injustices are experienced. [67] This implies criticism of neoliberal policies. Globalization has established the primacy of the economic and political over the social and ethical; it has removed the soul from ethical and cultural discourse.

Bioethics as a prophetic activity relies on the moral imagination. It accepts that human beings are the only creatures with the capacity for imagination. As *homo imaginens*, they can conceive alternative futures. Through this capacity, they can challenge the domination by rationalistic and bureaucratic forces. Imagination enables them to show that there are "more things in the universe than are dreamed of by the rationalist epistemologies and ontologies of science." [68] Introducing new metaphors and imaginary visions, bioethics can overcome the rule of the metaphors of the market: efficiency, profit, consumption, and competition.

Finally, in this last chapter, we argue that perhaps ethics is too demanding. Moral theories are asking more than most of us are capable of. For example, they request real altruism and sacrifices. Can we expect health professionals to be empathic all the time, to attend to the subjective experiences of patients, and take the opportunity to listen while often functioning in systems that emphasize efficiency, output, and results? Strict morality is not feasible in many practical circumstances. We need to recognize our moral limits. But if traditional moral theories do not provide a framework for daily life, what can be the framework? One reply is: decency. Decent moral action "recognizes that there are others in the world who have lives to live." [69] This answer articulates that we share the world, and that we must treat the interests of others as equal to our own. It expresses a sense of recognition of others, as well as solidarity with others. Similar ideas are elaborated by philosophers Margalit and Honneth. A decent society, according to Avishai Margalit, is one whose institutions do not humiliate people. Humiliation is injury of self-respect. Humans are treated as if they were not human, as is the case with racial prejudices in social life. Only human beings can produce humiliation. Respect, on the other hand, means that appropriate weight is given to the interests and values of people. [70] Axel Honneth highlights the role of social recognition. [71] The economic order promoted by neoliberal policies has led to the moral impoverishment of the social life-world. It has multiplied experiences of injustice, especially of humiliation and disrespect. Because recognition is refused or withdrawn, moral injuries will result. Dignity, integrity, equality, and honor are not respected. The normative assumptions of social interaction are violated, and people will react with indignation and anger. These forms of disrespect should be addressed in an ethics of decency and reciprocal recognition. If bioethics mobilizes the moral imagination in order to expand the scope of moral concern by applying the human capacity to empathize, it crucially contributes to social life and civilization. In this perspective, it is important and urgent to engage in renewal of education in medicine and bioethics, that is developing a new approach focused on a holistic view on human beings and a global view on bioethics. In this engagement, several disciplines could be involved to offer a deeper and richer process of education for future healthcare professionals.

## References


1 Sherwin B. Nuland, *The soul of medicine. Tales from the bedside* (New York: Kaplan Publishing, 2010).
2 Jerome Groopman, *How doctors think* (Boston: Houghton Mifflin, 2007).
3 Atul Gawande, *Being Mortal. Medicine and what matters in the end* (New York: Metropolitan Book/ Henry Holt and Company, 2014), 128.
4 Peter McCann, "Suffering and empathy in the stories of Anton Chekhov and their relevance to healthcare today," *Hektoen International. A Journal of Medical Humanities* 6, no. 1 (2014); Jack Coulehan, ed., *Chekhov's Doctors. A collection of Chekhov's medical tales* (Kent and London: The Kent State University Press, 2003).
5 Tom Quinn, "The death of compassion in Louis-Ferdinand Céline's *Voyage au bout de la nuit*," *Irish Journal of French Studies* 1 (2001): 67–74.
6 Gunter Wolf, "Portrayal of negative qualities in a doctor as a potential teaching tool in medical ethics and humanism: *Journey to the End of Night* by Louis-Ferdinand Céline," *Postgraduate Medical Journal* 82 (2006): 154–156; David O'Connell, *Louis-Ferdinand Céline* (Boston: Twayne Publishers, 1976).
7 William Barrett, *Death of the soul. From Descartes to the computer* (New York: Anchor Books, Doubleday, 1986).
8 Phil Cousineau, ed., *Soul. An archaeology* (New York: HarperCollins Publishers, 1995).
9 Thomas Moore, *Care of the soul. A guide for cultivating depth and sacredness in everyday life* (New York: HarperCollins Publishers, 1992).
10 Thomas Moore, "Does America have a soul?" *Mother Jones* (September–October 1996): 26–32; Agnès Poirier, *Notre-Dame. The soul of France* (London: Oneworld Publications, 2020).

11 British Educational Research Association, "Most teenagers believe they have a soul," *Press Release* (14 September 2016).
12 The Telegraph, "Most people believe in life after death, study finds" (13 April 2009); www.telegraph.co.uk/news/religion/5144766/Most-people-believe-in-life-after-death-study-finds.html.
13 Pew Research Center, "Religious and/or spiritual people say they have a soul" (23 May 2018); www.pewforum.org/2018/05/29/attitudes-toward-spirituality-and-religion/pf_05-29-18_religion-western-europe-05-05/.
14 Maggy Fox, "Fewer Americans believe in God – Yet they still believe in afterlife," *NBC News* (21 March 2016).
15 Danie Botha, "Are we at risk of losing the soul of medicine?" *Canadian Journal of Anaesthesia* 64 (2017): 122–127.
16 Michel Accad, "How Western medicine lost its soul," *The Linacre Quarterly* 83, no. 2 (2016): 144–146.
17 Mark G. Kuczewski, "The soul of medicine," *Perspectives in Biology and Medicine* 50, no. 3 (2007): 410–420.
18 Lindsay F. Wiley, "The struggle for the soul of public health," *Journal of Health Politics, Policy and Law* 41, no. 6 (2016): 1083–1096.
19 Abigal Zuger, "Dissatisfaction with medical practice," *The New England Journal of Medicine* 350 (2004): 69–75.
20 Rachel N. Remen, "Recapturing the soul of medicine," *Western Journal of Medicine* 174 (2001): 4–5.
21 Melanie Neumann, Friedrich Edelhäuser, Diethard Tauschel, Martin R. Fischer, Markus Wirtz, Christiane Woopen, Aviad Haramati, and Christian Scheffer, "Empathy decline and its reasons: A systematic review of studies with medical students and residents," *Academic Medicine* 86 (2011): 996–1009.
22 Abraham Kahn, and Sarab Sodhi, "Professionalism sans humanism: A body without a soul," *Academic Medicine* 91, no. 10 (2016): 1331–1332.
23 Gilbert C. Meilaender, *Body, soul, and bioethics* (Notre Dame: University of Notre Dame Press, 2009).
24 Walter Glannon, "Tracing the soul: Medical decisions at the margins of life," *Christian Bioethics* 6, no. 1 (2000): 49–69.
25 Moore, *Care of the soul*, xv.
26 Dakin Andone, and Artemis Moshtaghian, "A doctor in California appeared via video link to tell a patient he was going to die. The man's family is upset," *CNN* (11 March 2019).
27 Stewart Goetz, and Charles Taliaferro, *Naturalism* (Grand Rapids and Cambridge: William B. Eerdmans Publishing Company, 2008).
28 Bruce Rogers-Vaughn, *Caring for souls in a neoliberal age* (New York: Palgrave Macmillan, 2019), 103.
29 Lynne Rudder Baker, *Naturalism and the first-person perspective* (Oxford: Oxford University Press, 2013); Dan Zahavi, *Subjectivity and selfhood. Investigating the first-person perspective* (Cambridge and London: The MIT Press, 2005); Steven J. Wagner, and Richard Wagner, eds., *Naturalism. A critical appraisal* (Notre Dame: University of Notre Dame, 1993).
30 Frederick A. Olafson, *Naturalism and the human condition. Against scientism* (London and New York: Routledge, 2001).
31 Warren S. Brown, Nancy Murphy, and H. Newton Malony, eds., *Whatever happened to the soul? Scientific and theological portraits of human nature* (Minneapolis: Fortress Press, 1998).

32 Max Weber, "Science as a vocation," *Daedalus* 87, no. 1 (1958): 111–134.
33 Arthur Mitzman, *The iron cage. An historical interpretation of Max Weber* (New Brunswick and Oxford: Transaction Books, 2005; original 1969).
34 Jane Bennett, *The enchantment of modern life. Attachments, crossings, and ethics* (Princeton and Oxford: Princeton University Press, 2001); Joshua Landy, and Michael Saler, eds., *The re-enchantment of the world. Secular magic in a rational age* (Stanford: Stanford University Press, 2009).
35 Sheila Jasanoff, *Can science make sense of life?* (Cambridge: Polity Press, 2019), 38.
36 Daniel Cohen, *Homo economicus, prophète (égaré) des temps nouveaux* (Paris: Albin Michel, 2012).
37 Antara Haldar, "Intrinsic goodness," *Times Literary Supplement* (2 November 2018): 10–11.
38 Alastair V. Campbell, *The body in bioethics* (London and New York: Routledge, 2009).
39 Renée C. Fox, *The sociology of medicine: A participant observer's view* (Englewood Cliffs: Prentice Hall, 1989).
40 Alasdair MacIntyre, *Dependent rational animals. Why human beings need the virtues* (London: Duckworth, 1999).
41 Jodi Halpern, *From detached concern to empathy. Humanizing medical practice* (Oxford and New York: Oxford University Press, 2010).
42 Saras Henderson, and Alan Petersen, eds., *Consuming health. The commodification of health care* (London and New York: Routledge, 2002); Nancy Tomes, *Remaking the American patient. How Madison Avenue and modern medicine turned patients into consumers* (Chapel Hill: The University of North Carolina Press, 2016).
43 Robin Downie, "Patient and consumers," *Journal of the Royal College of Physicians of Edinburgh* 47 (2017): 261–265; David J. Hunter, "The case against choice and competition," *Health Economics, Policy and Law* 4 (2009): 489–501.
44 Solomon Benatar, "Moral imagination: The missing component in global health," *PLoS Medicine* 2, no. 12 (2005): e400; doi.org/10.1371/journal.pmed.0020400.
45 Mary Midgley, *What is philosophy for?* (London: Bloomsbury Academic, 2018), 73.
46 John Dewey, *A common faith* (New Haven: Yale University Press, 1934); Steven Fesmire, *John Dewey and moral imagination. Pragmatism in ethics* (Bloomington and Indianapolis: Indiana University Press, 2003).
47 Mary Warnock, *Imagination* (Berkeley and Los Angeles: University of California Press, 1978); Thomas E. McCullough, *The moral imagination and public life. Raising the ethical question* (Chatham: Chatham House Publishers, 1991); Mark Johnson, *Moral imagination. Implication of cognitive science for ethics* (Chicago and London: The University of Chicago Press, 1993); Edward Tivnan, *The moral imagination. Confronting the ethical issues of our day* (New York: Simon & Schuster, 1995); Edward S. Casey, *Imagining. A phenomenological study* (Bloomington and Indianapolis: Indiana University Press, 2000); Richard Kearney, *The wake of imagination. Toward a postmodern culture* (London: Routledge, 2001).
48 Kari A. Leibowitz, Emerson J. Hardebeck, J. Parker Goyer, and Alia J. Crum, "Physician assurance reduces patient symptoms in US adults: An experimental study," *Journal of General Internal Medicine* 33, no. 12 (2018): 2051–2052.
49 Lauren C. Howe, J. Parker Goyer, and Alia J. Crum, "Harnessing the placebo effect: Exploring the influence of physician characteristics on placebo response," *Health Psychology* 36, no. 11 (2017): 1074–1082.
50 Halpern, *From detached concern to empathy.*

51 George L. Engel, "The need for a new medical model: A challenge for biomedicine," *Science* 196, no. 4286 (1977): 129–136.

52 Soma Hewa, and Robert W. Hetherington, "Specialists with spirit: Crisis in the nursing profession," *Journal of Medical Ethics* 16 (1990): 179–284.

53 Jo Marchant, *Cure. A journey into the science of mind over body* (New York: Broadway Books, 2016); Michael J. Balboni, and Tracy A. Balboni, "Reintegrating care for the dying, body and soul," *The Harvard Theological Review* 103 (2010): 351–364.

54 David B. Morris, "Narrative medicines: Challenge and resistance," *The Permanente Journal* 12, no. 10 (2008): 88–96; Rita Charon, "Narrative medicine. A model for empathy, reflection, profession, and trust," *JAMA* 286 (2001): 1897–1902.

55 Baker, *Naturalism and the first-person perspective.*

56 Margaret Jane Radin, *Contested commodities* (Cambridge and London: Harvard University Press, 2001).

57 Ralph Schroeder, "'Personality' and 'inner distance': The conception of the individual in Max Weber's sociology," *History of the Human Sciences* 4, no. 1 (1991): 61–78.

58 Elizabeth Anderson, *Value in ethics and economics* (Cambridge and London: Harvard University Press, 1993); Jonathan Baron, and Sarah Leshner, "How serious are expressions of protected values?" *Journal of Experimental Psychology* 6, no. 3 (2000):183–194.

59 Eva Illouz, *Cold intimacies: The making of emotional capitalism* (Cambridge: Polity Press, 2007); Eva Illouz, *Saving the modern soul. Therapy, emotions, and the culture of self-help* (Berkeley, Los Angeles and London: University of California Press, 2008).

60 Gregory A. Petsko, "'The blue marble'," *Genome Biology* 12 (2011):112; Denis Cosgrove, "Contested global visions: One-world, whole-earth, and the Apollo space photographs," *Annals of the Association of American Geographers* 84 (1994): 270–294. See also: Wolfgang Sachs, *Planet dialectics. Explorations in environment and development* (London: Zed Books, 2015).

61 Siep Stuurman, *The invention of humanity. Equality and cultural difference in world history* (Cambridge and London: Harvard University Press, 2017).

62 Moore, *Care of the soul*, 5.

63 Rogers-Vaughn, *Caring for souls in a neoliberal age*, 5, 103, 213.

64 Meilaender: *Body, soul, and bioethics*, x.

65 Webb Keane, *Ethical life. Its natural and social histories* (Princeton and Oxford: Princeton University Press, 2016), 42.

66 Henk ten Have, *Wounded planet* (Baltimore: Johns Hopkins University Press, 2019), 226–228.

67 M. Therese Lysaught, and Michael McCarthy, eds., *Catholic bioethics and social justice. The praxis of US health care in a globalized world* (Collegeville: Liturgical Press Academic, 2018).

68 Richard Jenkins, "Disenchantment, enchantment and re-enchantment: Max Weber at the Millennium," *Max Weber Studies* 1 (2000): 12.

69 Todd May, *A decent life. Morality for the rest of us* (Chicago and London: The University of Chicago Press, 2019), 29.

70 Avishai Margalit, *The decent society* (Cambridge and London: Harvard University Press, 1996).

71 Axel Honneth, *Disrespect. The normative foundations of critical theory* (Cambridge: Polity Press, 2007).

# 2 The erasure of the soul

Proclamations that the soul is dead, or at least irrelevant or at most illusion or metaphor, have been made in all scientific disciplines. This chapter will analyze such proclamations and their implications. First of all, the natural sciences assume that the behavior of human beings can perfectly well be explained without any recourse to the notion of soul. The soul is also banned from the scientific discipline that is supposed to study it. Psychology as the science of mental life considers the soul as a superfluous relic from prescientific philosophy. Even in theology, the concept of soul is no longer widely used. Theologians prefer to substitute the word "spirit" for soul. In philosophy, there is a long tradition of thinking about the soul and its relatedness to the body. In contemporary philosophy, the soul is ridiculed as the ghost in the machine. Nonetheless, the perennial mind–body problem is not resolved. In medicine and healthcare, the dominant materialistic worldview cannot allow that the mind has any power to heal or influence health. Medical technology and medication are the effective actors. Subjective experience is a distraction. The soul does not play any role in treating and healing the physical body. However, in care practices, mind and matter cannot be separated. Recent studies show the healing effects of the mind as well as the central importance of human aspects of care. Finally, the relatively new field of bioethics has eradicated the soul. It focuses on the application of rules and norms to guide the behavior of physicians and activities of researchers and policy-makers. It has evolved into an abstract system of applied ethics that does not need the notion of soul.

The second part of the chapter will be less descriptive and more explanatory. It will ask how it can be explained that the soul has disappeared from scientific discourses. The argument developed is that a specific scientific worldview is responsible for the soul's demise. This is the ideology of naturalism. It is the worldview that only natural things exist. Naturalism implies two claims. First, reality is what natural science says it is. This is an ontological claim about how the world is constituted and what should be regarded as real entities. In the universe, there is only matter and energy. Mental events are really physical events. Persons are bodies. The mind is the brain. Mental states such as sensations, thoughts, beliefs, desires, and acts of will should not be ascribed to an immaterial substance such as a soul, but are caused by and identical to physical and chemical events in the brain. In this perspective, any idea of soul, mind, or spirit should be avoided. Second, beliefs are only justifiable by the methods of science. This is an epistemological claim. Scientific explanations are regarded as the only valid ones. Science is the ideal of true knowledge. It embodies objectivity. Science is grounded in observations. With independent and impartial criteria, it determines the truth of statements. It produces knowledge that is not biased or prejudiced by cultural and personal circumstances. Scientific knowledge is open to refutation, falsification, and criticism. Results are tested by the community of scientists, and thus made intersubjectively acceptable. Since all facts in the world can be clarified in terms of scientific explanations, there is no need for first-person perspectives. These perspectives are either reducible to third-person perspectives or eliminable.

In contemporary medicine and healthcare, naturalism is a powerful ideology. Often, a more specific form of naturalism is endorsed, that is physicalism. Physics is the paradigm of natural science, although other sciences such as chemistry, biology, and genetics are important, too. But, basically, all events and states in the world can be explained in terms of physical processes and laws. Living organisms can be fully understood with the machine metaphor. Since human beings are vast conglomerates of nerve cells, brains, and genes, and thus molecules, physics can clarify how they function. This perspective assumes that any dualism between body and mind should be rejected. Everything that exists is composed of physical elements. For medical practice, this implies that there is no bifurcation between the person and the physical body.

Although the philosophy of naturalism has become dominant in science and medicine, it has been criticized since its inception. It is obvious that naturalism has serious implications for how we understand ourselves as human beings. One critique is that naturalism misrepresents our way of being in the world. Humans are in the world with other beings and entities. But world is not the same as nature conceived within a scientific perspective. We live in the world, and not in nature. This way of being-in-the-world cannot be understood on the model of physical systems. Another critique argues that human persons are not identical to material substances. Human beings are in the world but at the same time they transcend the natural order. Perception is an example how human beings transcend the body as a physical system. There is something outside of our bodies that is directly given or present to us. For humans, what is perceived is not simply physical sense perception as shared by all animals, but what is meaningful for them. Perceiving some object is not merely an event in the central nervous system. What we perceive is outside the body; the brain cannot perceive anything.

The final paragraph of the chapter locates the debate of what has happened to the soul within the long-standing philosophy of dualism. Dualistic discourse has been and still is influential in medicine. Dualism has emerged from a primordial phenomenon: the experience of the world as well as self-knowledge gained directly from our own particular perspective. First-person experience is the main reason for belief in the existence of a soul. As agents, we have privileged access to our mental states. We cannot deny that we have sensations and thoughts, feelings and hopes. We experience bodily events that cause brain events. We cannot explain how that occurs but this does not imply that it does not occur. The fact that we cannot clarify these interactions does not mean that they do not exist. The point is that mental events are distinct from physical events.

It is clear that most contemporary views reject substance dualism. Scientists usually defend hard materialism: material objects are the only substances; there are no mental events. According to this reductive materialism, the person is a physical organism and all experiences can be explained by the physical sciences. Others uphold soft materialism, arguing that mental events are different from brain events, even when the only substances are material entities.

However, ordinary experiences have not discredited dualism. Talking about persons is not the same as talking about bodies and their connected mental life. Persons are not the same as their bodies. Obtaining more knowledge about the body and its parts does not provide knowledge about the person. This means that there is more to me than my body. This view does not necessarily translate into an ontological distinction: the idea that there are two distinct substances, a body and a soul, that cannot be reduced to each other. An alternative view defends an anthropological perspective: the human person is a unity of two entities or qualities; mental states are not identical to physical states, nor can they be reduced to such states. This does not mean that there are two separate substances. There is only one substance. As human beings, we experience the unity of the self; we are aware that we are a mental subject with a body. Third-person descriptions therefore will not capture the first-person point of view. We will elaborate this view with the help of the traditions of philosophical anthropology and phenomenology to exemplify this way of thinking. Human beings exist in the natural world but at the same time they transcend the natural world and can detach from it.

## Proclaiming the death of the soul

Francis Crick, discoverer of the structure of DNA and Nobel laureate in 1962, argues that typical human qualities such as memories, ambitions, sense of personal identity, and free will are the result of the interaction of nerve cells and their associated molecules. The idea that people have souls is a myth; it is a form of superstition. He calls this view his "astonishing hypothesis." [1] In order to explain the behavior of human beings, there is no need for the concept of soul. This is in his opinion a religious concept, and "educated people" do not need this notion. They know that "soul" is a metaphor. [2] It seems that the world is located outside of us but in fact, as the advance of science has demonstrated, the neurons do the seeing, and they are inside our head. Science will clarify what has traditionally been attributed to the soul. Philosophy, in Crick's opinion, will not be of any help; it has a poor record. Similar ideas are expressed by his colleague James Watson. According to him, DNA is the "blueprint" of human beings. The genome determines who we are; it is what makes us human; our fate is in our genes. Life is just a matter of physics and chemistry. Now that the basic machinery of life is discovered, the mission of molecular biology is "to answer questions about ourselves and our origins as a species." [3] A legendary story reports that Harvard biologist Walter Gilbert, one of the initiators of the Human Genome Project (HGP), during his presentations showed the public a computer disk with genetic information, proclaiming: "Here is a human being, it's me." [4] Geneticist Lee Silver attributes opposition to biotechnology to fears that the soul of individual organisms will be infringed. This fear in his opinion is of course unsupported. The soul is not a useful concept, but because many people believe in it, it cannot be ignored. The best approach is to redefine the soul, and make clear that it is a metaphor. [5]

### *Genetics and neuroscience*

In practice, this redefinition has already occurred. Many people regard the human genome as the essence of the human person. From their analysis of popular and news media, Nelkin and Lindee conclude that in popular culture DNA is looked upon as a soul-like entity, just as the Christian soul in previous times. [6] Geneticists themselves argue that such genomic essentialism is flawed. The human person is more than an entity with a genome. Humanness is influenced but not determined by the genetic constitution. Arguing that the human genome is the manifestation of the individual soul is not a scientific but a metaphysical point of view. [7]

Modern neuroscience also promotes the idea that physical and chemical processes in the brain determine human behavior. The notion of soul can be rejected since all human qualities and experiences can be explained by studying the brain. Soul has now become a superfluous concept. Brain determinism, however, has implications: free will, moral responsibility, moral agency, and deliberation are illusions. [8]

The scientific discipline that is traditionally studying the soul and inner mental life is psychology. The Greek word "psyche" refers to "soul," "spirit," "mind," and "breath." Aristotle's treatise on the soul is commonly taken as the starting point. The term "psychology" first appeared in the 16th century. In the 18th century, the soul was evicted from psychology. The discipline was fundamentally transformed into an empirical science of the mind. The nervous system was considered as the crucial connection between the mental and physical realms. [9] William James' influential *Principles of Psychology* in 1890 argues that talk of the soul is a relic from prescientific philosophy. It is a theory of popular philosophy and scholasticism but completely superfluous. There is no need for it in order to account for the facts of conscious experience. It explains nothing. James concludes that he will discard the word "soul" from the rest of his book. [10] It is much better to speak of consciousness rather than soul. Consciousness is best understood as the functions of the physical brain. The mind is an object in the world of other objects and can be studied in an objective way. Later in life, James also regarded "consciousness" as a non-entity. This concept, and its associated emphasis on introspection as a source of knowledge, is not helpful to develop psychology into an experimental science. It is better to focus on behavior. However, this restrictive view is criticized by other psychologists. Carl Gustav Jung, for example, denounced the impact of scientific materialism, reducing the mind to an epiphenomenon of matter: brains, glands, hormones, instincts, or drives. In this perspective, the psyche does not exist. Thoughts are "secretions of the brain." [11] This narrows the field of psychology: "empirical boundaries are set to man's discussion of every problem, to his choice of purposes, and even to what he calls 'meaning.'" [12] According to Jung, it is also a typical Western theory that the seat of consciousness is in the head; for Pueblo Indians, it is in the heart; for African tribes, it is in the belly. [13] The consequences are particularly adverse in healthcare. In Jung's view, despite patients' needs, "the science of medicine has avoided all contact with strictly psychic problems." [14] Even when psychiatry and psychology are part of medicine, they often treat these problems with physical means, primarily medication.

### *Contemporary theology*

The term "soul" has furthermore almost disappeared from contemporary theology. While the term is still used in theology, many theologians have substituted the word "spirit" for soul. In this way, they can make a distinction between secular and spiritual aspects of human life. Rejecting radical dualism, separating the soul from the body, the opposite view of reductive materialism regarding the person as a merely physical organism is difficult to accept. Some theologians have therefore worked out a perspective of "non-reductive physicalism." This states that there is not a duality of substances but a duality of aspects. Brain, mind, and spirit are not separate entities but aspects of the same set of events. What is regarded as the soul is "a functional capacity of a complex physical organism, rather than a separate spiritual essence that somehow inhabits a body." [15] While the person is a psychobiological unity, human capacities once attributed to the soul are now regarded as functions of the brain. One of the benefits of dualism, as specified by Stephen Post, is that the presence of a soul confers equal moral worth on all human beings. Every self has a soul as the seat of equality. [16]

### *Cartesian dualism*

Philosopher Gilbert Ryle has argued that the official doctrine of minds, commonly attributed to Descartes, is a myth; it is one big logical mistake. He labeled this false theory as "the dogma of the Ghost in the Machine." [17] In Ryle's opinion, it is a philosopher's myth since it is based on a category-mistake. Facts of mental life are regarded as belonging to a special category, while in fact they belong to another. It is like somebody saying that his headache is green, or visiting the University of Padua, and having seen all the buildings, asking where the university is. Mental operations do not refer to the mind as a separate entity, but they are the workings of the mind; they show that people are able and prone to do certain sorts of things. When a person is acting intelligently, he is bodily active and mentally active but not synchronically active in two different "places"; there is only one activity that is not hidden but can be observed by ourselves and others. Mental operations are reflected in patterns of behavior. Mental concepts refer to dispositions to behave in certain ways. [18] Ryle prefers a behavior-oriented explanation of the mind rather than explanations in terms of internal events such as brain activities.

Philosophy, especially philosophy of mind, has been profoundly influenced by Ryle's thesis of the ghost in the machine. For most of the time, it was assumed that the human person is a composite of body and soul. According to Aristotle, everything that is alive has a soul. There are different kinds of soul. Human beings are characterized by the rational soul. Talking about the soul is not restricted to the domain of religion but refers to the essence of human beings. It is regarded as the principle of life. [19] As the source of moral judgment, deliberation, and self-control, the soul is not simply the conclusion of a philosophical theory but the product of human experiences. The challenge for philosophers has been how the soul is related to the body. The distinction between body and soul does not imply that they are different substances or entities. For Thomas Aquinas, there is only one fundamental substance, that is the individual human being, a unity of soul–body. Radically separating the body and the soul means not only that the body is "desouled" as a physical machine but also that the soul is reduced to the mind and out of reach for scientific examination.

Ryle's disqualification of dualism has removed the soul from mainstream philosophical discourse. The primary culprit, as will be discussed later in this chapter, is Cartesian dualism. The soul–body problem has been redefined as the interaction between mind and brain. The most common position is that mind and body are not fundamentally separated. Physicalism asserts that the mind may be reduced to physical activities of the brain. Behaviorism affirms that mental states are, in fact, publicly observable behaviors. Functionalism argues that mental states are caused by behaviors and other mental states. Herbert Feigl, for example, advanced the identity theory of the mind; there is only one reality that is expressed in two different concepts. [20] Dominating theories of the mind are monistic and materialistic. They emphasize that the world exists of material objects and physical events.

The paradox is that the soul might be lost in philosophy and science but that it persists in popular language and in experiences of human life. Philosophers may declare that the soul is a ghost in the machine but doing so means that things that really matter to human beings, such as thoughts, beliefs, desires, preferences but also values, are no longer real; they should be regarded as fictions and mistakes. However, the soul is not a theory; it is an experience. Many philosophers of mind deny the reality of this experience. A person has the capacity to conceive of himself as himself in the first person. The person, as first personal being, is an entity in the world, the genuine subject of experience. [21] Monistic and materialistic theories reject the experience that the self is the substantial subject of experiences. They wrongly assume that there is no distinction between first-person and third-person perspectives. [22]

### *Healthcare*

The soul does not play a significant role in contemporary healthcare. As noted in the previous chapter, physician-writers generally complain that the soul has been lost in medicine. The dissipation of soul is strongly felt in nursing, developed as a profession out of humanitarian concerns for patients, with compassion and empathy as basic values. Due to the increasing impact of medical technology and organizational bureaucracy, it is experiencing growing difficulties in maintaining human relationships, as treatments are focused on technology and bodily interventions, and care is regarded as a commercial service. [23] In medicine, the disappearance of the soul is manifested in several ways. First of all, the human body is treated as a mechanism that can be fully understood with the concepts and methods of the natural sciences. This is associated with the ideal of objectivity that dictates these sciences. Physicians should avoid subjective impressions and biases. They should not be moved by emotions or feelings, but they should be detached so that they can make an objective assessment of the patient's complaints. The mechanistic view of human beings is furthermore related to strong beliefs in technology and medication. Almost half of all Americans are on medication. Approximately 60% of adults older than 65 take five or more different drugs at any one time. [24] There is also a pervasive narrative of miracle drugs. People believe that there will be a continuous stream of "magic bullets" that can overcome diseases, like antibiotics and corticosteroids in the past. Another manifestation that medicine has become a soul-less activity is its specialization and fragmentation, making it impossible to practice holistic care. Finally, the organizational context of modern medicine has exorcized its soul. Healthcare is approached as a business. Time to see patients is limited and communication should first of all be effective, that is producing a diagnosis and suggesting a treatment, preferably with medication.

The tendency in medicine to neglect the soul is not a recent phenomenon. In his dialogue *Charmides*, Plato already commented that in his days it is a great error in the treatment of the human body that physicians separate the soul from the body. [25] Another example is the controversy in the 13th century between Maimonides and Nahmanides, both physicians and rabbis. They each prioritized one of the two dimensions of medicine: the cognitive one based on objective knowledge and disease, and the expressive one based on subjective relations with the patient. [26] In modern medicine, dominated by a materialistic worldview, the erasure of the soul had two effects. One is that the mind has no longer any power to influence health or the power to heal. The other is that subjective experiences are a distraction; empathy, social support, and hope do not play a significant role in dealing with patients. Both effects contribute to the dissatisfaction with current medicine. They are also contrary to evidence that increasingly becomes available. We do better, have less pain and sickness if we feel safe, cared for and in control. In her book *Cure*, Jo Marchant describes the benefits of a holistic approach to medicine. Recent studies show the healing effects of the mind. [27] They also demonstrate the effects of social conditions such as loneliness, lack of social relations, and poverty on health. Marchant concludes that the true ingredients of successful treatment are empathy, care, social support, and hope. Essential are the humane aspects of care. The focus on the physical condition of the body and the dominance of biology in medicine is, in fact, a major source of dysfunction, especially in American healthcare. [28] The United States spends more than many other countries on healthcare, but Americans are not healthier than the citizens of these countries. There is a need to refocus to another type of interventions, not investing in more medicine but improving on social and behavioral risk factors.

### *Bioethics*

Finally, the soul has disappeared from bioethics. Bioethicist Gilbert Meilaender argues that the development of bioethics has not been "entirely benign." [29] The soul, which he defines as "attention to the meaning of being human," is easily lost in bioethical discourse because it no longer examines fundamental questions about who we are as human beings. [30] One reason is that doctors are primarily regarded as skilled technicians who are guided by internal morality, that is norms generated within the practice of medicine itself. They used to learn a particular way of professional life, often reflecting on the goals of medicine and the good of patients. Bioethics, however, emphasizes external morality, requesting the application of external rules and norms. In this normative setting, a major focus is on respect for patient autonomy, rejecting professional paternalism. The only person to determine what should be done is ultimately the patient himself or herself. Bioethics also has defined itself as a pragmatic discipline. It should assist physicians and policy-makers to make decisions and to solve problematic cases. Its focus is on regulation, public policy, and social consensus rather than normative judgment. In this perspective, reflection on background beliefs about human nature and destiny is often not relevant. Meilaender argues that bioethics should go back to "its earlier self," that in his view implies concern with "humanity." [31]

That the soul cannot be neglected in bioethical discourse is illustrated in the debate on what defines life and death. If the soul highlights what is essential to human beings, it explains why they have moral status and dignity. It determines what makes humans into persons. When exactly the soul comes into existence is the subject of vigorous ethical debates, especially regarding the beginning and end of human life. [32] Fundamental values concerning humanity furthermore play a role in public and popular debates on ethical issues. Bioethical issues are nowadays taken up by various social movements and patient advocacy groups around the world. An example is the Save Charlie movement. When pediatricians in London decided that it was better for Charlie Gard, a baby with a rare genetic disorder and brain damage, to die, his parents started a movement on social media to save him and allow him to try an experimental treatment in the United States. The courts denied this treatment and Charlie died. But on social media there was a huge number of people involved in the ethical debate. It demonstrated that the agenda-setting of bioethics is no longer controlled by bioethics professionals. [33]

## The scientific worldview of naturalism

How can it be explained that the soul is lost in science, psychology, theology, philosophy, healthcare, and bioethics? Usually, it is explained that the culprit is naturalism. It is broadly defined as "a theory that relates scientific method to philosophy by affirming that all beings and events in the universe (whatever their inherent character may be) are natural." [34] However, the term is not precise and can have various meanings. It refers to a broad metaphysical thesis with specific claims about what exists and does not exists in the world. Its unifying factor is the rejection of supernatural entities. The basic constituents of the universe are physical or material. A self-proclaimed naturalist such as John Dewey, for example, states that there is no dichotomy between nature and human beings: "human affairs . . . are projections, continuations, complications of the nature which exists in the physical and pre-human world." [35] There is no duality between mind and body, nature and society, or between secular and sacred. There is nothing more than the natural world; no God, no soul, no immortality.

### *Ontological and epistemological naturalism*

A distinction is made between ontological and epistemological naturalism. Ontological naturalism is a view about how the world is constituted and what should be regarded as "real entities." Epistemological naturalism is a view about the best ways to obtain knowledge and justify beliefs.

The first component of naturalism assumes that "there is nothing more to the mental, biological and social realms than arrangements of physical entities." [36] It is often, but not necessarily, combined with materialism, considering human beings as identical to material substances. A species of naturalism is physicalism. [37] This is the thesis that everything is physical. The ancient philosopher Thales, for example, was convinced that the basic constituent of nature is water. Since everything is physical, there is physical explanation for all facts. The second component of epistemological (or methodological) naturalism assumes that philosophical explanation should use the same methods of investigation as the natural sciences. [38] Scientific explanations are the only valid ones. First-person perspectives should be eliminated. Everything in the world is impersonal. Religious commitments are not relevant for obtaining knowledge about the natural world.

In practice, ontological and epistemological naturalism are often combined. Both components regard science as the ideal of knowledge. In the scientific worldview of naturalism, only those things are real that are within the scope of a purely scientific description and explanation of the world. Morality, values, and normativity are not part of the natural order. [39]

### *Reductive and non-reductive naturalism*

Naturalism can furthermore be reductive or non-reductive. A reductive approach analyzes a concept in other terms. All entities are reduced to physical or material entities. An example is the view that mental states are brain states. Thomas Nagel has called this the "orthodox view": a conception of the world that combines reductionism, materialism, and physicalism in a scientific approach that describes and analyzes everything with the concepts and methods of physics, chemistry, and biology. [40] In response to reductionism, non-reductive versions of naturalism have been developed. [41] They assert that the mental is irreducible. It cannot be reduced to behaviors or brain states. It is a significant dimension of reality. At the same time, everything that exists is physical, so that mental states are physical states. The mind is not a separate entity. Between mind and brain is functional dependency. There is no change in the mental without change in the physical, but this does not imply reducibility. Mental phenomena such as consciousness are higher-level or emergent properties of the brain. Mental properties "supervene" on physical properties. The supervenience thesis is used to explain that mental properties are multiply realizable by different kinds of physical properties. They arise from the basic constituents of physical systems. Knowledge of these systems is therefore not sufficient to explain the emergent properties.

A recent example of naturalism is Nagel's expanded or liberal naturalism. [42] He proposes a specific form of naturalism that is broader in scope, stating that the basic constituents of the universe are not merely physical or material, but that is still naturalistic. In his view, the basic constituents are "protomental elements"; the physical is also mental. [43]

Non-reductive naturalism still faces the problem of mental causation. It is not clear how consciousness can have a causal effect on the physical world. At the same time, it escapes the threat to human autonomy posed by reductive naturalism. It safeguards that human beings are free agents who can act on the basis of reasons.

### *Medicine and healthcare*

Naturalism is a powerful ideology in medicine and healthcare. The biomedical model is specifically based on physicalism. The assumption is that biological phenomena can ultimately be explained with the sciences of physics and chemistry. Human beings are regarded as complicated biological machines. Physicalism implies that they can be empirically studied, subjected to experiments, and manipulated or repaired by technical interventions. Diseases, suffering, disabilities, and bodily dysfunction can be explained in terms of physical processes and laws. Fatigue, for example, is a subjective experience, but it is real because it is a bodily, material phenomenon, correlated to a physical state of the brain. Conditions such as addiction and obesity can be explained by neuroscience, independent of immaterial explanations such as will power or free choices. This approach has ethical consequences: it de-stigmatizes such conditions and removes moral responsibility. Naturalism is also reflected in philosophical explanations of disease as abnormal functioning of bodily systems. Diseases are regarded as deviations from the natural functions of organ systems and can be determined in an objective, scientific way. There is no need for any value judgments. Similar views are expressed in genetic determinism. Molecular biology ultimately explains human behavior and medical disorders.

### *Naturalist ethics*

Naturalism integrates ethics into the worldview of science. Moral facts are like other scientific facts in the world and do not exist as a separate category. They can be discovered and objectively studied like other entities in the world. One approach is to eliminate them as relevant factors. A more common approach is to reduce them to natural facts (such as pain or pleasure). They can be regarded as synonymous with natural facts. A third approach is irreducibility. Moral properties are natural but not reducible; they supervene on natural properties. [44] Moral naturalism is often connected with moral realism. As natural entities, moral facts and values are real and objective; they can be examined with empirical methods. [45] This is an attractive view since moral properties and facts are therefore not subjective and a matter of opinion, emotion, or construction. According to Nagel, there are objective values in the world, independent of our judgments. These values not only are detected but also motivate us to act. [46]

### *Problems with naturalism*

Naturalism is a metaphysical perspective about the world claiming that only the natural exists. But "natural" is an elastic and ambiguous concept. There is no consensus about the concept in naturalism. Are natural facts empirical facts, extended in space, material, or physical facts? There is agreement that the "natural" is everything within the domain of the natural sciences. But again, there is no agreement on what a natural science is: physics, chemistry, biology, geometry, geology, genetics, psychology? There is no unified account or common methodology of the sciences. [47] Why should we assume that there are only physical events in the world? [48]

Naturalism has implications for how human beings understand themselves. It is argued that naturalism misrepresents our way of being in the world. Human beings are in the world with other beings and entities. But world is not the same as nature conceived within a scientific perspective. We live in the world, and not in nature. What is typical for human beings is that they transcend the natural order. This way of being-in-the-world cannot be understood on the model of physical systems. [49] An example how humans transcend the body as a physical system is perception. Something outside of our body, for instance the computer that we use to write this book, is present to us and directly given as an object in the world. Naturalism regards the perception of the computer as an intra-mental event; it is an event in the central nervous system. However, the brain cannot perceive anything; what we perceive lies outside our bodies and brains. Perception is a function of the whole human body and not just of a part of it. For human beings, the world presents entities that are not in their minds.

This criticism is related to the objection that naturalism does not do justice to human experience. This point was first advanced by Edmund Husserl, the founder of phenomenology. For him, naturalism threatens a proper understanding of ourselves as human beings. It ignores that human experience is the ground of scientific investigation. Because of this, we no longer ask the most important questions: " questions of the meaning and meaninglessness of the whole of this human existence." [50] It is important, Husserl points out, to return to experience, and thus defeat naturalism. For him, human subjectivity is not an object like other entities in the natural world. Consciousness is a condition for the possibility of having any experience at all. Naturalism also is a misconstruction of science. Science is a human accomplishment. Somebody had to develop scientific procedures and methods. Science is not merely discovering and describing objective facts in the world. The sciences are achievements of humans who are engaged in cognitive encounters with the lifeworld. This means that subjective presuppositions play a necessary role in developing scientific approaches. Naturalism therefore wrongly assumes that the world exists independent from being perceived by a subject, even if the universe is much older than humanity. Separating nature and world, naturalism has alienated science from the human lifeworld. The lifeworld is the world of prereflexive experience. The problem with naturalistic science is that it does not recognize that science is a human effort. The history of geometrics, for example, shows that Galilei in his mathematical approach assumed that he discovered and described the real world, while in fact it is used as what Husserl calls a "Ideenkleid" (a dress of ideas). [51] Science uncovers mathematized nature but it obscures the concrete lifeworld of human experiences. Scientism has forgotten that every scientific activity is preceded by encounters with the world.

Correlating subject and object is based on the concept of intentionality. Human beings are intentional beings. Mental states such as thinking, perceiving, and imagining are directed toward states of affairs; they are about something. Physical states do not have intentionality. Consciousness is being conscious *of* something, and objects in the world are objects *for* consciousness. The knowing subject is part of the world. He or she is in an intentional relation with the world. According to Husserl, human beings are objects in the world and at the same time subjects for the world. Subjectivity is a condition for the possibility of objective knowledge. [52] Intentionality is crucial for the relation between physician and patient. Illness is primarily experienced by patients but also physicians. It is not an objective entity but a form of life. [53] Caring for patients requests more than analyzing abstract disease. A relationship with the patient needs to be established directed to understanding and healing. [54] Intentionality means that healthcare should be focused on the patient and his or her suffering.

Another element of Husserl's critique of naturalism has further implications for healthcare. Naturalism implies that first-person perspectives are reducible to third-person perspectives or can be eliminated. What exists in reality are individuals and their properties. All the facts about an individual can be explained with a scientific approach; they can be expressed in the third person. But these last perspectives cannot capture our first-person point of view. Baker defines the first-person perspective as "the capacity to think of oneself . . . as the object of one's thought." [55] It exhibits self-consciousness. I, as a first personal being, am a subject of experience. The world has a real and personal dimension that cannot be eliminated. [56] Experiencing involves a subject of experience. [57] Denial of the reality of subjective experiences has consequences. Without first-person perspectives there are no persons, no agency, no moral responsibility. In medical practice, it means that subjective experiences are eliminated or incorporated in a scientific understanding of what is wrong with the patient.

### *Problems with moral naturalism*

Naturalism argues that consciousness and the self are illusions. It also denies that values exist. The main problem with naturalism is prescriptivity. This is a crucial element of morality. Certain facts in the world provide a reason to act. [58] This is the normativity of ethics. Moral facts are different from empirical facts because they motivate human beings to do something. Reductive naturalism regards prescriptive properties as natural properties. But in that case, the concept of natural is overstretched since descriptive facts, as basically material or physical facts, do not have normativity. An alternative is to argue that moral facts have no prescriptivity. They do not provide reasons to act. Whether or not they provide such reasons depends on the attitudes, desires, and preferences of a particular agent. This perspective denies that ethics aims at telling agents what they ought to do. Non-reductive naturalism faces the same dilemma. Understanding moral properties as supervening natural properties does not imply that moral properties themselves are natural properties. They are either natural (overextending the concept of the natural) or they are not. In both cases, it is not clear why they are prescriptive. Even Nagel's expanded naturalism cannot escape this dilemma. [59]

## Dualism

What has happened to the soul and its eradication from scientific, philosophical, and ethical discourse is connected to the traditional debate of dualism between body and mind. Most contemporary views reject substance dualism – the view that body and soul/mind are separate substances. Hard materialism is a common position: material objects are the only substances. The person is a physical organism; all experiences can be explained by the physical sciences. Soft materialism is another position: mental events are different from brain events. Persons also have mental properties, even if the only substances are material objects. According to this non-reductive physicalism, it is not necessary to postulate the existence of a metaphysical entity such as the soul. [60]

The discourse of dualism has been and still is influential in medicine. Descartes is usually blamed for separating the soul and the body. According to Descartes, human beings are composed of two fundamentally different substances. He defined substance as "a thing which so exists that it needs nothing else in order to exist." [61] His argument for the existence of spiritual substance is the phenomenon of thinking (I am aware of something). Material substance is essentially characterized by being extensive in space. The result is that a human being is a composite of *res cogitans*, a thinking thing, and *res extensa*, an extended thing. These substances are each other's opposites and entirely different; they are not reducible to one another. [62] This conception of matter, and thus also the body, has important consequences. Matter has merely quantitative aspects, which may be described through mathematics. Anything that takes place in the material world can be reduced to a change in spatial proportions. Every natural phenomenon manifests itself according to the laws of movement, that is mechanically. Nature may therefore be comprehended in purely mechanical terms. Bodily processes can also be examined and explained mathematically and physically. Descartes himself demonstrates this in detail in the fifth part of his *Discours de la Méthode*. The movement of the heart and the circulation of the blood are completely explicable by the principles and laws of mechanics. The human body can best be compared with ingenious artifacts, robots manufactured by technicians. Descartes had in mind the hydraulically operated statues, which he had seen in the royal gardens at Saint-Germain-en-Laye:

> Indeed the nerves of the automaton that the body is can be compared with the tubes of the robots by those fountains, the muscles with the spiral springs and the vital spirits with the water that sets them in motion and of which the heart is the source. [63]

The body, then, is an intricate machinery, which should be explained as a mechanism. The Cartesian image of human beings has developed into the "philosophical substratum of contemporary medicine." [64] Descartes himself saw the main benefit of his new philosophy in the field of medicine. He compared philosophy with a tree of which the roots are formed by metaphysics, the trunk by physics, and the branches by medical science, mechanics, and morals. In the last part of his *Discours de la Méthode*, Descartes points out how his philosophy can make man understand reality and thus enable him to become the master of nature. The conservation of health could benefit from this; he believes that "if anything may make people wiser and more sensible than they have been so far, . . . it could only be in medicine where one ought to look for it." [65] Medicine at that time did not have much to offer; but when practiced by the methods formulated by Descartes, it promised great results, such as protection from numerous diseases and decay in old age. In the 17th century, Cartesianism inspired the iatrophysical school in medicine, first in Holland where he lived for 20 years, and later at Padua university. [66] This school sought mechanical explanations of physical functioning, as well as health and illness. It culminated in the discovery of blood circulation by William Harvey in 1628. [67]

In the longer run, Cartesian philosophy permeated medicine as a scientific approach. Descartes had an optimistic view on the advancement of human knowledge. The future of medicine shall be bright, as he wrote in October 1645 to the Marquis of Newcastle: "The conservation of health has always been the principal object of my studies, and I do not for a moment doubt that it will be possible to acquire vast medical knowledge that has remained unknown until the present." [68] His philosophy encouraged a mathematical and quantitative way of representing things and measuring them. It also promoted an experimental approach. Furthermore, it articulated a distinction between objective and subjective realities. The knowing subject and knowable objects are separated. While the world initially included the knowing subject, it has now become an objective reality apart from the subject. It is no longer that which we experience every day, the reality familiar to human beings and full of meaning, but that has been stripped of any subjectivity. The knowing subject takes a position of observation and registration; it no longer participates in events taking place in the world. The soul has been banned from the objective, material world. For medicine, this scientific approach has important consequences. The human body is reconceptualized as an intricate material machinery, not different from other things in the world. Descartes prefers to compare it with a clockwork. Medical cases are therefore of a technical nature and in principle solvable.

One fundamental problem of mind–body dualism is the causal question: How do mental and physical states interact? In human beings, soul and body are actually united. We know from experience that one substance can influence the other. When I want to move my hand, it moves; when something pricks the skin of my finger, I feel pain. In principle, the influence from one substance on the other cannot be a causal influence, for both substances are essentially different. Strictly speaking, one cannot localize the soul in some place inside or outside the body or the brain. But how can the factual connection between body and soul be explained? Already in Descartes' lifetime, the question was asked how the soul as only a thinking substance can influence the body. [69] Descartes poses a solution that is not very satisfactory. Although the soul is joined to all parts of the body, there is one place in which it exercises its functions more particularly than elsewhere. The pineal gland is taken to be the seat of the human soul. This tiny structure in the brain is the only one that is not duplicated, and is therefore appropriate to function as a switchboard connecting body and soul. In particular, acts of the will are given a motor effect there. This solution at most clarifies where body and soul come into contact, but how this interaction takes place remains obscure.

Critical analysis of Descartes' writings has clarified that the usual interpretation of his philosophy is seriously flawed. He regarded the human being as a "substantial union" of two substances: rational soul and sentient body. [70] In a dualistic approach, the soul has been removed from the medical domain, so that subjective experiences have been eliminated. This has also been a problem for Descartes. [71] In his view, the soul does not take a position in the body like a pilot in his ship. This is an experience that we do not learn from our rational or imaginative faculty, but from our feeling:

> Simply by living and in daily conversation, by not occupying oneself with meditation and with studying things that appeal to the imaginative faculty, one learns to form an idea of the unity of soul and body; . . . the unity that everyone always experiences in himself when not philosophizing. [72]

The unity of soul and body is essential for humans and not something of minor importance. By not recognizing this unity, philosophical thinking has dissociated itself from daily experiences. It has inspired a new conception of nature – what Husserl has called "geschlossenen Körperwelt." [73]

Ordinary experiences have not discredited dualism. [74] Talking about persons is not the same as talking about bodies and their connected mental life. Obtaining more knowledge about the body and its parts does not provide knowledge about the person. This means that there is more to me than my body. Dualism has emerged from a primordial phenomenon: the experience of the world as well as self-knowledge is gained directly from my own particular perspective. First-person experience is the main reason for belief in the existence of a soul. As agents, we have privileged access to our mental states. We cannot deny that we have sensations and thoughts, feelings, and hopes. We experience bodily events that cause brain events. We cannot explain how that occurs but from this we cannot conclude that interactions do not occur. The fact that we cannot explain these interactions does not mean that they do not exist. The point is that mental events are distinct from physical events. As Richard Swinburne points out: being in pain is not the same as firing brain fibers. [75] He defends substance dualism: since talk about persons is not analyzable in terms of talk about bodies and their connected mental life, the most natural way to make sense of this fact is talking about persons as consisting of two parts.

However, the difference between body and soul does not necessarily translate into an ontological distinction: the idea that there are two distinct substances, a body and a soul, that cannot be reduced to each other. This is the view of Thomas Aquinas. The soul and body are not two substances but constitute one actually existing substance, the human person. The fundamental substance is the individual human being. People are not bodies plus soul, but ensouled bodies. A bodiless soul therefore is no person. The soul as essence is diffused in every part of the body. The soul occupies the body but is not located within it. The soul is present in every part of the body. Since the body is essential in human life, "my soul is not I," as Thomas concluded. Bodily continuity is required for personal identity.[76] A contemporary view defends an anthropological perspective: the human person is a unity of two entities or qualities; mental states are not identical to physical states, nor can they be reduced to such states. There is only one substance. As human beings, we experience the unity of the self; we are aware that we are a mental subject with a body. We do not only have a body but are a body. Third-person descriptions therefore will not capture the first-person point of view. [77]

The anthropological tradition in philosophy of medicine exemplifies this way of thinking. [78] Many advocates of anthropologically oriented medicine have been practicing physicians who became prolific writers with a broad interest in the humanities. Their main interest was to redefine and reinterpret medicine as a science of human beings. In philosophically rethinking medical activities, they used ideas from several contemporary philosophical schools, particularly phenomenology (Husserl, Merleau-Ponty), existentialism (Marcel, Sartre), and philosophical anthropology (Scheler, Gehlen, and Plessner). They clearly rejected Cartesian dualism. Any demarcation between body and mind is artificial. The idea that there is an objective, real world, independent from an isolated, individual subject was also not acceptable to them. A human being cannot relate himself or herself to the world as a neutral observer. The methodology of the natural sciences therefore is not fully appropriate in the context of healthcare. This does not imply that causal thinking and technical approaches of the natural sciences should not be allowed in medicine; on the contrary, they are highly valuable and useful; but medical thinking and practicing should not restrict itself to these scientific methods. In the words of Viktor von Weizsäcker: "Medicine is not technology; it is technology, too." [79] Instead of rejecting scientific methods, they should be considered according to their relative value. The problem is that such methods cannot grasp what is essential to human beings. As a living organism, every person constitutes a whole, a meaningful entity, which is disconnected and disintegrated by abstract, analytical approaches. To examine the living being, we should participate in life, and focus upon the purposeful coherence and interrelationships, the significance of experience and conduct. If medicine wants to evolve into a science of the human person, it should overcome the usual distinction between the objective and subjective. This means that the subject should be introduced into medicine. If medicine is not objective, it is impossible; if medicine is only an objective science, it is inhuman. [80] Anthropologically oriented physicians furthermore argued that a comprehensive understanding of disease is necessary. The conception of disease, current in modern medicine, is incomplete. The reason is not that the science of pathology is insufficient and not fully developed, but that pathology operates with inadequate notions and assumptions. Focusing on the causal mechanisms of disease, medicine cannot fully understand the ill person, because explaining disease also refers to the problem of the significance of a symptom, the meaning of a particular complaint. Science-based medicine, in fact, hinders the insight that disease has meaning; in its approach, the only relevant question concerns the pathogenesis and pathophysiology of the disease; the anthropological question that many patients face "Why here and now" is irrelevant. Our argument is not that medicine should address the psychological dimensions of disease. Since dualistic thinking is rejected, one cannot say that both the body and the mind are involved in the disease process; it is impossible to find out where the disease started, thereby recognizing the primacy of body or mind. Disease gives voice to a threatened existence. Being ill primarily is an existential category; only secondarily, we can make any differentiation between organic and psychic suffering. Being ill is a way of being a human person. When I not only have my life, but also give expression to it, when I not merely have my body, but also am my body at the same time, then it is also the case that I am not only having my disease and suffering it, but also make my disease. Thus, being ill is a response of the person to his or her own individual existence. In this perspective, disease is not a merely negative event, a blind fate, waiting to be eliminated from the world; the important thing is what we make of it, whether we examine it as an occasion to reconsider and improve our life. [81]

The tradition of anthropological medicine had a limited impact; it has mainly been influential in Germany and the Netherlands. [82] Nowadays, it is revived in phenomenological approaches to medicine and healthcare. [83] It affirms that the basic experience of the world is gained directly from our own particular perspective; science is the second-order expression. Explaining illness therefore requires first-person perspectives.

One fundamental question is whether these perspectives really overcome Cartesian dualism. It seems that anthropological medicine and other holistic approaches such as psychosomatic medicine still start from a dualistic way of thinking, attempting to explain the interaction between body and soul. They presuppose the existence of different components human beings are composed of. This question will be discussed in Chapter 6.

## Conclusion

This chapter has examined how the soul has been eradicated from the discourses of science, psychology, theology, philosophy, medicine, and bioethics. It has attempted to explain why the soul has disappeared from these discourses. The scientific worldview of naturalism is regarded as responsible for the soul's demise. According to this view, only natural things exist. Naturalism implies an ontological claim about the constitution of the world. Mental events are really physical events. Perceptions, thoughts, or desires should not be subscribed to a soul, but are caused by physical and chemical events in the brain. Naturalism also implies an epistemological claim. Science is the only source of valid explanations. Science is grounded in objectivity and it determines the truth of statements. The knowledge it produces is not distorted by personal, cultural, or religious opinions. All facts in the world can be explained in scientific terms. There is no need for first-person perspectives. However, naturalism and physicalism are not scientific theories. They are theses about the nature of the world, thus worldviews that question the presuppositions of everyday life. [84]

The chapter indicates that naturalism, and especially physicalism, is an influential ideology in medicine and healthcare. It is assumed that living organisms are conglomerates of nerve cells, brains, and genes, and thus molecules; physics can explain how they function and how diseases and disorders emerge and can be treated. Obtaining and applying medical knowledge does not require any bifurcation between the person and the physical body. Although the philosopher Descartes is usually blamed for separating soul and body, he emphasized the unity of body and mind. However, the long-term effect of his philosophy was that the soul has been removed from the medical domain, and that the body was reduced to a complex of mechanistic, organic processes.

The chapter finally relates the dominant scientific worldview to philosophy of mind, and particularly the debate on dualism. Separating body and soul has enormously promoted the advancement of medical science. At the same time, it has removed the soul from healthcare practice. Nonetheless, ordinary experiences cannot simply be discarded, especially not when they concern health, disease, illness, and suffering. Human beings and world are principally connected. They do not live in an abstract world, neither in a pure inner world. Philosophers like Edmund Husserl have argued that human beings exist in the natural world but at the same time they transcend the natural world and can detach from it. This is what Helmuth Plessner has called the "excentricity" of human beings: they are not fixated on daily existence but are distanced from themselves since they are included in wider perspectives of culture and humanity. [85] Being in the world also means coexisting with other beings. Subjectivity is intersubjectivity. Husserl's project criticized natural sciences as offering a too limited perspective. The problem is that these sciences and their technological applications have thoroughly penetrated our everyday lifeworld, although they have lost their meaning for our life. This is the result of the emergence of a new social order, especially in Western societies and cultures, that has created a new type of human being. The world has become knowable, predictable, manageable, and malleable by human beings. In principle, there is nothing magical or mysterious in the world. This will be the subject of the next chapter.

## References

1 Francis Crick, *The astonishing hypothesis. The scientific search for the soul* (New York: Simon & Schuster, 1994).
2 Crick, *The astonishing hypothesis*, 7, 258.
3 James Watson, *DNA. The secret of life* (New York: Alfred A Knopf, 2003), 258.
4 Hugh Miller, "DNA blueprints, personhood, and genetic privacy," *Health Matrix. The journal of Law-Medicine* 8, no. 2 (1998): 180.
5 Lee M. Silver, "Biotechnology and conceptualizations of the soul," *Cambridge Quarterly of Healthcare Ethics* 12 (2003): 335–341.
6 Dorothy Nelkin, and M. Susan Lindee, *The DNA mystique: The gene as a cultural icon* (New York: W. H. Freeman and Company, 1995), 41.
7 See: Alex Mauron, "Is the genome the secular equivalent of the soul?" *Science* 291 (2001): 831–832; Alex Mauron, "Renovating the house of being. Genomes, souls, and selves," *Annuals of the New York Academy of Sciences* 1001 (2003): 240–252.
8 Jesse Lee Preston, Ryan S. Ritter, and Justin Hepler, "Neuroscience and the soul: Competing explanations for the human experience," *Cognition* 127 (2013): 31–37.
9 Fernando Vidal, *The sciences of the soul: The early modern origins of psychology* (Chicago and London: Chicago University Press, 2011).
10 William James, *Principles of Psychology* (University of Chicago: Encyclopedia Britannica, Inc, 1990; original 1890), 225.
11 Carl Gustav Jung, *Modern man in search of a soul* (New York: Harcourt, Brace and Company, 1933), 178.
12 Jung, *Modern man in search of a soul*, 174.
13 Jung, *Modern man in search of a soul*, 184.
14 Jung, *Modern man in search of a soul*, 221.
15 Warren S. Brown, Nancy Murphy, and H. Newton Malony, eds., *Whatever happened to the soul? Scientific and theological portraits of human nature* (Minneapolis: Fortress Press, 1998), xiii.
16 Stephen G. Post, "A moral case for nonreductive physicalism," in *Whatever happened to the soul?* eds. Warren S. Brown, Nancy Murphy, and H. Newton Malony (Minneapolis: Fortress Press, 1998), 195–212.
17 Gilbert Ryle, *The concept of mind* (Harmondsworth: Penguin Books, 1949), 17ff.
18 ". . .'my mind' does not stand for another organ. It signifies my ability and proneness to do certain things and not some piece of personal apparatus without which I could or would not do them." Ryle, *The concept of mind*, 161. See also: William Lyons, *Gilbert Ryle. An introduction to his philosophy* (Brighton: The Harvester Press, 1980).

19 In the 12th century, Hildegard van Bingen affirmed: "The soul is breath of living spirit, that with excellent sensitivity, permeates the entire body to give it life." See: Phil Cousineau, ed., *Soul. An archaeology* (New York: HarperCollins Publishers, 1995), 38.
20 Herbert Feigl, *The 'mental' and the 'physical'. The essay and a postscript* (Minneapolis: University of Minneapolis Press, 1967).
21 Lynne Rudder Baker, *Naturalism and the first-person perspective* (Oxford: Oxford University Press, 2013), 82.
22 Stewart Goetz, and Charles Taliaferro, *A brief history of the soul* (Chichester: Wiley-Blackwell, 2011), 19.
23 Soma Hewa, and Robert W. Hetherington, "Specialists with spirit: Crisis in the nursing profession," *Journal of Medical Ethics* 16 (1990): 179–284.
24 Jo Marchant, *Cure. A journey into the science of mind over body* (New York: Broadway Books, 2016), 253.
25 Plato, *Charmides*, 156e–157a; http://classics.mit.edu/Plato/charmides.html.
26 Henri Zukier, "The soul in medicine: Rabbinic and scientific controversies," *Journal of Religion and Health* 55 (2016): 2174–2188.
27 Marchant, *Cure*, 217 ff.
28 Robert M. Kaplan, *More than medicine. The broken promise of American health* (Cambridge and London: Harvard University Press, 2019).
29 Gilbert C. Meilaender, *Body, soul, and bioethics* (Notre Dame: University of Notre Dame Press, 2009; original 1995), ix.
30 Meilaender, *Body, soul, and bioethics*, x.
31 Meilaender, *Body, soul, and bioethics*, 32, 36.
32 Walter Glannon, "Tracing the soul: Medical decisions at the margins of life," *Christian Bioethics* 6, no. 1 (2000): 49–69.
33 Natasha Hammond-Browning, "When doctors and parents don't agree: The story of Charlie Gard," *Bioethical Inquiry* 14 (2017): 461–468.
34 Encyclopedia Brittanica, "Naturalism" (2019); www.britannica.com/topic/naturalism-philosophy.
35 John Dewey, "Half-hearted naturalism," *The Journal of Philosophy* 24, no. 3 (1927): 58. See also: Steven M. Cahn, ed., *New studies in the philosophy of John Dewey* (Hanover: The University Press of New England, 1977); Richard J. Bernstein, "Dewey's naturalism," *The Review of Metaphysics* 13, no. 2 (1959): 340–353.
36 David Papineau, "Naturalism," *The Stanford Encyclopedia of Philosophy* (Winter 2016 edition), ed. Edward N. Zalta; https://plato.stanford.edu/archives/win2016/entries/naturalism.
37 Daniel Stoljar, "Physicalism," *The Stanford Encyclopedia of Philosophy* (Winter 2016 edition), ed. Edward N. Zalta; https://plato.stanford.edu/archives/win2017/entries/physicalism. Daniel Stoljar, *Physicalism* (London and New York: Routledge, 2010).
38 "Naturalism in its epistemological form takes natural science as a paradigm of justified belief." Steven J. Wagner, and Richard Wagner, eds., *Naturalism. A critical approach* (Notre Dame: University of Notre Dame Press, 1993), 212. "Epistemological naturalism is the view that epistemological questions . . . are to be investigated empirically . . . Methodological naturalism is the view that the methods of philosophy should be restricted to the methods of science." Baker, *Naturalism and the first-person perspective*, 5.
39 Wagner, and Wagner, *Naturalism*, 1–21.

40 "This naturalistic program is both metaphysical and scientific. It holds both that everything in the world is physical and that everything that happens in the world has its most basic explanation, whether we can come to know it or not, in physical law, as applied to physical things and events and their constituents." Thomas Nagel, *Mind and cosmos: Why the materialist Neo-Darwinian conception of nature is almost certainly false* (Oxford: Oxford University Press, 2012), 43.

41 Stuart Silvers, "Nonreductive naturalism," *Theoria: An International Journal for Theory, History and Foundations of Science* 12, no. 1 (1997): 163–184.

42 Elke Elisabeth Schmidt, "The dilemma of moral naturalism in Nagel's Mind and Cosmos," *Ethical Perspectives* 25, no. 2 (2018): 203–231.

43 Nagel, *Mind and cosmos*, 87.

44 Schmidt, "The dilemma of moral naturalism in Nagel's Mind and Cosmos, 211 ff.

45 Mattew Lutz, and James Lenman, "Moral naturalism," *The Stanford Encyclopedia of Philosophy* (Fall 2018 edition), ed. Edward N. Zalta; https://plato.stanford.edu/archives/fall2018/entries/naturalism-moral.

46 Nagel, *Mind and cosmos*, 112, 122.

47 Schmidt, "The dilemma of moral naturalism in Nagel's Mind and Cosmos," 210–211.

48 Stoljar argues that the notion of physicalism is as problematic as that of naturalism. It lead to many different questions and debates: "it is far from clear what 'physical' means in the context of physicalism." Stoljar, *Physicalism*, 28.

49 Frederick A. Olafson, *Naturalism and the human condition. Against scientism* (London and New York: Routledge, 2001).

50 "In unserer Lebensnot . . . hat diese Wissenschaft uns nichts zu sagen. Gerade die Fragen schlieszt sie prinzipiell aus, die für den in unseren unseligen Zeiten den schichsalvollsten Umwälzungen preisgegebenen Menschen die brennenden sind: die Fragen nach Sinn oder Sinnlosigkeit dieses ganzen menschlichen Daseins." Edmund Husserl, *Die Krisis der europäische Wissenschaften und die transzendentale Phänomenologie. Eine Einleitung in die phänomenologische Philosophie* (Hamburg: Felix Meiner Verlag, 1977), 4–5. See also: Gregory A. Trotter, "Toward a non-reductive naturalism: Combining the insights of Husserl and Dewey," *William James Studies* 12, no. 1 (2016): 19–35.

51 "In der geometrischen und naturwissenschaftlichen Mathematisierung messen wir so der Lebenswelt – der in unserem konkreten Weltleben uns ständig als wirklich gegebenen Welt – in der offenen Unendlichkeit möglicher Erfahrungen ein wohlpassendes Ideenkleid an . . ." Husserl, *Die Krisis der europäische Wissenschaften und die transzendentale Phänomenologie*, 55.

52 Dermot Moran, "Husserl's transcendental philosophy and the critique of naturalism," *Continental Philosophy Review* 41 (2008): 401–425.

53 Havi Carel, "Phenomenology as a resource for patients," *Journal of Medicine and Philosophy* 37 (2012): 96–113.

54 See, for example, Shawn D. Whatley, "Borrowed philosophy: Bedside physicalism and the need for a *sui generis* metaphysic of medicine," *Journal of Evaluation of Clinical Practice* 20 (2014): 961–964; Rothlyn P. Zahurek, "Intentionality: The matrix of healing creates caring, healing presence," *Beginnings (American Holistic Nurses' Association* (April 2014): 6–9.

55 Baker, *Naturalism and the first-person perspective*, xix.

56 "Conscious subjects and their mental lives are inescapable components of reality not describable by the physical sciences." Nagel, *Mind and cosmos*, 41.

57 Dan Zahavi, *Subjectivity and selfhood. Investigating the first-person perspective* (Cambridge and London: The MIT Press, 2005).
58 Nagel, *Mind and cosmos*, 102 ff.
59 This is the argument of Schmidt, "The dilemma of moral naturalism in Nagel's Mind and Cosmos," 217 ff.
60 See, for example, Brown, Murphy, and Malony, eds., *Whatever happened to the soul?*
61 René Descartes, *Oeuvres de Descartes*, publiées par Charles Adam and Paul Tannery (Paris: Vrin, 1897–1913), Vol. IX–1: 47.
62 Henk ten Have, "Medicine and the Cartesian image of man," *Theoretical Medicine* 8 (1987): 235–246.
63 Descartes, *Oeuvres de Descartes*, Vol. XI: 130–131.
64 Edmund D. Pellegrino, and David C. Thomasma, *A philosophical basis of medical practice* (New York: Oxford University Press, 1981), 99.
65 Descartes, *Oeuvres de Descartes*, Vol. VI: 62.
66 Gerrit A. Lindeboom, *Descartes and medicine* (Amsterdam: Rodopi, 1979).
67 Ten Have, "Medicine and the Cartesian image of man," 240–242.
68 Descartes, *Oeuvres de Descartes*, Vol. IV: 329.
69 Lindeboom, *Descartes and medicine*, 57 ff.
70 Gordon Baker, and Katherine J. Morris, *Descartes' dualism* (London and New York: Routledge, 1996).
71 See, for example, Cornelis A. van Peursen, *Lichaam – ziel – geest. Inleiding tot een fenomenologische antropologie* (Utrecht: Erven J. Bijleveld, 1970, 4th edition), 22 ff.
72 Descartes, *Oeuvres de Descartes*, Vol. III: 692, 694. See also: Grant Duncan, "Mind-body dualism and the biopsychosocial model of pain: What did Descartes really say?" *Journal of Medicine and Philosophy* 25, no. 4 (2000): 485–513.
73 Husserl, *Die Krisis der europäische Wissenschaften und die transzendentale Phänomenologie*, 65.
74 Eric Austin Lee, and Samuel Kimbriel, eds., *The resounding soul. Reflections on the metaphysics and vivacity of the human person* (Eugene: Cascade Books, 2015).
75 Richard Swinburne, *The evolution of the soul* (Oxford: Clarendon Press, 1997, revised edition; 1st edition 1986).
76 Brian Davies, *The thought of Thomas Aquinas* (Oxford: Clarendon Press, 1992), 216; Denys Turner, *Thomas Aquinas. A Portrait* (New Haven and London: Yale University Press, 2013); see also: Goetz and Taliaferro, *A brief history of the soul.*
77 James P. Moreland, and Scott B. Rae, *Body & Soul. Human nature & the crisis in ethics* (Downers Grove: InterVarsity Press, 2000).
78 Henk ten Have, "The anthropological tradition in philosophy of medicine," *Theoretical Medicine* 16 (1995): 3–14.
79 Viktor von Weizsäcker, "Medizin, Klinik und Psychoanalyse," in *Zwischen Medizin und Philosophie*, eds. Viktor von Weizsäcker and Dieter Wyss (Göttingen: Vandenhoeck & Ruprecht, 1957; original 1928), 32.
80 Frederik J. J. Buytendijk, "De relatie arts-patiënt," *Nederlands Tijdschrift voor Geneeskunde* 103 (1959): 2504–2508.
81 Viktor von Weizsäcker, "Psychosomatische Medizin," in *Zwischen Medizin und Philosophie*, eds. Viktor von Weizsäcker and Dieter Wyss (Göttingen: Vandenhoeck & Ruprecht, 1957; original 1949), 92.
82 Phillip Honenberger: *Naturalism and philosophical anthropology. Nature, life, and the human between transcendental and empirical perspectives* (Houndmills: Palgrave Macmillan, 2016).

83 Fredrik Svenaeus, *Phenomenological bioethics. Medical technologies, human suffering, and the meaning of being alive* (London and New York: Routledge, 2018); Havi Carel, *Phenomenology of illness* (Oxford: Oxford University Press, 2016). See also: Fred Dallmayr, "The return of philosophical anthropology," in *Philosophy and anthropology: Border crossing and transformations*, eds. Ananta Kumar Giri and John Clammer (London: Anthem Press, 2013), 357–364.
84 Stoljar, *Physicalism*, 13, 15.
85 Helmuth Plessner, *Levels of organic life and the human. An introduction into philosophical anthropology* (New York: Fordham University Press, 2019; original 1928).

# 3 The disenchantment of the world

The disappearance of the soul in modern times is the manifestation of a wider phenomenon that sociologist Max Weber has called the "disenchantment of the world." With the expansion of modernity, traditional agricultural societies are replaced by other economic and social arrangements. This new social order has encouraged the emergence of a novel type of human being. The historical process studied by Weber produced an understanding of the world and all areas of human experience that is less mysterious and magical. The world has become knowable and predictable by humans. This chapter will analyze the disenchantment thesis and its implications.

Weber argues that rationalization and intellectualization are characteristics of our times. This thesis has two dimensions. One is the decline of magic. The other dimension is increasing rationalization and also bureaucratization. Both processes imply that the sciences, according to Weber, become more powerful but cannot ask or answer questions of meaning and value. Technical means and calculations are what they can provide. Disenchantment is a universal and inevitable process that will only become stronger and will dominate all spheres of life.

The disenchantment thesis proclaims that modernity is ruled by instrumental rationality but also by formal rationality that has emerged through bureaucracy and industrialization. This last type of rationality uses means–end calculations referring to abstract and universally applied rules, laws, or regulations. It creates a form of domination that is impersonal. The consequence is that we live in what Weber calls the Iron Cage.

The next section of the chapter examines disenchantment in medicine and healthcare. Dissatisfaction with modern medicine, as mentioned in previous chapters, is often the result of disenchantment. Medical science tells us what we must do if we want to master life but it disregards the question whether it makes sense to do so. Medicine is permeated with the ideal of systematic observation, distinguishing sharply between objectivity and subjectivity. Physicians learn how to see the body in a specific and similar way. This "clinical gaze" is the result of training and technology, especially visualizing instruments. Contemporary medicine is furthermore permeated with the market language of providers, services, and industry. Medicine as technological production is mechanistic, reproducible, and measurable. These images of medicine as a science as well as industry have disenchanting consequences: the personal and the professional are separated. Healthcare providers are abstract categories, not concrete individuals, just as patients have become clients, thus files and cases.

Disenchantment has furthermore affected the discipline of bioethics. This will be explored in the subsequent paragraph of the chapter. Disenchantment, in the view of Weber, is the eclipse of the moral universe of the premodern world. The moral and interpretative unity of this world is lost and fragmented. It has moved from the public realm into the private sphere of personal relationships. This can be regarded as liberation from irrational external forces. The result is that social concerns are displaced into personal moral ones. Consensus is impossible; the only option is mutual agreement based on the free choice of individuals consenting with others. This implies that the role of bioethics is limited. While medical science and technology can tell us what to do but not why and how to use them, bioethics has emerged as a response to human suffering and issues of meaning. But by associating with the instrumental and formal rationality of medicine, bioethics itself cannot make sense of what patients are experiencing. Moral values now have become the subject of empirical observation, measurement, comparison, and testing.

The final part of this chapter focuses on re-enchantment. Weber assumed that disenchantment is a universal phenomenon that will only become stronger in all spheres of life. However, many scholars have observed that there is no decline in relevancy of values, religion, and spirituality since Weber formulated his thesis. In postmodernity, there seems to be widespread acceptance of mystery, ambiguity, and contingency, rejecting scientism and eliciting responses of wonder, reverence, and sacramentality of things. There are many responses challenging the domination of rationalization, intellectualism, and bureaucratization. They put emphasis on the soul: on human capacities, sensibilities to nature, connectedness with other people, affective human communication, alternative lifestyles, and spirituality.

## The disenchantment thesis

Weber argues that rationalization and intellectualization are characteristic of our times: "there are no mysterious incalculable forces that come into play, but rather . . . one can, in principle, master all things by calculation." He concludes: "This means that the world is disenchanted." [1] Magic and mystery as instruments to salvation have been eliminated.

The first dimension of Weber's thesis identifies the process of secularization. God is no longer present in the world and has become a transcendent power. That means a new sense of human abilities; it produced the movement of humanism. It also means that the individual is on its own. Marcel Gauchet has explained this process as the retreat of religion, considered as the understanding of the universe as a sacred order, from public space. Religious attitudes accept that what gives meaning to human existence comes not from us but from different beings *before us*. [2] Whatever causes and justifies the visible human sphere is outside this sphere. The decline of religion in the face of modernity, and the emphasis on the transcendence of God, brings the individual back to its own resources: "As God withdrew, the world changes from something *presented* . . . to something to be *constituted*". [3] This process created a new sense of human challenges and abilities. Religion is dis-embedded from public life and relocated in the private sphere of individual life. Disenchantment therefore is not simply the extension of processes of rationalization and intellectualization. It is, in the words of Sam Han, "a reconfiguration in the traditional layout of the relations between humans, nature and God." The priority goes to the human and to humanism. The realm of nature and that of humans are kept free from divine intervention. [4]

The second dimension assumes that the world becomes increasingly subjected to approaches of science and rational government but at the same time it becomes more and more impersonal. The sciences, according to Weber, should be value-free. They cannot ask or answer questions of meaning and value. Technical means and calculations are what they can provide. The implication is that what is needed is intellectual analysis; social commitment is not possible. In Weber's theories, different types of rationality are at work. Most important is instrumental rationality. This determines means–end types of social action. It is concerned with the most effective and expedient means to accomplish certain ends. The preferable ends are determined by the pragmatic and selfish interests of individuals. Substantive rationality, focused on values as ends of action, has become impossible as social action. [5]

The main research concern of Weber was how to explain the origin and effects of modern capitalism. What have been the conditions for the emergence of capitalism as use of wealth to gain profit in commerce? And how has this impacted and transformed the self-understanding of human beings? Disenchantment has occurred through different stages: from primitive societies (with emphasis on magic), to traditional societies (emphasizing religion and the transcendent idea of the sacred) to modern societies (with the predominance of science). Weber witnessed significant changes in society and culture. [6] Traditional agricultural societies are replaced by industrial and capitalist arrangements. For example, Berlin transformed from a provincial city into a cosmopolitan and modern metropole. The rise of bureaucratic states was associated with increasing administration and industrialization, with specialization and division of labor. But at the same time a new culture emerged where feelings, emotions, and experiences played a major role. The economic mode of analysis became most attractive in many spheres of life. A new type of rationality became dominant: efficient, means–end calculation with planning and manipulation. Rationalization is especially manifested in four spheres of life: religion, science, economy, and state. [7]

Capitalism is joined with the ideal of technical progress. This ideal can be achieved with standardization of activities: instrumental action and control of conditions of existence. [8] All things can be mastered by calculation. Capitalism is not so much characterized by the desire for profits but is the expression of rational ethics; in the words of Weber: "The ethic of duty and honor in one's vocation produced and maintains that Iron Cage, through which economic activity nowadays acquire its special character and fate." [9]

Weber's interest in the rise of capitalism as a change in economic structures is linked to his interest in culture. Economic transformation is associated with social changes and transitions in political authority. Weber famously connected capitalism and protestant ethos. Especially, puritanism regarded work as a vocation; it must be done. The ethics of ascetism that was peculiar for monastery life moved out of the medieval monasteries into vocational life. It came to determine the lifestyle of all people, not only those engaged in economic transactions and labor. [10] Protestantism presumes that the world exists to serve the glorification of God. People live to honor God; only some are predestined and chosen for eternal life. This implies the loneliness of the individual. Magical means to salvation are not available. There is no atonement, grace, or forgiveness. What is required is constant self-control and a rationally planned regulation of life in accordance with God's will. This worldly asceticism requires strict regulation of conduct: modesty, not showing luxury, and also duty and work ethos. [11]

Weber wants to understand the historical process of disenchantment, not criticizing it. The process is regarded as a liberation of the mind: it progressively eliminates magic and irrationality from social life. The world can be reconstructed on a rational basis. But the process simultaneously and radically alters everyday life and human experiences. It constricts imagination, and introduces a new logic into civilization. [12] Disenchantment is a universal and inevitable process that will only become stronger and will dominate all spheres of life. That implies loss of values. In regard to science, Weber has, in fact, a paradoxical view. He recognizes that it produces benefits and progress, but at the same time he regrets its effect on modern culture. [13] Since no change is possible, Weber has a pessimistic and melancholic attitude toward disenchantment. He concludes: "the ultimate and most sublime values have retreated from public life either into the transcendental realm of mystic life or into the brotherliness of direct and personal human relations." [14] The world has become meaningless. What remains are specialists without spirit.

## The Iron Cage

Modernity, according to Weber, is ruled by instrumental as well as formal rationality, creating a form of domination that is impersonal. This is framed by Weber as "the Iron Cage." Scholars have discussed what is exactly meant by this imagery. A better translation of the original German term "stahlhartes Gehäuse" might be "shell as hard as steel" that defines the living space in which human activity, choices, and valuing take place. It is the constraining structure that is a component of the very existence of individuals. [15] People are trapped in a rationalistic, bureaucratized system that restricts their freedom and creativity – an order of things that cannot be altered. This is not an external prison but a predicament that has become part of the human frame. Human beings themselves behave in impersonal, calculative, and formalized ways. It means that individuals in modernity have a limited degree of autonomy. [16]

In this view, the modern world is characterized by impersonal structures of domination. At the same time, the self is marked by the quest for autonomy and self-expression. A new type of human species has emerged but retreated in the private sphere. The consequence is the creation of a soul-less social world. Shared norms for social life have been eliminated, and human beings are increasingly subjected to abstract, anonymous, and routine forms of external power. Only two choices are possible according to Weber: resignation and submission to the demands of modern society, or preservation of a sense of individuality, maintaining some "inner distance" to the depersonalizing forces of the modern world. [17]

## Disenchantment of medicine

Dissatisfaction with modern medicine, as mentioned in previous chapters, is often the result of disenchantment. Weber himself refers to medicine as a highly developed "practical technology" aimed at maintaining life and diminishing suffering. But medical science does not ask whether life is worth living. It tells us what we must do if we want to master life, health, and disease but it disregards the question whether it makes sense to do so. [18] Disenchantment in medicine has been animated by Cartesianism. Balthasar Bekker, a Dutch minister and follower of Descartes, published in 1691 a bestselling book, *De Betoverde Weereld* (The World Bewitched) in which he criticized spiritual phenomena and denied the existence of angels, devils, spirits, ghosts, and witches. His main concern was that true faith needs to be distinguished from superstition. Immaterial substances such as ghosts cannot influence bodies. [19]

Disenchantment is visible in medicine in at least two aspects: the emphasis on objectivity, and the impact of bureaucracy and economy. Modern medicine is infused with the ideal of systematic observation, making a clear distinction between objectivity and subjectivity. The basic assumption is that scientific observation is not contaminated by theories, cultural and social context, or subjective biases. Systematic observation therefore is the basis for a scientific approach to medicine. [20] Physicians have to learn how to see the body in a specific and similar way. This way of observing and examining is the result of training and technology, especially visualizing instruments. Michel Foucault has introduced the notion of "clinical gaze." He argues that in the final part of the 18th century a mutation in medical discourse took place, enabling doctors to see what really matters to patients. Medicine based on symptoms changed into anatomo-clinical medicine – a medicine of organs, sites, and causes. Pathological anatomy became the basis for clinical medicine. Symptoms were explained with reference to lesions in the body. Locating illnesses inside the body, physicians must "abstract the patient": to know the illness, they should relate symptoms to pathological facts. [21] Pathology provided an objective and real foundation for describing diseases. With this conceptual and methodological approach, medicine transformed into an applied science. The mutation in the conceptual framework of medicine made the body of the individual person into an object of scientific investigation and analysis. The physician should look through the surface into the depth of the body and its tissues.

His primary concern is the correct diagnosis. The clinical gaze therefore makes the invisible visible. Clinical symptoms are not the most significant manifestation of illness but refer to lesions. The gaze requires meticulous examination. The doctor is using specific methods such as auscultation and percussion, and finally autopsy, to clarify the underlying pathology. The clinical gaze also requires the collection of written reports, files, documents, and records in order to facilitate statistical analyses. The result is that each individual is made into a case of a specific disease. [22]

In the perspective of Foucault, the new framework is not merely a reorganization of the medical discourse. It creates the possibilities for a scientific discourse about disease. Clinical experience became possible, opening the individual to the language of rationality. The precondition for this mutation is death. Through integrating death into medical discourse, death is no longer contrary to nature but incorporated into the living body of individuals. It is the precondition for medical discourse. [23] The clinical gaze translates the inherent finitude of human beings into a basic explanation of subjective experiences. The implication is that such objectification makes human beings into subjects of science and disciplinary power. In this sense, it is argued that modern patients are the result of the clinical gaze. They are medical constructs. Patients have receded from the medical narrative. Their voices have disappeared. [24] What is important is how patients are perceived by doctors. Another implication articulated by Foucault is that this mutation is only possible through an institutional setting such as the establishment of hospitals and clinics but also the professionalization of medicine. In the past, patients have been cared for by families and relatives. Patients have not been dominated by doctors; they shopped around, and often disregarded doctor's advice.

Contemporary medicine is furthermore permeated with the market language of providers, services, and industry. The result is, in the words of Blythe and Curlin, that the practice of medicine is regarded as "the technological production and bureaucratically administered provision of goods and services to be used according to the individual's preferences." [25] Medicine as technological production is mechanistic, reproducible, and measurable. These images of medicine as a science as well as industry have disenchanting consequences: the personal and the professional are separated. Healthcare providers are presented as abstract categories, not concrete individuals, just as patients have become clients. As a result, patients with existential questions about life, death, and suffering feel like objects, and health professionals as functionaries within bureaucratic organizations and management systems. [26] Disenchantment as the triumph of instrumental reason leads to dehumanization and alienation in medical interactions. [27] Market metaphors direct the imagination in specific directions: efficiency, consumption, and competition. Nowadays, the clinical gaze is often linked to, or even superseded by, the economic gaze focused on productivity and economic growth. The individual is viewed as vital because of his or her contribution to economic welfare. [28]

Disenchantment in healthcare has two effects: elimination of subjectivity, and priority of technical production. The emphasis on instrumental reason makes it hard to discuss the goals of medical analysis and intervention. The dead body is in fact the ideal body. Knowledge is acquired for control over the natural order of diseases, and no longer appreciated for understanding why patients are suffering. From the perspective of patients, this approach is not satisfactory. Many patients have questions about the meaning of life, death, and suffering. But medicine cannot answer such questions. Medicine demonstrates technical mastery but impotence concerning existential troubles. It may be using case histories and personal narratives but these are not really subjective. The critique is that in medical practice, science and human values cannot be separated; patients cannot merely be defined as contracting clients. [29]

## Disenchantment of bioethics

Disenchantment has also affected the discipline of bioethics. According to Weber, science is the dominant source of rational understanding and knowledge of the world. Science is a value-free enterprise. Disenchantment means that something of great value is lost. Ultimate values have retreated in the private sphere of personal relationships, so that we have to accept that the world is pointless. The effect of this process is first that social concerns are difficult to address. They are displaced into private moral ones. The second effect is that the role of bioethics is limited. The ability of secular bioethics to resolve moral controversies is constrained. Consensus can only be accomplished by mutual agreement, thus through the free choices of individuals consenting with others. Any appeal to ultimate foundations for ethical decisions is impossible. [30] Nonetheless, there is a continuous tension between the sacred and the secular in modern medicine. Many technologies are available but they cannot guide us how to use them. Ethical studies repeatedly emphasized that the fact that technologies are at hand should not dictate their applications. Their use depends on the goals, needs, and values of patients. What is needed therefore is reflection on relevant goals and values. This is the reason why bioethics as a new discipline has emerged decades ago. It was a response to the power of scientific and technological medicine, arguing that values of patients should guide this power. The focus should be on ameliorating human suffering, and not merely on the possibilities of technical interventions or medical treatments. Careful demarcation and limitation of medical action still is a major consideration in many bioethical debates. This is, for instance, evident in ongoing discussions about experiments with human beings. Especially in times of a pandemic, when there is an urgent need for new and effective medication, debates focus on whether protection of the interests of patients should have priority over the interests of science and society. However, with its formal approach, bioethics has difficulties in addressing issues related to the meaning of suffering. It cannot make much sense of patients' experiences. [31]

Another effect of disenchantment is the so-called "empirical turn" in bioethics during the last two decades. Quantitative and qualitative methods (e.g. case studies, surveys, questionnaires, interviews, and participatory observation) are increasingly used in ethics. The purpose is to obtain empirical information and to map the medical reality. Examples are studies to clarify the attitudes of nurses toward euthanasia, or analyses of quantitative data about conflicts of interests in pharmaceutical research. The recent upsurge of empirical ethics has several explanations. [32] One is the dissatisfaction with the methods of mainstream bioethics. Ethical theories and principles are applied without sufficient attention to the practical realities of healthcare. Actual experiences and social and cultural contexts are not taken into account. A second factor is the development of clinical ethics, that is the application of ethical analysis within clinical settings with a focus on specific patient cases. Ethics consultation begins with an examination of the practicalities of the case as well as the encounters between patient and healthcare providers. This type of consultation has become a clinical service in many hospitals, especially in the United States and Canada. Consultants can have different backgrounds: medicine, nursing, social work, law, and chaplaincy. The majority are practicing healthcare professionals. They are not necessarily experts in ethics. This has raised at least issues of qualification and education. [33] Against this background, the American Society for Bioethics and Humanities (ASBH) has launched a Code of Ethics and Professional Responsibilities for Health Care Ethics Consultants based on core competencies. It has also inaugurated a certification and accreditation program for healthcare ethics consulting with examinations and tests. [34] The role of consultants is to assess factual information, to analyze the ethical questions, and to evaluate the outcomes of the consultation. This bedside role is primarily pragmatic, facilitating clinical decision-making. However, there is no agreement on the goals of ethics consultation. A third explanation for the growth of empirical ethics is the current emphasis on evidence-based approaches. This has stimulated evidence-based ethics, arguing that ethical decisions should be based on medical scientific evidence, integrating empirical data into ethical decision-making. [35] A final explanation is related to funding of ethics research. In 1990, the HGP started research activities focused on the Ethical, Legal, and Social Implications (ELSI) of emerging life sciences. Three percent of the HGP budget (projected budget of $3 billion over 15 years) was allocated to ELSI, which made huge resources available for ethical research. In 1994, the European Union started its own funding initiative, the Ethical, Legal and Social Aspects (ELSA) program. This type of research requires that bioethical analysis is combined with empirical and participatory approaches. Empirical evidence is needed to develop policies. Funding of ELSI or ELSA research seems to promote a research agenda that is empirically driven. [36]

Empirical bioethics has raised several concerns. First is methodological diversity. Many data are generated but it is often not clear how different results can be synthesized and interpreted. It is also not obvious how empirical findings may be used. It is pointed out that they "inform" ethical reasoning but that leaves open many possible applications. [37] Others argue that ethical "meaningful" information can be gained when we know the attitudes, moral beliefs, reasoning, and behavior of people, so that this can "enrich normative arguments and make ethical discourse more context sensitive and comprehensive." [38]

More fundamental problems concern the relationship between empirical data and normative reflection. When moral values become the subject of empirical observation, measurement, and testing, the risk is that the normative content is obscured. [39] A survey among bioethics researchers in 12 European countries shows that the majority (87.5%) is using empirical methods but only a minority has integrated empirical data with normative analysis, although their projects entailed a normative question. [40] Prescriptivity is also an issue. Research describes what people do but not what they ought to do. It is relevant to examine the actual conduct of people, how policies are implemented, to recognize ethical issues that have escaped attention, to know opinions and reasoning patterns, and to make ethics more context-sensitive or realistic. This information can enhance the practical feasibility and potential effectiveness of bioethics. But it still leaves open the question of normativity of ethics discourse. Mapping the moral domain is important but cannot be in itself prescriptive. Empirical approaches wrongly assume that the facts described and identified are neutral, and are not presupposing values. [41] As a result, the role of the ethicist is that of interpreter, facilitator, Socratic guide, educator, and mediator but he or she "is not to give ethical judgments or justifications." [42]

## Re-enchantment

Weber regarded disenchantment as a ubiquitous experience that will only become stronger in all spheres of life. However, as a cultural phenomenon and historical process, disenchantment is seriously questioned and disputed. In the postmodern era, there is growing interest and acceptance of mystery, ambiguity, and contingency, emphasizing responses of wonder and miracle. The ideologies of scientism and naturalism are increasingly criticized and rejected. Since Weber formulated his thesis, there is no obvious decline in relevancy of values, religion, and spirituality. [43] Weber also underestimated the capacity of human beings to resist bureaucratic rationalities, and to circumvent formal rationality through informal practices. Scholars, moreover, doubt whether there ever was a unified and homogenous world that has increasingly fragmented in modern times. For example, the civilizing process described by Norbert Elias indicates that world views and practices have become more unified over time. [44] Nowadays, processes of globalization are making the world more homogenous. All over the globe, there are many responses challenging the domination of rationalization, intellectualism, and bureaucratization. What they have in common is articulation of qualities of the soul: they emphasize the significance of human capabilities, sensibilities to nature and biodiversity, connectedness to other people, honest and affective human communication, spirituality, and the search for meaningful lifestyles. [45] Questioning the disenchantment thesis has resulted in highlighting re-enchantment. Examining historical processes and cultural developments learns that disenchantment is most often accompanied by recurrent or new processes of enchantment.

### *Science and ethics*

One characteristic of Weber's approach is idealization of science. His thesis explains why and how the soul has disappeared from the modern worldview. He argues that human beings live in a fully rationalized world without mystery or magic, with science and technology as the driving forces of rationalization and bureaucratization. However, science is not as neutral and value-free as Weber suggests. As discussed in the previous chapter, science with its ideology of naturalism assumes that physics alone can explain what the world is like. In this perspective, questions about values, meaning, love, and morality can be answered according to science in a relatively simple way. They are illusions. In practice, that means that scientists often take a normative stance. They promote a particular way of interpreting human life and are convinced that this is a superior view. Scientists assume that they have the authority to determine how life should be manipulated and improved. Scientists, as Sheila Jasanoff argues, are "myth-makers." [46] They advance the idea that science is pure, disinterested, and not embedded in society and industry, asserting that it should be free of external controls and regulate itself. This is not the value-neutral approach that Weber advocated. On the contrary, it seems that science and technology have transformed into a magical, mysterious, and transcendent worldview that claims superiority and dominance as the only rational framework to attribute meaning to contemporary life. Weber's insistence that scientists must refrain from evaluative statements is also paradoxical. In his work, he emphasized the importance of culture. Scientific knowledge is produced by culture. It refers to what is possible rather than being a natural way of knowing the world. Weber is not a naturalist. He points out: "belief in the value of scientific truth is a product of specific cultures and is not given in nature." [47] The concept of culture is a value concept. It a sphere of disagreement; it needs interpretation. [48] Weber's idea of scientific value-neutrality is difficult to maintain nowadays. Today, science frequently leads to contradiction, controversy, and confusion. It is based on a "beautiful lie," that is that scientific progress is the result of "the free play of free intellects." [49]

The 1999 World Conference on Science, jointly organized by UNESCO and the International Council for Science (ICSU) in Budapest (Hungary), devoted special attention to the issue of ethical principles and responsibilities in the practice of science. At the opening session, Joseph Rotblat in his keynote address plainly stated: "I hope that this World Conference on Science will finally convince the scientific community that modern science must take human values into account." He drew an analogy with ethical codes of conduct for medical practitioners (e.g. the Hippocratic Oath), and argued that the pursuit of science requires a similar code to "generate awareness and stimulate thinking on the wider issues among young scientists." [50] Rotblat, a Polish physicist, worked on the Manhattan Project during the Second World War but became concerned about nuclear weapons. He was one of the founders of the Pugwash Conferences on Science and World Affairs in 1957 – an international organization of scientists and public figures aimed at reducing the risk of armed conflicts. In 1995, he shared the Noble Peace Prize.

Rotblat's call for a code was positively received. The ICSU published an empirical study in 2002, analyzing 115 ethical standards for science (39 international and 76 national), and showing that the number of standards over the years has increased exponentially from mere 6 existing before the 1970s to more than 40 being issued during the last 5 years of the second millennium. Discussions accelerated since the September 2001 terroristic attacks in the United States. Especially the anthrax letters reactivated the concerns about possible dual use of scientific knowledge and technologies. At the level of the United Nations, it was stated that ethical codes of conduct for scientists and engineers should be encouraged, and that ethics of science education and awareness should be promoted. UNESCO and its World Commission on the Ethics of Scientific Knowledge and Technology (COMEST) launched feasibility studies and consultations for a possible declaration on science ethics. The protracted policy debate finally resulted in the adoption by UNESCO member states of the *Recommendation on Science and Scientific Researchers* in 2017. [51]

Over the past few decades, research integrity has emerged as a major concern. This is the reason why many national and international scientific organizations have developed codes of conduct and ethical regulations, not waiting for a global framework. Integrity became an issue because numerous cases of falsification, deception, and misconduct in scientific research were revealed that shocked the scientific community and the general public. It furthermore became evident that many publications cannot be trusted because they could not be replicated, contained manipulated information, or were ghost-written. A new genre of journals had come into existence.

After an examination of research integrity in China, the journal *Science* concluded that there is a flourishing black market in publications. [52] For fees ranging from $1,600 to $26,000, authorship in Science Citation Index (SCI) journals is for sale. Shady companies are trading in SCI papers. Chinese regulatory agencies are concerned about global influence and the reputation of Chinese science. They have taken initiatives to cultivate research ethics through education and codes of conduct. [53] SCI papers are the basis of promotion in many universities; they also lead to privileges and financial rewards. In her study on bioethics governance in China, Zhang noticed that some Chinese scholars recall the impact factor of their publications but not the name of the journals in which they appeared. [54] This situation is not exceptional. It occurs in many other countries. One of the underlying mechanisms is the blind faith in quantitative measures for scientific output. Scientists are considered as "knowledge producers"; the more publications the better. The emphasis is also on individual researchers rather than institutional research teams, encouraging competition and rivalry. Now that research budgets are declining, and competition for grants is ferocious, scientific misconduct is rampant. But the holy grail of the impact factor is at least one factor that encourages misconduct. It can be argued that the use of the journal impact factor as indicator of scientific quality is contrary to the ethics of science. It suggests reputation and prestige, while there is no experimental data supporting this suggestion. What has been invented as a bibliographic tool for librarians and publishers is misused for the quantitative assessment of researchers and their research. It violates, as Moustafa argues, the ethical rules of scholarly citation since it does not primarily refer to original work. [55] Review journals and articles have the highest impact factors. Editorial policies are distorted since editors may invite senior authors to submit "citable" manuscripts that boost the impact of their journal. Furthermore, the myth of the journal impact factor also leads to university ranking systems that use one biased criterion to compare heterogeneous systems in different countries. Finally, it reshapes the research agenda, promoting preference for popular topics that might result in fast publications in high-impact journals. The question therefore is: Why is such an unscientific approach to measure scientific quality used? Why is it not more severely criticized from the point of view of science ethics? The alternative approach to assessing the quality of research is peer review. This is used not only for review of unpublished materials, but also for rating published work (e.g. in tenure-track decisions for academic positions) and for assessing research proposals. The focus of this review is on the content and quality of scientific work. Submitted manuscripts are evaluated by two or more outside reviewers. The underlying idea is that scientific progress in a specific discipline occurs through original scientific studies in peer-reviewed journals. In order to make sure that information can be trusted, that knowledge is new and based on sound methods, experts in the same field are asked to evaluate the manuscripts before publication. Peer reviewers actually have two functions. One is "filtering"; they make recommendations to assist the editors in deciding about publication. The other is quality assurance; they review the manuscripts following the standards of the field, provide comments and constructive criticism, and make suggestions for improvement. However, peer review is not a scientific process. Reviewers often do not agree with each other; they make different recommendations. Whether or not decisions of journal editors are influenced by recommendations of peer reviewers depends on the type of recommendation. If reviewers agree that a manuscript should be rejected, their recommendation is generally followed by the editors. [56] For other recommendations, the degree of concordance is modest. Another finding in the literature is that the quality of reviews is often quite different. Some reviewers are tough, others are more lenient. Some reviewers are extremely tardy, while others are swift and effective. Editors may know the style of the reviewer. Since editors tend to follow the most critical recommendations, they may influence the fate of a manuscript by the choice of particular reviewers. The final decision about a manuscript is often not influenced by the quality of the review or the seniority of reviewers, at least according to a study of Vintzileos and colleagues. [57] Reviewers as well as editors might also be influenced by the so-called Dunning–Kruger effect. [58] This refers to the notorious Rumsfeldian "unknown unknowns." Reviewers could be relatively ignorant about the topic; they might not be aware of their ignorance; they could act as if they were experts. Since disciplines are evolving rapidly and becoming more subspecialized, it is safe to assume that reviewers have less knowledge about a particular topic than the authors of a manuscript. The same applies to editors. [59]

The *Declaration of Helsinki* requires that the results of research be published; this is an ethical obligation. [60] Publishing has different purposes: it disseminates the results of academic work, it promotes discussion and debate, it encourages the formation of new ideas and views, it solicits feedback and comments. This demonstrates the basic value of science: sharing of knowledge and participating in a community of scholars. Science essentially is not an individual affair but a collaborative effort based on the global good of knowledge. It is therefore governed by scientists themselves as global commons. Young scholars should learn not only how to write articles and to get published but also how to deal with rejections and how to respond carefully and diplomatically to reviewers' criticism. [61] Truly innovative research might never pass the peer review system, as illustrated by Noble laureates who saw their publications rejected by prestigious journals. [62]

Scientific publishing is compromised nowadays. There is an expanding "false academy." [63] Fraudsters are operating everywhere and at all stages of scientific research. In these times of "fake news" and "alternative facts," as a scientist one can no longer trust "colleagues." One of the hot topics of the moment in science and publishing are "predatory journals." [64] Editors and commentators have called this phenomenon "an emerging threat to the medical literature," "the worst thing in publishing, ever," "another nail in the coffin of academics," or simply "academic nightmares." [65] Predatory journals are characterized by a very weak or absent peer review process in combination with publication fees. They heavily spam potential authors. All us are receiving frequent invitations to contribute manuscripts or join editorial boards. On their websites, there is insufficient contact information. The listing of editorial boards is incomplete. The major focus is on quick publication without serious review after payment of a fee. [66] The business model is "pay and publish". The result is "bogus research." [67] This is the real danger of predatory publishing: these publications pollute the pool of scientific knowledge and undermine the reliability of research results. They are, for example, included in databases such as PubMed. [68] Bypassing the traditional peer-review process, they produce weak, unreliable, and questionable knowledge. [69]

Research integrity is recognized as fundamental value of science nowadays because it is essential for trust. This is generally regarded as a basic value in healthcare and science. Without trust, physicians will not be able to provide for their patients. Scientists will no longer be supported when they have lost the trust of the general public. If scientific publications are not reliable, the readership will lose confidence in the data produced by researchers. The notion of scientific integrity refers to honesty, commitment to truth, independence, freedom of inquiry, and impartiality. [70] These are the foundations for the trust of society in science. Integrity and trust are important not only for personal action but also for professional activity. One of the major contributors to declining trust is that the context of science and research has changed significantly. Science nowadays is conceptualized as a commercial enterprise, or at least closely connected to entrepreneurial and business activities. That means the demarcations between science and other activities have been obliterated. Scientists often have conflicts of interest. As researchers, they are concerned with finding out the truth and reliable information. At the same time, they have to obtain grants and funding, and often have to earn their own salaries. [71] They are also encouraged to obtain patents and protect intellectual property rights. Bioethics discourse rarely addresses this biopolitical context; it is even more uncommon that it critically scrutinizes it. Often, it is simply assumed that this context cannot be examined because it is not within the remit of ethical discourse. Ethics prefers to concentrate on individual decisions on whether and how to use new clinical and research opportunities without asking questions about the social, economic, and political conditions within which such decisions are made.

### *Historical analysis*

Scholars have questioned the historical studies on which Weber has based his thesis of disenchantment. Weber regarded the Protestant Reformation as a milestone toward the triumph of rationalism over superstition in the Age of Enlightenment. Protestantism, according to Weber, implies a fundamental rejection of sacramental magic; numinous forces are removed from everyday life so that it is de-sacralized. But it is argued that this thesis is too simple. [72] The Reformation did not play a crucial role in the processes that Weber describes. During the Age of Reason, strong beliefs in miracles, providence, ghosts, angels, and demons persisted. Belief in magic, the supernatural, and an invisible world did not disappear after 1700. In Protestantism, the sacred is still assumed to intervene in the world; many events are interpreted as divine intervention. On the other hand, the picture of the Middle Ages as dark ages is not correct. Medieval religion was not in terminal decline. The supposition of the disenchantment thesis that religion is fading away is not corroborated by contemporary research. Besides the loss of influence of established churches in Western countries, many processes of sacralization are at work, with new ideals and ideas, as argued by German philosopher Hans Joas. [73] Religion should be analyzed not only at the level of institutions and dogmas but also at the level of practices and experiences. Human beings have retained their power to develop new perspectives on the world through extraordinary and transcendent experiences. Modernization has not resulted in the downfall of the sacred, but in multiplication of perspectives on the sacred and new forms of spirituality.

Disenchantment interpreted as the eclipse of the moral universe is also problematic from a historical perspective. It is questionable whether there ever was a unified and homogeneous traditional world with unity of moral views that has now become fragmented. On the contrary, it seems that world views have become more unified. Sociologist Norbert Elias elaborated a theory of the civilizing process in European countries. [74] In the course of centuries, standards of human behavior changed considerably. Individual behavior was pacified, with increased regulation of affects, and more self-control and self-restraint. Elias discusses examples such as table manners, attitudes toward natural functions (e.g. defecating and coughing), nose-blowing, spitting, and aggressive conduct. People have become more sensitive to social conduct. The private, intimate sphere was more and more segregated from the public sphere but this does not necessarily lead to fragmentation of morals. Human relationships shifted, especially between men and women, and with children. This transformation of behavior and psychical habitus was connected to changes in the structure of society. A hierarchical social order emerged, and physical violence was monopolized by centralizing states.

Elias' theory specifies that during the last few centuries a uniform process has affected at least European countries where similar values have been interiorized by increasing parts of populations. The notion of "civilization" is indicative: it articulates what is common to human beings. The distinction with barbarism and uncivilized populace necessitates higher thresholds of embarrassment, shame, and for what is offensive and repugnant. [75] Later, in Chapter 6, we will argue that contemporary processes of globalization result in more homogeneous values across the world, promoting a sense of global consciousness in which people share the same challenges. That does not mean that there is uniformity. The dissemination of global approaches is associated with local divergencies, and in fact triggers the articulation of differences. Convergence and fragmentation are not mutually exclusive but occur at the same time.

Similar questions are raised about the supposed decline of magic. Weber argues that "principally there are no mysterious incalculable forces. . . . One need no longer have recourse to magical means." [76] The term "magic" is used as the prototype of superstition, the opposite of rationality and rational calculation. In this broad sense, it coincides with religion, mystery, and sacredness. But in this sense, there is little evidence for the decline of magic. [77] The idea that today's societies are myth-less is itself a myth. [78] Mysteries have not vanished. There is a wide range of substantial re-enchantments: alternative lifestyles, religious fundamentalism, spiritual traditions, dreams of alterity. There are also secular enchantments in the shape of futures, ideologies, rituals, symbols, and myths. Many people challenge the dominant world view of science, and are skeptical about the progress of medicine. There is no longer a unified framework for understanding the natural world, even when the ideology of naturalism is still prevalent. It is not helpful to equate enchantment and magic. Enchantment is the experience that there is more to life than the material, the visible, and the explainable. This sense of enchantment has not declined. The world has never been disenchanted, although there are strong forces of disenchantment. David Greaves has applied this perspective to Western medicine. In his opinion, any system of medicine must necessarily embody a mysterious quality. Mystery is an element of indeterminacy and uncertainty that characterizes medicine as a science and art. Medicine therefore is a mixture of rational and mysterious qualities. [79]

## *New forms of enchantment*

Several scholars advance the thesis that progressive disenchantment of the world is accompanied from the start by progressive re-enchantment. There is a variety of strategies for re-enchantment, not only from religious but also from secular perspectives. Rather than an antithesis between enchantment and disenchantment, with the first as a relic from the past, modernity involves contraries, oppositions, and contradictions: rationality and wonder, secularism and religion coexists. Modern science is extirpating mysteries from the natural world and at the same time restoring mysteries. It is promising power, wisdom, and salvation. [80] An example of a secular approach to enchantment is the work of Jane Bennett. She claims that the contemporary world retains the power to enchant human beings. Modern people wonder about minor experiences, everyday marvels, mysteries, and miracles. In her words: "To be enchanted is to be struck and shaken by the extraordinary that lives amid the familiar and the everyday." [81] Enchantment is not confined to the religious or transcendental. There is also enchanted materialism. The material world is not inert matter. There are more than two options: disenchanted materialism or enchanting cosmology. Matter, as demonstrated in nanotechnology, can design itself, generate, and evolve forms of matter. Matter is animated and active. Nature enchants but also do artifacts and synthetic devices such as robots. [82]

Others argue that re-enchantment is encouraged by the domination of rationalistic forces in present-day society. The doctrine that calculative, procedural, and formal rationality is the best way to proceed is resisted and often rejected. Many people believe, as stated by Jenkins, that there are "more things in the universe than are dreamed of by the rationalist epistemologies and ontologies of science." [83] They see such re-enchantment in the significance of values and the surge of spirituality, alternative healing practices, and new age movements. The focus on entrepreneurialism (rather than on management and bureaucracy) is also an example, with its impetus to innovation, change, and lateral thinking, not separating the person from the office or function. In many cases, these examples refer to the soul: the need to unfold human capacities, develop sensibilities to nature, a sense of connectedness with other people, and affective human communication. [84]

Disenchantment of the world, according to Weber, has transformed civilization and introduced a new logic. It has made social life meaningless and impersonal. At first sight, it has created a depressive world in which change is not possible. [85] Social concerns have been displaced into personal ones. Nonetheless, the total picture is mixed. On the one hand, opposing rationalization to non-rational, traditional thinking ignores that there are competing truth claims about the world. It denies that religion and technoscience are both ways of knowing the world. The effects of science and technology are interpreted as "disindividualizing force" leading to massification and de-spiritualization, degrading the human spirit and eliminating the soul. [86] Human beings are turned into what philosopher Gabriel Marcel has called "technical man"; estranged from an awareness of his inner reality and assimilated to the world of objects, he loses touch with himself. [87] Human beings are treated, and view themselves, as machines subjugated to a spirit of abstraction. [88]

On the other hand, modern capitalism has created a new kind of being. In response to a culture that has grown abstract, calculating, rational, material, and instrumental, the individual self has become more inward orientated and focused on interiority. The impersonal forces of contemporary culture have stimulated the growth of subjectivism. This has generated a more positive assessment of the process of disenchantment. While the self has withdrawn from the world, a new language of the self has emerged. Subjectivity is what characterizes human beings; it is crucial for how we understand and relate to ourselves as humans. Subjectivity is therefore continuously redefined, constructed, observed, and recorded.

The upshot is that the soul is not an illusion. [89] But subjectivity is not merely personal. The idea that the public sphere is a-emotional, and can be separated from the private emotional sphere, no longer holds. Emotions play a role in economic transaction. Social arrangements are often at the same time emotional arrangements.

The new emphasis on subjectivity, however, has a price. It has produced a therapeutic worldview. This means that emotional life follows the logic of economic relations and exchange. [90] Intimate feelings and passions are transformed into measurable and calculable objects. While subjective life has intensified, there is at the same time increasing objectivization of the means to express and exchange emotions. Dis-embedded from concrete and particular actions and relationships, they are no longer entangled within social bonds. Communicating emotions means, as Eva Illouz points out, taking the position of an abstract speaker. [91] Another implication of this worldview is an ethics of self-improvement. Communication is regarded as a major technology of self-management, based on the proper government of emotions. It requires introspection, self-monitoring, and elucidation of one's self-image. Human beings have to learn how to manage themselves. Emotional competence is needed to control emotions, to motivate oneself, to show empathy, and to handle relationships. This competence is guided by the ideal of health. Self-development and health are regarded as similar challenges. The therapeutic culture of the self is not the consequence of external forces but the result of subtle disciplining so that subjects are fabricated that are governable. [92] Modern citizens shape their lives through the choices they make about lifestyle, family life, and personality.

## Conclusion

Supposedly, for his disenchantment thesis, Weber was inspired by the German physician and poet Friedrich Schiller. In his poem *Die Götter Griechenlands* (The Gods of Greece), Schiller bemoaned the "die Entgötterte Natur" and the vanishing of mythology. [93] He wanted to respiritualize the world. [94] However, Schiller did not use the term "Entzauberung." The source of the term in Weber's work is therefore not clear. In fact, disenchantment is not a linear and uniform development but rather a cultural diagnosis that encompasses, as Joas affirms, at least three distinct processes: diminishing belief in magic, de-sacralization, and weakening of the idea of transcendency. [95]

This chapter has explained disenchantment as the practices and mechanisms of rationalization, intellectualization, and bureaucratization in Western culture that have removed magical and mysterious forces as relevant ingredients to understand and explain the world. The soul and spiritual elements have gradually been eliminated. In principle, according to Weber, human beings will be able to control everything by means of calculation. Science is the predominant way to shape and enhance human existence. In the chapter, the implications of these processes have been highlighted. Ultimate values have retreated from public life. Scientific knowledge has become fragmentated and specialized. Science is conceptualized as value-free with rational knowledge as a neutral instrument. Action is rational when it is technical, focused on efficiently using means to accomplish ends. In this rationalized context, a new type of person has emerged: an independent, self-reliant individual but isolated and on its own.

We have argued in this chapter that the disenchantment thesis, although influential for the self-interpretation of modern culture, is nowadays seriously criticized. Science is not simply a rational and value-free approach. It is founded on fundamental values such as integrity that are often compromised and instigate continuous debates about the values implicated in scientific work and the need to (re)articulate them in everyday research practices and education. The historical and cultural analyses on which Weber grounded his disenchantment thesis are furthermore questioned and problematized. More subtle and nuanced processes are at work that do not allow for straightforward conclusions. Finally, new forms of enchantment are continuously explored and elaborated, rehabilitating the discourse of the soul.

Disenchantment has affected healthcare and bioethics. This chapter gives examples such as the clinical gaze and empirical ethics. The effect is that subjectivity has been disqualified in medical and ethical discourse. The naturalistic ideology and the disenchantment thesis have produced a scientific worldview that determines how human beings and their illnesses, as well as moral values that are important for human existence, are perceived and interpreted in healthcare encounters. Communications between patients and health professionals are often governed by metaphors and images without soul. This will be the topic of the next chapter.

## References

1 Max Weber, "Science as a vocation," *Daedalus* 87, no. 1 (1958): 117.
2 "The underlying belief is that we owe everything we have, our way of living, our rules, our customs, and what we know, to beings of a different nature . . . everything governing our daily lives was handed down to us." Marcel Gauchet, *The disenchantment of the world. A political history of religion* (Princeton: Princeton University Press, 1997), 23–24.
3 Gauchet, *The disenchantment of the world*, 95.
4 Sam Han, "Disenchantment revisited: Formations of the 'secular' and 'religious' in the technological discourse of modernity," *Social Compass* 62, no. 1 (2015): 76–88.
5 Stephen Kalberg, "Max Weber's types of rationality: Cornerstones for the analysis of rationalization processes in history," *American Journal of Sociology* 85, no. 5 (1980): 1145–1179.
6 Lawrence A. Scaff, *Fleeing the iron cage. Culture, politics, and modernity in the thought of Max Weber* (Berkeley, Los Angeles and London: University of California Press, 1989).
7 Ian H. Angus, "Disenchantment and modernity: The mirror of technique," *Human Studies* 6, no. 2 (1983): 141–166.
8 Scaff, *Fleeing the iron cage*, 100.
9 Max Weber, *Gesamtausgabe* (Tübingen: J. C. B. Mohr (Paul Siebeck), 1984), I/15: 356–357.

10 "This style of life embodied an ethos of vocation, of systematically disciplined inner-worldly accomplishment capable of remaking an entire "world" – the world of bourgeois society." Scaff, *Fleeing the iron cage*, 89.
11 Dirk Käsler, *Max Weber. An introduction to his life and work* (Chicago: The University of Chicago Press, 1988).
12 H. C. Greisman, "Disenchantment of the world: Romanticism, aesthetics and sociological theory," *The British Journal of Sociology* 27, no. 4 (1976): 495–507.
13 Ralph Schroeder, "Disenchantment and its discontents: Weberian perspectives on science and technology," *The Sociological Review* 43, no. 2 (1995): 227–250.
14 Weber, "Science as a vocation," 133.
15 David Chalcraft, "Bringing the text back in: On ways of reading the iron cage metaphor in the two editions of *The Protestant Ethic*," in *Organizing modernity. New Weberian perspectives on work, organization and society*, eds. Larry J. Ray and Michael Reed (London: Routledge, 1994), 16–45; Arthur Mitzman, *The iron cage. An historical interpretation of Max Weber* (New Brunswick and Oxford: Transaction Books, 2005; original 1969); Peter Baehr, "The 'Iron cage' and the 'Shell as hard as steel': Parsons, Weber, and the Stahlhartes Gehäuse in the Protestant Ethics and the Spirit of Capitalism," *History and Theory* 40, no. 2 (2001): 153–169.
16 Mitzman, *The Iron Cage*; Philip A. Woods, "Rationalisation, disenchantement and re-enchantement. Engaging with Weber's sociology of modernity," in *The Routledge International Handbook of the Sociology of Education*, eds. Michael W. Apple, Stephen J. Ball, and Luis Amando Gandin (London and New York: Routledge, 2010), 121–131.
17 Ralph Schroeder, "'Personality' and 'inner distance': The conception of the individual in Max Weber's sociology," *History of the Human Sciences* 4, no. 1 (1991): 61–78.
18 Weber, "Science as a vocation," 122.
19 Balthasar Bekker, *De betoverde wereld* (Amsterdam: Daniel van den Dalen, 1691). See also: Han van Ruler, "Minds, forms, and spirits: The nature of Cartesian disenchantment," *Journal of the History of Ideas* 61, no. 3 (2000): 381–395.
20 Lorraine Daston, "On scientific observation," *Isis* 99, no. 1 (2008): 97–110; Lorraine Daston, and Peter Galison, *Objectivity* (New York: Zone Books, 2010).
21 Michel Foucault, *The birth of the clinic. An archaeology of medical perception* (New York: Pantheon Books, 1973), 8.
22 The conceptual transformation of medical discourse ". . . gave to the clinical field a new structure in which the individual in question was not so much a sick person as the endlessly reproducible pathological fact to be found in all patients suffering in a similar way;" Foucault, *The birth of the clinic*, 97.
23 Jeffrey P. Bishop, *The anticipatory corpse. Medicine, power and the care of the dying* (Notre Dame: University of Notre Dame Press, 2011).
24 Nicholas D. Jewson, "The disappearance of the sick-man from medical cosmology, 1770–1870," *Sociology* 10, no. 2 (1976): 225–244.
25 Jacob A. Blythe, and Farr A. Curlin, "'Just do your job': Technology, bureaucracy, and the eclipse of conscience in contemporary medicine," *Theoretical Medicine and Bioethics* 39 (2018): 432.
26 The provider is "the anonymous locus of a certain set of competencies," Blythe, and Curlin, "'Just do your job'," 442.
27 Alan S. Astrow, "On the disenchantment of medicine: Abraham Joshua Heschel's 1964 address to the American Medical Association," *Theoretical Medicine and Bioethics* 39 (2018): 483–497.

28 See, for example, Devi Sridhar, "Health policy: From the clinical to the economic gaze," *The Lancet* 378 (2011): 1909.

29 Devan Stahl, "Patient reflections on the disenchantment of techno-medicine," *Theoretical Medicine and Bioethics* 39 (2018): 499–513; Joel James Shuman, "Re-enchanting the body: Overcoming the melancholy of anatomy," *Theoretical Medicine and Bioethics* 39 (2018): 473–481.

30 "Without God, morality is contingent, culturally and historically conditioned. As a result, it shatters into numerous incommensurable perspectives." Mark J. Cherry, "The scandal of secular bioethics: What happens when the culture acts as if there is no God?" *Christian Bioethics* 23, no. 2 (2017): 89.

31 ". . . the secular stance of bioethics limits its ability to fully respond to the challenging existential and moral questions that emerge in medicine and medical research." Raymond De Vries, "Good without God: Bioethics and the sacred," *Society* 52 (2015): 439.

32 Pascal Borry, Paul Schotsmans, and Kris Dierickx, "The birth of the empirical turn in bioethics," *Bioethics* 19, no. 1 (2005): 49–71.

33 George J. Agich, "Education and the improvement of clinical ethics services," *BMC Medical Education* 13 (2013): 41; See also: Cynthia M. A. Geppert, and Wayne N. Shelton, "A comparison of general medical and clinical ethics consultations: What can we learn from each other?" *Mayo Clinic Proceedings* 87, no. 4 (2012): 381–398.

34 The ASBH first published the Code in 1998; a 2nd edition was published in 2011. Rachel Yarmolinsky, "Ethics for ethicists? The professionalization of clinical ethics consultation," AMA *Journal of Ethics* 18, no. 5 (2016): 506–513; Anita Tarzian, Lucia D. Wocial, and the ASBH Clinical Ethics Consultation Affairs Committee, "A code of ethics for health care ethics consultants: Journey to the present and implications for the field," *American Journal of Bioethics* 15, no. 5 (2015): 38–51.

35 Terri L. Major-Kincade, Jon E. Tyson, and Kathleen A. Kennedy, "Training pediatric house staff in evidence-based ethics: An exploratory controlled trial," *Journal of Perinatology* 21 (2001): 161–166.

36 Clair Morrisey, and Rebecca L. Walker, "Funding and forums for ELSI research: Who (or What) is setting the agenda?" *AJOB Primary Research* 3, no. 3 (2012): 51–60.

37 Daniel Strech, Matthis Synofzik, and Georg Marckmann, "Systematic review of empirical bioethics," *Journal of Medical Ethics* 34 (2008): 471.

38 Kimberley A. Strong, Wendy Lipworth, and Ian Kerridge, "The strengths and limitations of empirical bioethics," *Journal of Law and Medicine* 18, no. 2 (2010): 317–318.

39 Strong, Lipworth, and Kerridge, "The strengths and limitations of empirical bioethics," 318.

40 Tenzin Wangmo, and Veerle Provoost, "The use of empirical research in bioethics: A survey of researchers in twelve European countries," *BMC Medical Ethics* 18 (2017): 79.

41 Rob de Vries, and Bert Gordijn, "Empirical ethics and its alleged meta-ethical fallacies," *Bioethics* 23, no. 4 (2009): 193–201.

42 Guy Widdershoven, Tineke Abma, and Bert Molewijk, "Empirical ethics as dialogical practice," *Bioethics* 23, no. 4 (2009): 248. See also: Donald S. Kornfield, "What is the role of a clinical ethics consultant?" *The American Journal of Bioethics* 16, no. 3 (2016): 40–42.

43 Woods, "Rationalisation, disenchantement and re-enchantement," 121–131; Richard Jenkins, "Disenchantment, enchantment and re-enchantment: Max Weber at the Millennium," *Max Weber Studies* 1 (2000): 11–32; Jane Bennett, *The enchantment of modern life. Attachments, crossings, and ethics* (Princeton and Oxford: Princeton University

Press, 2001); Joshua Landy, and Michael Saler, eds., *The re-enchantment of the world. Secular magic in a rational age* (Stanford: Stanford University Press, 2009).

44 Norbert Elias, *The civilizing process. Sociogenetic and psychogenetic investigations* (Malden: Blackwell Publishing, 2017, revised edition; original 1939).

45 Patrick Sherry, "Disenchantment, re-enchantment, and enchantment," *Modern Theology* 25 (2009): 369–386.

46 Sheila Jasanoff, *Can science make sense of life?* (Cambridge: Polity Press, 2019), 38.

47 Max Weber, *Gesammelte Afsätze zur Wissenschaftlehre*. Edited by J. Winckelmann (Tübingen: J. C. B. Mohr, Paul Siebeck, 1968, 3rd edition), 213.

48 Scaff, *Fleeing the iron cage*, 85.

49 Daniel Sarewitz, "Saving science," *The New Atlantis* 49 (Spring–Summer 2016), 6.

50 Henk ten Have, "The need and desirability of an (Hippocratic) Oath or Pledge for scientists," in *New perspectives in academia*, eds. Jüri Engelbrecht and Johannes J. F. Schroots (Amsterdam: KNAW; ALLEA Biennial Yearbook 2006, 2007), 19–30.

51 UNESCO, *Recommendation on science and scientific researchers* (2017); https://unesdoc.unesco.org/ark:/48223/pf0000263618.

52 Mara Hvistendahl, "China's publication bazaar," *Science* 342 (2013): 1035–1039.

53 Wei Yang, "Research integrity in China," *Science* 342 (2013): 1019.

54 Joy Y. Zhang, *The cosmopolitanization of science. Stem cell governance in China* (Houndmills: Palgrave/Macmillan, 2012).

55 Khaled Moustafa, "The disaster of the impact factor," *Science and Engineering Ethics* 21 (2015): 139–142.

56 Richard L. Kravitz, Peter Franks, Mitchel D. Feldman, Martha Gerrity, Cindy Byrne, and William M. Tierney, "Editorial peer reviewers' recommendations at a general medical journal: Are they reliable and do editors care?" *PLoS One* 5, no. 4 (2010): e10072. Luciano A. Sposato, Bruce Ovbiagle, S. Claiborne Johnston, Marc Fisher, and Gustavo Saposnik, "A peek behind the curtain: Peer review and editorial decision making at *Stroke*," *Annals of Neurology* 76 (2014): 151–158.

57 A. M. Vintzileos, C. V. Ananth, A. O. Odibo, S. P. Chauban, J. C. Smulian, and Y. Oyelese, "The relationship between a reviewer's recommendation and editorial decision of manuscripts submitted for publication in obstetrics," *American Journal of Obstetrics & Gynecology* 211 (2014): 703.e1–5.

58 Sui Huang, "When peers are not peers and don't know it: The Dunning-Kruger effect and self-fulfilling prophecy in peer-review," *Bioessays* 35 (2013): 414–416.

59 T. Jefferson, M. Rudin, F. S. Brodney, and F. Davidoff, "Editorial peer review for improving the quality of reports of biomedical studies," *Cochrane Database of Systematic Reviews* 18, no. 2 (2007): MR000016; Christopher J. Lortie, Stefano Allesina, Lonnie Aarssen, Olyana Grod, and Amber E. Budden, "With great power comes great responsibility: The importance of rejection, power, and editors in the practice of scientific publishers," *PLoS One* 8, no. 12 (2013): e85382.

60 World Medical Association, *Declaration of Helsinki* (2013).

61 Kirti Nath Jha, "How to write articles that get published," *Journal of Clinical and Diagnostic Research* 8, no. 9 (2014): XG01–XG03; Sandra V. Kotsis, and Kevin C. Chung, "Manuscript rejection: How to submit a revision and tips on being a good peer reviewer," *Plastic and Reconstructive Surgery* 133 (2014): 958–963; Fujian Song, Yoon Loke, and Lee Hooper, "Why are medical and health-related studies not being published? A systematic review of reasons given by investigators," *PLoS One* 9, no. 10 (2014): e110418.

62 Editorial, "Coping with peer rejection," *Nature* 425 (2003): 645.

63 Stefan Eriksson, and Gert Helgesson, "The false academy: Predatory publishing in science and bioethics," *Medicine Health Care and Philosophy* 20, no. 2 (2017): 163–170.
64 Jeffrey Beall, "Predatory journals threaten the quality of published medical research," *Journal of Orthopaedic & Sports Physical Therapy* 47, no. 1 (2017): 3–5; L. Shamseer, D. Moher, O. Maduekwe, L. Turner, V. Barbour, R. Burch, J. Clark, J. Galipeau, J. Roberts, and B. J. Shea, "Potential predatory and legitimate biomedical journals: Can you tell the difference? A cross-sectional comparison," *BMC Medicine* 15 (2017): 28; Chandler W. Carroll, "Spotting the wolf in sheep's clothing: Predatory open access publications," *Journal of Graduate Medical Education* 8, no. 5 (2016): 662–664; Lenche Danevska, Mirko Spiroski, Doncho Donev, Nada Pop-Jordanova, and Momir Polenakovic, "How to recognize and avoid potential, possible, or probable predatory open-access publishers, standalone, and hijacked journals," *Contributions, Section of Medical Sciences* 37, no. 2–3 (2016): 5–13; Jeffrey Beall, "Dangerous predatory publishers threaten medical research," *Journal of Korean Medical Science* 31 (2016):1511–1513.
65 H. B. Harvey, and D. F. Weinstein, "Predatory publishing: An emerging threat to the medical literature," *Academic Medicine* 92 (2017): 150–151; Chad Cook, "Predatory journals: The worst thing in publishing, ever," *Journal of Orthopaedic & Sports Physical Therapy* 47, no. 1 (2017): 1–2; Pradeep Kumar, and Deepak Saxena, "Pandemic of publications and predatory journals: Another nail in the coffin of academics," *Indian Journal of Community Medicine* 41, no. 3 (2016): 169–171; Sonya E. Van Nuland, and Kem A. Rogers, "Academic nightmares: Predatory publishing," *Anatomical Sciences Education* 10, no. 4 (2017): 392–394.
66 Van Nuland, and Rogers, "Academic Nightmares: Predatory publishing"; Danevska, Spiroski, Donev, Pop-Jordanova, and Polenakovic, "How to recognize and avoid potential, possible, or probable predatory open-access publishers, standalone, and hijacked journals."
67 Mehdi Dadkhah, and Giorgio Bianciardi, "Ranking predatory journals: Solve the problem instead of removing it!" *Advanced Pharmaceutical Bulletin* 6, no. 1 (2016): 1–4.
68 Harvey, and Weinstein, "Predatory publishing."
69 Cook, "Predatory journals."
70 Maria do Ceu Patrão Neves, "On scientific integrity: Conceptual clarification," *Medicine, Health Care and Philosophy* 21, no. 2 (2018): 181–187.
71 Daniel Sperling, "(Re)disclosing physician financial interests: Rebuilding trust or making unreasonable burdens on physicians?" *Medicine Health Care and Philosophy* 20, no. 2 (2017): 179–186.
72 Alexandra Walsham, "The Reformation and 'the disenchantment of the world' reassessed," *The Historical Journal* 51, no. 2 (2008): 497–528.
73 Hans Joas, *Die Macht des Heiligen. Eine Alternative zur Geschichte der Entzaubering* (Berlin: Suhrkamp Verlag, 2017).
74 Elias, *The civilizing process*.
75 ". . . the general direction of the change in conduct, the "trend" of the movement of civilization, is everywhere the same. It always veers towards a more or less automatic self-control, towards the subordination of short-term impulses to the commends of an ingrained long-term view, and towards the formation of a more complex and secure "super-ego" agency." (Elias, *The civilizing process*, 380). Also: "No society can survive without a channelling of individual drives and affects, without a very specific control of individual behaviour." (Elias, *The civilizing process*, 443).
76 Weber, "Science as a vocation," 117.
77 Jenkins, "Disenchantment, enchantment and re-enchantment," 18.

78 Jason Ā. Josephson-Storm, *The myth of disenchantment. Magic, modernity, and the death of the human sciences* (Chicago and London: The University of Chicago Press, 2017). Kelly, Crabtree, and Marshall examine a range of example of human capacities that cannot be accounted for in physicalism. The worldview of physicalism in their views cannot account for the full spectrum of human experiences. See; Edward F. Kelly, Adam Crabtree, and Paul Marshall, eds., *Beyond physicalism. Toward reconciliation of science and spirituality* (Lanham, Boulder, New York and London: Rowman & Littlefield, 2015). See also: Wouter J. Hanegraaf, "How magic survived the disenchantment of the world," *Religion* 33 (2003): 357–380.
79 David Greaves, *Mystery in Western medicine* (Aldershot: Avebury, 1996).
80 See: Landy, and Saler, *The re-enchantment of the world.*
81 Bennett, *The enchantment of modern life*, 4.
82 "Enchantment as a state of openness to the disturbing-captivating elements in everyday experience." We encounter phenomena ". . . that surprise, fascinate, disturb, and provoke wonder." Bennett, *The enchantment of modern life*, 131.
83 Jenkins, "Disenchantment, enchantment and re-enchantment," 12.
84 Woods, "Rationalisation, disenchantement and re-enchantement," 121–131.
85 H. C. Greisman, "Disenchantment of the world: Romanticism, aesthetics and sociological theory," *The British Journal of Sociology* 27, no. 4 (1976): 495–507.
86 Han, "Disenchantement revisited," 81.
87 Gabriel Marcel, *Man against mass society* (South Bend: St. Augustine's Press, 2008; original 1952), 55.
88 "In our contemporary world it may be said that the more a man becomes dependent on the gadgets whose smooth functioning assures him a tolerable life at the material level, the more estranged he becomes from an awareness of his inner reality." Marcel, *Man against mass society*, 41.
89 Eva Illouz, *Saving the modern soul. Therapy, emotions, and the culture of self-help* (Berkeley, Los Angeles and London: University of California Press, 2008); Nikolas Rose, *Governing the soul. The shaping of the private self* (London and New York: Free Association Books, 1999).
90 Eva Illouz has introduced the term "emotional capitalism" for this new mode of sociability. Eva Illouz, *Cold intimacies: The making of emotional capitalism* (Cambridge: Polity Press, 2007).
91 Illouz, *Cold intimacies*, 38.
92 "The citizens of a liberal democracy are to regulate themselves, government mechanisms construe them as active participants in their lives." Rose, *Governing the soul*, 10.
93 Friedrich Schiller, *Die Götter Griechenlands* (1788): 168.
94 E. S. Gerhard, "Schiller's 'Die Götter Griechenlands'," *The German Quarterly* 15, no. 2 (1942): 86–92. See also: Matthew Vest, and Ashley Moyse, "Understanding modern, technological medicine: Enchanted, disenchanted, or other?" *Theoretical Medicine and Bioethics* 39 (2018): 407–417; Steven Grosby, "Max Weber, religion, and the disenchantment of the world," *Sociology* 50 (2013): 301–310; Angus, "Disenchantment and modernity," 141–166.
95 Joas, *Die Macht des Heiligen*, 141 ff.

# 4 The lost soul – images without soul

Sociologist Max Weber has introduced a powerful narrative of cultural progression from magic to religion to science. In previous chapters, we have argued that this narrative is associated with the scientific world view of naturalism. The combined forces of disenchantment and naturalism have extirpated the soul from present-day discourses. At the same time, we pointed out that these forces do not represent scientific theories but play a more fundamental role as views about the nature of the world and human beings. Philosopher Thomas Nagel has called naturalism "a heroic triumph of ideological theory over common sense." [1] The disenchantment thesis as well as naturalism therefore present a specific ideological point of view. An ideology is a coherent conglomerate of ideas, beliefs, and values that determines how realities are interpreted. It is a crucial concept in social sciences but also in philosophy. Theodore Adorno defined it as "an organization of opinions, attitudes, and values – a way of thinking about man and society." [2] The notion of ideology has practical and political implications. As a pattern of thoughts and values, an ideology influences political behavior and is therefore concurrent with a set of practices. As a worldview that describes, organizes, and interprets the world, it guides the actions of individuals within the world, and accordingly seeks to mold the world to conform to its vision. An ideology is the "nexus between ideas and actions." [3]

Jürgen Habermas argues that science and technology present an ideology, precisely because they claim to be an objective and value-neutral enterprise, which is going beyond ideology. They provide technical solutions for human problems, depoliticize social issues, and legitimize domination. But, contrary to these claims, they are not separated from values and social norms. [4]

Ideologies play a significant role in healthcare. The recent movement of refusing vaccination, for example, is driven by the political ideology of conservatism. Parents' unwillingness to vaccinate children is not primarily the result of a deficit of knowledge but of a specific world view that influences their perception of safety and risks. This value orientation is related to lower levels of trust in medical experts, particularly government experts. Official information sources are therefore no longer reliable for these parents. Providing more information will not help them to overcome their skepticism. [5]

For our argument, it is important to note that ideology is not only discourse but is often using images and symbols to frame popular consciousness. Visual representations are communicated to promulgate these discourses and reiterate messages through various types of media. They disseminate specific sets of values. An example are the images of the blue marbles, which will be further discussed in Chapter 6. Another example are images of Shanghai, which has changed from a small fishing village not too long ago into a booming metropole, illustrating the power of China, the fastest growing economy in the world. The District of Pudong is an iconic landmark of the contemporary economic order based on market ideology. In healthcare, images are used in advertisements and popular health magazines to show that the patient as a consumer has a wide range of choices among treatment options. Images are a powerful way to express ideologies but also to show their failings and deformities. Especially in this era of social media, they are more impressive than texts. Images arouse emotions. They go beyond the level of discursive argumentation and reinforce the strengths or weaknesses of the ideologies they illustrate. An example of this are the recent pictures of drowned immigrants. More than written texts, they denounce the ideology of nationalism and closed borders.

In this chapter, we will argue that the dominant scientific worldview, the naturalistic ideology, and the view of the world as disenchanted propagate specific images and metaphors that predetermine the normative debate of bioethical issues. Subsequently, discussion will focus on the image of the human person as *homo economicus*, the human body as mechanism, the individual person as a lone ranger, the physician as an expert with detached concern, and the patient as a consumer and client. These images are the expressions of current ideologies within society in general and healthcare in particular, but they are now more and more criticized. The main point is that they are images without soul.

## *Homo economicus*

The superhero of mainstream economics is *homo economicus*. This is the image of the human being as only concerned with his own material self-interest. He is not committed to do anything good. Rationality is synonymous with selfishness. [6] The human person is first of all a rational self-interested individual motivated by minimizing costs and maximizing gains for himself. Greed and selfishness are determinatively motivating human behavior. References are frequently made to the notorious statement of Adam Smith that we can have our dinner because the butcher and baker are regarding their self-interest, not because they are benevolent persons. [7] This statement is used to justify self-interest. The common interpretation is that the invisible hand of the market morally justifies the pursuit of individual interests because this will result in the good of society as a whole. Studies of Smith' writings clarify that he used the invisible hand argument only for the economic sphere, not as a moral principle. The basis for morality, according to Smith, is sympathy with the feelings of other people. Smith was critical of business people; they pursue their interests at the expense of the public interest; they deceive and oppress the rest of society, for example by seeking monopolies. [8] Self-interest as a moral principle was particularly promoted by the philosophers of neoliberalism. Ayn Rand, for example, advocated rational egoism. Human beings must not sacrifice themselves to others but live for their own sake. Trade is the basic ethical principle for all human relationships. [9] Political scientist Friedrich von Hayek used the notion of "market" as a metaphor for the organization of social life. Only within his framework, individual liberty and freedom can flourish. Competition is the core value, making the individual responsible for his or her actions, which will work for the benefit of all. [10] Economist Milton Friedman elaborated rational choice theory in policy recommendations. The theory assumes that social behavior is the result of rational decisions of individuals that are guided by individual preferences, driven by calculations of maximizing expected utility. Friedman used the invisible hand argument to claim that businesses have the positive moral obligation to only pursue their own interests: "The social responsibility of business is to increase its profits." [11]

The image of *homo economicus* has three assumptions about human behavior. First is that preferences are outcome-regarding; they are focused on the goods and services that can be acquired, consumed, and possessed. Second, preferences are self-regarding; agents are only concerned with their own experiences and welfare. Third, preferences are only changing through exogenous influences, that is external impacts. Nowadays, it is recognized that all assumptions are incorrect. Preferences are process-regarding as well; people care about how they treat others and how they are treated by others. Moreover, preferences are other-regarding; agents care about the well-being of other persons. Finally, preferences are under endogenous influences; they are formed in social interaction. [12] Many studies show that regarding the human being as *homo economicus* is a reductive view. It presents, as Amartya Sen has formulated it, the human as a "social moron." [13]

A famous experiment in behavioral economics is the ultimatum game. Two players have a sum of money. They play under conditions of anonymity. One of them is asked to offer money to the second player. The proposer can make only one offer; the responder can either accept or reject this offer. If the offer is accepted, both players share; if it is rejected, both players receive nothing. If self-regard is determinative, the proposer will offer the minimum possible amount; the responder will accept any positive amount. However, in the play, the self-regarding outcome is never attained. Proposers routinely offer substantial amounts to share. This outcome is true for various societies. In all of them, proposers and responders behave with reciprocity.

Similar outcomes were obtained with experiments with free riding. Findings consistently indicate that cooperation is much more frequent than expected on the basis of the economic model of *homo economicus*. The conclusion is that most people are not selfish but fair-minded and reciprocal. In the experimental conditions, they care about fairness. They reward people who are willing to cooperate, and punish others who do not cooperate. [14] This phenomenon of reciprocity, fairness, and altruism is difficult to explain from the perspective of naturalism. Evolution theory would predict that non-selfish behavior toward non-kin will lead to extinction in the longer run. But this is not necessarily true since these behaviors can lead to mutualism and cooperation. The experiments, however, do not provide any indirect or long-term benefits. Real altruism is not an exchange of advantages and disadvantages. The image of the *homo economicus* is therefore erroneous and pathological. Rational choice theory is deficient since it ignores that human beings are, in fact, moral superior to this fictional image. They are motivated by other things than greed and material self-interest. They are sensitive to the approval and disapproval of other human beings. They are inclined to cooperation and have an aversion to inequality. For most of them, morality is a stronger motive to act than self-interest. [15] An example is collective action in global bioethics. Civil rights movements are opposing authoritarian regimes, although this is often dangerous and cannot be explained in terms of self-interest. [16] A recent study reveals a high level of civil honesty around the globe. Lost wallets with varying amounts of money were often returned. This is not only a matter of altruism; people do not want to be regarded as thieves. [17] Human conduct is determined not merely by instrumental rationality but also by what Gintis calls "social rationality." [18] Voting is an example. Why do people vote? Not because of the personal or social consequences but because it is the right thing to do as a citizen. My own vote will not change anything, and will not determine the outcome of an election.

Another deficiency of the standard assumptions of economic theory is what economists label as computational inferiority. Human beings lack complete information and self-control. Human actions are often flawed and faltering, for example because we get angry or frustrated. From the perspective of rational choice theory, this is irrationality. But in everyday interaction selfish calculations do not play a major role.

### *Social and ethical impact of neoliberalism*

Neoliberalism and its dominating image of *homo economicus* have an enormous impact on social and ethical discourses. They promulgate a specific view of human interactions and society. A kind of Darwinian logic is promoted, according to which the weak are losing and the stronger prosper. Shared communal life is disintegrating. Vulnerability is primarily an individual affair.

The emphasis in this view is on the individual chooser, while the community is absent. He or she only relates to others through market exchanges. The "market" is used as a metaphor for social life. Of all forms of social organization, the market is the most fair and efficient one. For Rand, it is the basic social principle. As a self-regulating force, the market will give room to self-actualizing individuals whose productivity and creativity will work for the benefit of all. There is no need for protection or regulation. Everything should be transformed into a commodity or service and transacted in a market. Each individual is responsible and accountable for his or her action, including care. The free market, therefore, is a recipe for the problems of the world. At the same time, this is not regarded as a moral position. Economics sees itself as a value-neutral science such as physics. It has nothing to do with emotions and ethics. [19] Although more nuanced and sophisticated theories of economics have been developed, most still proceed with the underlying assumption that human behavior is basically guided by self-interest. [20]

These views have far-reaching implications for the ethical debate. First of all, the neoliberal assumption that people are amoral is wrong. People are generous and civic-minded. Ethical motives are guiding human behavior in virtually all human populations. Moral and economic values cannot be separated. [21] There are also a number of practical implications. The image of *homo economicus* facilitates commercialization and commodification. Advocates of the free market prefer that many areas of life are subjected to free market principles. Healthcare is not an exception. Health services should be competitive and offer a range of choices for rational, self-interested individuals. Also, the body and its parts should be treated as commodities that can be exchanged, sold, and purchased. [22] Second, neoliberal policies should remove constraints on free market competition. Government interference must be reduced as much as possible. Deregulation, privatization, and reduction of public expenditures and taxes are encouraged. The consequence is that vulnerabilities and inequalities have multiplied. But this result is to be expected since people are different but all have the power, if they want, to ameliorate their condition. The idea is that rational egoism will improve not only their individual condition but also that of society as collection of individuals. The suggestion that human beings are characterized because they cooperate, as nowadays confirmed by recent studies in behavioral economics, evolutionary biology, and social thinking, is not acceptable in these views. [23] Another implication, which will be discussed in Chapter 6, is reductive interpretation of values. The image of *homo economicus* is connected to preferences. The rational individual is making choices according to what he or she desires or values most. Critics argue that equating values and preferences is misleading. Values are different; they are not mere preferences but deeply ingrained in the individual's life and not easily changeable. Values constitute who we are. A further implication is the phenomenon of crowding out. When human interactions are monetized and become transactions, the meaning and character of interactions change. The involved human beings are no longer engaged. Monetary incentives can be counterproductive; they often crowd out ethical motives such as generosity, reciprocity, and trust. An illustrative example is the introduction of fines for prolonging length of stay in hospitals in Norway. This led to a significant increase in hospital length of stay. [24] A much-debated example in bioethics is the donation of blood. This is an altruistic act, but when donors are paid, less blood is donated. Richard Titmuss has argued that creating a market in blood is dehumanizing. [25] A paid donor system is unjust and exploitative. A privatized blood market produces greater risks. More importantly, it leads to morally impoverished relations between individuals, regarding them as self-interested profit maximizers. The picture of the rational chooser transforms the motives that used to guide people in donating blood for altruistic reasons. Introducing market thinking changes the meaning of human interactions. [26] For many people, transactions like this are repugnant and inappropriate since they devalue public goods and affront human dignity. [27]

***Emphasis on individualistic subjectivity***

The neoliberal subject is epitomized in the image of *homo economicus*. It is redefined as new subjectivity, as discussed in the previous chapter. The contemporary citizen is focused on the government of life. This is not an empirical statement but a normative requirement for good citizens. They should maximize corporeal existence and do everything to maintain their health. The emphasis is on responsible conduct and self-regulation. The individual should achieve self-management. [28] We earlier referred to the work of Eva Illouz, who demonstrated the role of emotions in economic transactions. With the cultural pervasiveness of neoliberalism, a new mode of sociability has emerged characterized by a therapeutic emotional style ("emotional capitalism"). [29] The present-day citizen is supposed to be a self-governor: rational, responsible, predictable, and well-versed in communication skills. He or she should continuously aim at self-improvement. The dominating model of citizenship is entrepreneurship. As entrepreneurs, human beings not only make calculations on the basis of data but also select goals and seek to achieve these. Maximization of accomplishments is one thing, but choice is more important. The entrepreneur is involved in discovery, detection, and exploration of opportunities. He collects information, is using his capacities, speculates, learns, and adapts himself. He monitors and evaluates himself. In other words, he is *homo agens*: active, creative, and constructive. [30] His agency is guided by instrumental rationality. Existential problems such as illness and unhappiness, but also social problems such as poverty are failures of self-management. Responsible citizenship, in this view, requires unceasing performance; individuals have constantly to work on themselves. This is essential for the functioning of economies but the precondition is a redefinition of the self. This was properly formulated by Margaret Thatcher: "Economics are the method; the object is to change the heart and soul." [31] Ironically, neoliberal policies of globalization have made individual self-management more complicated and onerous since they multiplied vulnerabilities and produced a new precariat. [32]

Mainstream bioethics articulates respect for individual autonomy as one of the fundamental ethical principles. It elaborates issues as informed consent, ownership of the body, personal responsibility, and rational decision-making. Doing so, it mimics the main tenets of neoliberal ideology within healthcare. [33] The image of *homo economicus* is transformed into, and perfectly aligned with, the corresponding image of the autonomous person. Bioethics has therefore difficulties in addressing neoliberalism as one of the major sources of present-day ethical problems such as exploitation, trafficking, and inequality. As long as it is captured in the normative framework of neoliberalism, it cannot really criticize the context within which many bioethical problems arise. If the world cannot be changed, or is not seriously scrutinized, the only option is to change oneself.

Rogers-Vaughn has pointed out that the notion of soul may help provide a broader ethical perspective. It may counter the radical individualism of neoliberal ideology. It can also overcome the neoliberal suppression of transcendence, calling attention to other values that are more ultimate than rationality, competition, and self-interest. Soul also restores voice to the suffering that is usually privatized and silenced. [34] It relocates the emphasis from private self-mastery to intersubjective dialogue.

## Body mechanism

The body plays a central role in medicine. At the same time, it is radically separated from the soul or mind. Persons are regarded as bodies without soul. The human person in contemporary medicine is a disembodied rational agent. This view of the body promotes a mechanistic approach in healthcare. Since medicine identifies itself as a natural science, it is proceeding with a "mechanical model." Diseases are defects of the biological machinery of the body. Medical knowledge is derived from empirical experience; data is collected by observation, tested in experiments, and verified or falsified by others. Medical problems therefore require rational and objective biological approaches. [35]

Viewing the body as a mechanism exemplifies the process that Dutch historian of science Eduard Dijksterhuis has called the "mechanization of the world picture." Scientific thinking, especially in the natural sciences, and particularly in physics, has become dominated by the metaphor of mechanism. The aim of modern science is to discover and describe mechanisms. This metaphor has permeated philosophical and cultural thinking, as well as ordinary language. It has become a "world picture" (Weltanschauung), a comprehensive view of the world and human life. The universe is regarded as an enormous mechanism. Natural phenomena operate in a mechanical way, like a clockwork or automaton. The advantage of this perspective is that it allows the use of mathematics and thus quantification and calculation. It furthermore enables practical control and mastery of nature. Regularity and predictability are characteristic for mechanisms. A mechanism can be replicated and imitated in a model. It invites the use of tools. At the same time, it is persuasive and attractive because it has visibility. Experiments can show the correspondence between thought constructions and physical reality. Dijksterhuis describes how mechanization has emerged in antiquity and culminated in the work of Isaac Newton in 1687. He argues that a mechanism is different from a machine. A mechanism can be studied without deeper questions concerning origin and purpose, while a machine is interesting since it refers to not only how it is constructed but also who has constructed it. [36] Mary Midgley has accentuated that the main point of the mechanism metaphor is that it produces continuity with the surroundings. Human beings are not fundamentally different from the rest of the natural world, and can be studied in the same way as other entities in nature. [37] This explains the attractiveness of naturalism and genetic determinism in particular. Genes are the basic units of the human mechanism. They provide detailed instructions for repairing defects in the mechanism and for designing similar, and even better, mechanisms. Simultaneously, they elucidate why there is no need for the soul: they define the essence of the person, and they have substituted the traditional role of the soul. [38]

The world view of mechanization has profoundly influenced medicine. Descartes presented the image of a tree with physics as the trunk and mechanics, medicine, and morals as branches. The body is matter. It is geometrically characterized by extensiveness. In his view, the material world, following mechanical rules, has been created by God. He has set it in motion and then it moves as clock. The body and its functions can therefore be examined and analyzed as a mechanism. A healthy human is like a well-made clock. [39] This methodological approach does not require the concept of a soul. God as the active designer of the mechanism or machine also disappeared as relevant factor. Mechanisms have become important in the biological sciences, especially molecular biology and neurobiology. Discovering and describing the mechanisms underlying a phenomenon means explaining the phenomenon, that is understanding how it works and how it is produced. [40]

The image of the body as a mechanism is connected to the ideology of the market, turning the body (and its parts) into a commodity, an object that can be objectified, isolated, and exchanged. The body is the private property of the individual person. It is alienable: it can be traded, given away, or sold. It is also fungible: interchangeable with other goods without any loss in value; and it is commensurable: it can be ranked in value according to a common scale. Property language acknowledges the importance of personal autonomy. It provides persons control. People have an interest in what happens to their bodies and body parts. [41]

From the beginning, considering the body as a mechanism is criticized as a reductive view. It is an abstraction precisely because human persons are perceived as bodies without soul. [42] Bodies have only value as economic assets. In this approach, something essential is missing.

Philosophers argue that the image of mechanism presents a simplistic view of the relation between human beings and bodies. We all have experience of our own body. The body is not abstract but always the body of someone. It is experienced as a whole, a unity. The body is individuated: it is distinctive in shape, look, and ways of moving. It has plasticity since it changes over time. The body also has the power of self-healing. It is furthermore pointed out that bodily characteristics such as upright posture, sight, smell, and taste determine what persons can do, not as biological organisms but as beings-in-the-world. [43] At the same time, the body can be used as a tool; it is the instrument with which we act upon the world. Because embodiment allows acting, and therefore moral agency, it is fundamentally related to ethics. Being an embodied person consists in the exercise of virtues. An example is self-respect. This affective virtue is necessary to incorporate one's body as one's own body. Otherwise, one is alienated from the body, and the person's embodiment is impaired. [44] It is also important to note that we experience the body as weak and vulnerable; it can make us dependent; it can be an impediment to what we will and desire; it can be ugly and misshapen, and thus an embarrassment. These paradoxical experiences of the body are unique for human beings.

Roger Scruton has elaborated on the experience that in humans, personhood and animality are united. [45] As subjects, they have first-person perspectives. But, characteristically, they are embedded in a web of interpersonal relationships that gives rise to second-person perspectives. Because we enter into relationships with other persons, we know ourselves in the first person. Moral concepts such as responsibility and blame emerge in the interaction between these perspectives. The second-person perspective is in fact incorporated into the first-person perspective so that my actions are accountable to others and we can give reasons for what we do. The reasons we give to justify ourselves do not depend on our preferences or desires but must be reasons that the other will accept, in other words referring to what we share. Scruton correctly concludes that personhood is not a way of being but a way of becoming. Because of our relatedness, we are continuously called to account: "I am answerable to you for what I say and do, and you likewise to me." [46] As embodied beings, it is our body that brings us into relationships and situate us in the world. Scientific theories that classify persons as the other objects in the world cannot explain human nature.

Similar ideas are asserted by Richard Swinburne. [47] Human beings are of a very different kind from inanimate physical substances. Bodies have physical properties, and brains and other body parts are physical objects. Without a body, humans will not be able to interact with other people and the physical world. The activities of the body are public events: they are accessible to all human beings. But the body or the brain is not who we are. We have consciousness. Mental events (sensations, beliefs, thoughts, intentions, and desires) can only be experienced by the person himself or herself. He or she has privileged access to these events, making it his or her experience. Swinburne argues that we are essentially souls. That is why, we treat human beings and machines differently. According to him, the physical properties of our body are crucial but not essential for our existence. It is logically possible that we can exists without a body or brain. In our opinion, this view is too restrictive and dualistic. For human persons, the body is essential. As argued in Chapter 2, the person is a unity of body and soul. This is why, the image of the body as mechanism is insufficient and disregarding the essential part of what makes us human persons.

Policy-makers and public health professionals have emphasized a different point. Regarding the body as mechanism guides healthcare in specific directions. Medical rationality requires first of all a correct diagnosis. It is important to know what is impaired or deficient in the bodily mechanism before it can be repaired. This is the appeal of genetic determinism and molecular medicine. Nowadays, physicians can identify what is wrong in the basic components of the mechanism and explain the symptoms of the patient. Then rational treatment and clinical intervention can follow. Many studies have shown that this approach has perverted effects. Health and life expectancy are not related to healthcare expenditures, as the declining life expectance in the United States since 2017 illustrates (as argued in Chapter 2). [48] The focus on diagnostics gives priority to biomarkers rather than health outcomes. High blood pressure and cholesterol are "treated" with blockbuster drugs, while the question is whether such interventions extend lives and improve the quality of life. Another example is colorectal cancer. Successful treatment could add 12 years of life to adults with this cancer. But this will only add 1 week to average life expectancy. Valuable interventions for individual patients do not help the overall population. [49] Faith in clinical research into bodily mechanisms is also not warranted. Positive results from clinical trials are rare. [50] Social determinants of health are often more determinative of health than healthcare. The appropriate answer in health policies will be to shift from investments in healthcare to investments in health, for example efforts to reduce poverty and inequality, and to increase the impact of education. People with a graduate degree generally live longer. [51] However, the United States invests currently $0.55 for non-medical social services for each $1 spent on medical care. In other member countries of the Organisation for Economic Co-operation and Development, this is on average $2 on non-medical services for each dollar spent on medical care. [52] Research programs of social determinants of health are very limited. The National Institutes of Health in the United States, which is the largest government funder of biomedical research in the world, spend less than 5% of their budget to behavioral and social sciences research. [53] Examining research inputs and outputs provides a distorted picture as well. Research investments have tremendously increased over the past five decades but they have had comparatively little clinical relevance. More than 1 million new biomedical publications are produced annually. But novel therapeutics, improvements of health, and gains in life expectancy have been proportionally smaller. More research is resulting in more publications but is less focused on benefitting health and preventing disease. [54] In these circumstances, there is a growing movement of medical nihilism. It signals that the effectiveness of many medical interventions is doubtful. Benefits are systematically overestimated, and harms underestimated. This is the result of belief in magic bullets that can quickly repair and restore the functions of the bodily mechanism. What is needed, however, is fewer medical interventions, more lifestyle modifications, and more care. [55]

Additionally, the application of market thinking on the human body is more seriously scrutinized. The body is a symbol of the whole person. Although it is a tool and part of the natural world, it has not merely instrumental value. The human body demands respect, independent from its instrumental uses. Commodifying the body implies a reductionistic view of values. In an economic perspective, all things that people value can be subject of market exchange. All values are commensurable, and can be expressed and compared in monetary terms. However, as will be argued in Chapter 6, this is not the way how people value things. [56] The body does not have a price but has dignity because it cannot be separated from the person. The body is regarded as an integral part of the person. I can only be the person I am because I am embodied in this particular body. Without this body, I would no longer be the person I am. Perhaps, it can be admitted that there are limited property rights with regard to particular parts of the body because they have similarity to ownable objects. This unity of person and body implies that the concept of self-ownership of the body is problematic. If the self is embodied, how can the self be autonomous and separated from the body? [57] Who in fact owns the body? The idea that human beings are their own masters does not imply that they are owners of themselves. Besides these philosophical questions, the body as commodity raises practical challenges. Transforming bodies, tissues, and cells into commodities can generate a range of ethical problems: violation of bodily integrity, exploitation of vulnerable populations, distortion of research agendas, undermining trust in science, and conflicts with community values. [58]

Medical doctors and patients use other arguments to demonstrate that the image of the body as mechanism is deficient. A repeated point is the healing power of the mind. The human body has the ability to deal with illness. It was already affirmed by Hippocratic physicians that doctors cure but nature heals. In healing, the charisma and personality of the healer are important for success. Humanistic qualities such as integrity, respect, and compassion are essential for physicians. David Greaves argues that healing is the soul of medicine. Dealing with issues such as suffering and subjective experiences are inexplicable to science. Some dimension of mystery is therefore a crucial part of medicine. In the healing process, it is not possible to separate science from magic, religion, and spirituality. [59]

Recently, more attention is given to the positive links between health, religion, and faith. Connecting body and soul is regarded as a way toward better healthcare. This attention goes against the general habit of strictly separating biomedicine and religious healing. It is argued that spiritual support for patients will lead to less aggressive care, slower disease progression, longer survival, and better quality of life, especially when life nears death. [60] However, in everyday practice, these issues are commonly not addressed. Although physicians in the United States are more religious than the general population, they treat faith as a private concern and do not connect with their patients in exploring spiritual concerns. [61] Nowadays, religious healing practices are more popular. [62] One explanation is that many patients need psychosocial and spiritual support, nor merely medical care. Religious approaches put need and suffering in a broader perspective and can thus provide meaning. Another explanation is that religion mobilizes emotions, imagination, memory, perception, and senses, which influence the body. [63] Many studies have focused on examining the effects of prayer. This is a rather common practice. In the United States, 35% of people use prayer for health concerns. [64] Other research found that more than 79% of patients prayed for their own health. [65] Studies show mixed results of praying. Scientists are skeptical and prefer to set up randomized double-blind trials. When there are effects, they attribute it to meditation. Different forms of meditation have resulted in psychological and biological changes that are associated with improved health, for example they boost the immune response, reduce anxiety and pain, and enhance the quality of life. Spiritual meditation is also superior to secular meditation. [66] Prayer, regarded as a special form of meditation, diminishes stress, quiets the body, and promotes healing. It is also associated with the placebo response and spontaneous remission. [67] Studies have focused on the possibility of divine intervention. For distant intercessory prayer, clinical trials have been used to determine its efficacy. When rigorous methodologies are applied, no positive therapeutic findings can be reported. [68] However, when people pray for healing, they are usually not remote but close to the person they know or the person himself is praying. For such proximal and personal prayer, double-blind studies are not the best research method. [69] Religion, and specifically prayer, is not medicine. It is a spiritual search for meaning and hope in life. The majority of people praying for health concerns do that for wellness, less for specific health conditions. [70] Prayer is connecting and deepening the relationship with God and other persons. That prayer has no effect on curing illnesses does not mean it is a pointless activity. It has other purposes, for example openness to transcendent experiences, contemplation, and compassion. Praying is different from bargaining, and God is not primarily a provider of health benefits. In answering to prayers, God is not acting like a medicine to cure a disease. While medication causes chemical reactions in our body, prayers will not cause God to act but He freely chooses to grant or not grant our prayer request. If God is viewed in this way, the efficacy of prayer cannot be measured with empirical tests.

Other arguments against the mechanism image refer to psychosomatic medicine. This field of medicine studies the interactions between social, behavioral, and psychological dimensions of life with bodily processes and diseases. It emerged in the 1930s as a movement to counter the influence of the mechanistic image of human beings. The idea is that diseases manifest themselves in the body but are actually caused by psychological factors and life events. Older examples are ulcerative colitis, essential hypertension, and bronchial asthma. Nowadays, new illnesses such as burnout, chronic fatigue syndrome, and fibromyalgia are regarded as psychosomatic. For many physicians, psychosomatic disorders are in fact pseudo-diseases. They agree that in medical practice there are many patient complaints that cannot be explained (estimations are that 10%–15% of all patients visiting the general practitioner have unexplained complaints; most of them are women). [71] The image of the body as mechanism, nowadays, has directed medical thinking toward the new discipline of neuroscience. Psychiatry is gradually replaced by neurobiology. In this perspective, mental causation can ultimately be explained if more is known about the interaction of the brain with the rest of the body. [72] Mental phenomena do not require a special and different approach.

A different type of argument against the image of body as mechanism relates to studies of the dying process. Patients who have been clinically dead have recollections of the period of unconsciousness. They report experiences of seeing a tunnel, a bright light, beautiful landscapes, deceased relatives, and pleasant feelings. Some have out-of-body experiences where they observe what is happening when they are "dead." Eben Alexander, neurosurgeon in Harvard, tells the story of his out-of-body experiences during an almost lethal 7-days coma due to rare bacterial meningitis. During this time, he journeyed through an ultra-real spiritual world with light, music, and love. [73] These near-death experiences were first described in 1975 by Raymond Moody. They have been confirmed in many subsequent publications. When cardiac arrest occurs, cerebral functions are severely impaired or even absent, and consciousness is lost. But how can it be explained that in such conditions patients are aware of these experiences? Near-death experiences therefore seriously question the significance of brain processes for consciousness. When the brain is not functioning, consciousness seems to continue, at least in some cases. [74] The continuation of conscious experiences after the death of the body is an argument in favor of the persistence of a disembodied self, or soul. [75]

Other interesting data refers to patients in so-called "vegetative states." Until recently, it was assumed that such patients have no brain activity. These patients are awake but not aware. They are clinically unresponsive and cannot communicate. Recent studies using EEG and functional MRI showed that 15% of patients responded with brain activity to spoken commands. [76] Some remnant of consciousness, or "covert consciousness," should be present. Other studies found that even 40% of such patients are fully aware. Professional societies have issued new guidelines in 2008. They suggest to abandon the notion of persistent vegetative state, and use "prolonged disorders of consciousness" instead. More accurate diagnoses and better assessment of these patients are needed. These guidelines have important practical consequences since food and fluids are usually withdrawn after some time, and pain medication is not provided. [77]

The conclusion from the above-mentioned arguments is that medicine is in need of humanization. [78] It is necessary to overcome the dominant reductionism and physicalism and to put the experiencing person in the center of medical activities and concerns. In Chapter 6, we will argue that other images can help in humanizing medicine.

## The lone ranger

Another powerful image is individualism. Through our bodies, we are situated in the world as independent selves and we can act on our surroundings. Individual capacities determine what people make of their lives. This is the image of the autonomous subject that is dominant in mainstream bioethics. Respect for individual autonomy means non-interference. Our decisions and actions should be respected as long as we do not harm other human beings. The main challenge for bioethics is how to empower the individual through an emphasis on rights and capabilities. Individual self-determination is a compelling force against medical paternalism. It has inspired social movements against slavery and racism, and galvanized the development of human rights. [79]

Individualism is the ideology that human beings are independent and self-reliant. This ideology is often expressed in the image of the lone ranger. It has become a Western icon, as the daring and adventurous individual who is facing challenges and breaking frontiers. Individualism is commonly opposed to collectivism. Nobody, no state, no community can tell us what to do. The life of an individual belongs to himself or herself, choosing his or her own values, and having the right to live as he or she would like, being his or her own master. The ethical foundation for individualism is the moral worth and dignity of the individual. Individualism articulates the uniqueness of people, their independence but also separateness as individual persons. No two people are the same. Individualism is related to the above-mentioned images of *homo economicus* and body as mechanism. Some argue (e.g. Ayn Rand) that individualism implies ethical egoism. It frequently also entails that individuals own their bodies and can dispose of them as they like. It is even argued that individuals create their own soul. [80]

The focus on the individual is one of the driving forces of Weber's process of disenchantment. It is argued that the concept of the individual is a central notion in Weber's work. [81] The spirit of capitalism requires a particular way of conducting life (*Lebensführung*), that is fashioning oneself as a distinctive kind of individual. This way of life is stimulated, according to Weber, by Protestant beliefs such as Calvinism, Pietism, and Baptism. They require a rational inner-worldly ascetism. The individual is placed by God in a specific station of life and should make the best of it by self-discipline. He alone can strive for salvation; nobody else can help him. His life should be alert, not focused on pleasures, greed, and luxury but should be serious, rational, and controlled. But the individual also lives in an Iron Cage. Moral values have retreated in the private sphere. Each individual is therefore lonely and isolated, on his or her own. [82] Paradoxically, as argued in Chapter 3, autonomy and self-expression are, in Weber's view, the inner core of the person against the impersonal nature of social life.

There is a distinction between individualism and individuality. While every human being is an individual with its own characteristics, not everybody is individualistic. The concept of individuality has developed into the ideology of individualism over the last centuries.

Individuality has two dimensions: separated and demarcated from other organisms, and being oneself and distinct. It claims that only individuals as indivisible singular samples of the species have real existence, in distinction to relations, wholes, or traits. [83] Individuality means uniqueness: not merely being oneself but not being someone else.

The notion of "individual" has become the organizing principle in the West. It was shaped by Christian beliefs making it possible that liberal secularism developed in this part of the world. [84] In ancient times, there was no notion of individuality. Human beings were defined by family, tribe, or city. Christianity promoted the idea that human beings have access to the deepest reality as individuals. Being human means being a rational and moral, thus responsible agent. In canon law, for example, from the 12th to the 15th century, the sphere of personal responsibility was redefined as the sphere of personal autonomy, emphasizing inner conviction and self-discipline. [85] The term "individual" has become current in the 15th century. [86]

Since a long time, bioethics has been criticized for its limited moral vocabulary, centered on the value complex of individual rights, self-determination, and privacy, at the expense of social responsibility and social justice. [87] It is argued that the individual is not independent from his context and that we are not "unencumbered selves." [88] Individualism has been called a "myth" precisely because it separates personal lives from the social environment and assumes that our self is not constituted by social processes (e.g. education and media influences) and informed by community values. [89] One consequence of this image is that human vulnerability is denied or translated into impairment or deficiency of the person's capacity to make autonomous decisions. [90] Another consequence is that the interconnectedness of human life is lost. It is, in fact, the interaction with other people that makes us into autonomous individuals. What is lost is the significance of dependency, networking, and cooperation. Jasanoff, for example, refers to the personification of scientific achievements. Discoveries and innovations are presented as eureka moments and the work of individual geniuses. The contributions of teams and networks in knowledge-making, which are crucial for science today, are simply erased. [91] Another consequence of this loss of connectedness concerns human relationships with the environment. Human beings are embedded not only in society and culture but also in the natural world of animals and plants. That implies the starting point for ethical discourse should be different: rather than the individual patient or professional, it is important to recognize that individuals can only flourish when conditions exist that promote and sustain autonomous life. They depend on biodiversity for clean air, safe water, adequate nutrition, effective drugs, and protection from infectious diseases. The notion of "environment" is inadequate to express this fundamental interconnection. Human beings are not just surrounded by an environment but included within a diverse and living world. "Biodiversity" more appropriately indicates that nature and culture cannot be separated but are intimately connected. Furthermore, human beings themselves cannot be opposed to nature. Humans are part of nature, and can only be healthy when ecosystems are healthy. The consequence of both considerations is that an ethical perspective is needed that transcends the usual dichotomies between humans, nature, and culture. For example, Dirk Lanzerath, in his studies on the ethics of biodiversity, has argued for an "anthroporelational ethics." [92] In fact, the same broad idea inspired Potter's coining of the term "global bioethics." [93]

In the ethical critique of individualism, two issues are advanced. One is the loss of connectedness. [94] The argument is that the individual is conceived as an isolated abstract entity. Community, tradition, history, social practices, and culture are only relevant secondarily. Societies are regarded as mere collections of individuals. This perspective ignores that human beings are a social product. They are not abstract beings but become concrete and individual within a communal context. This point is particularly advanced in the philosophy of communitarianism. [95] African philosophers, for example, argue that the person is defined by the community. [96] Without the community, the person has no existence. His or her relatedness makes that he or she is there. Community and individuality are not options that the individual can choose. This point of view entails another view of society. It is aptly expressed by Léopold Senghor, the first president of Senegal: African society is "a communion of souls rather than an aggregate of individuals." [97] A similar point of view is presented in the philosophy of personalism. It emphasizes the uniqueness, dignity, and subjectivity of the human person but at the same time the person is a social being, that is intrinsically situated and embedded in the context of community and society. [98]

Communitarianism and personalism, as ethical philosophies, are particularly underlined as alternative approaches to mainstream bioethics. Daniel Callahan has argued that individualism presents moral queries as individual problems, and therefore does not address the social and cultural context of such problems. It has a bias toward technological solutions and neglects the common good. [99]

Personalism has been especially prominent in European approaches in bioethics. Paul Schotsmans, bioethicist from Belgium, points out that personalism provides a philosophy that is most appropriate for medicine that is a relational, healing profession. The human being is open to other human beings and involved in cooperation. The focus on individual autonomy therefore is too limited for medical-professional practice. [100] In light of such criticisms, feminist philosophers, in particular, have reconceptualized autonomy as "relational autonomy." Rather than an individualistic conception of autonomy, they have stressed the significance of interdependency and embeddedness in family, community, and society. The effect is that besides self-determination, other values are important, such as responsibility, care, cooperation, and trust. [101]

The criticisms of communitarianism, personalism, and feminism against individualism will be elaborated later in Chapter 6 because they appeal to the moral imagination in a different way than mainstream bioethics, and produce images that may revitalized the soul of healthcare and ethics. They articulate the fact of dependency and vulnerability, regard relatedness as a necessary condition for personal identity, and argue that embeddedness in communities is a precondition for moral agency. They also affirm another point that will be elaborated in the next paragraph: the role of emotions in ethics and medicine. The dominant concept of the autonomous individual assumes that the person is rational and is able to control emotional experiences in the decision-making process. This assumption, however, is questionable.

A second issue that is advanced in the ethical critique of individualism is the notion of progress. The image of the lone ranger evokes prospects of frontiers and progress. Human beings are confronted with borderlines and limitations but these can be passed and overstepped. The idea that the future will always be better is particularly strong in scientific discourse, and the idea of progress is equally vigorous in popular media. Science will only grow. It does not have inherent limitations. Scientific progress is therefore unstoppable. Every attempt to limit science and technology is doomed to failure. In the near future, personalized medicine will offer precise, targeted, and individualized treatments. [102] Age-old ailments and suffering can be eradicated. Genetic technologies will be used to enhance and perfect human beings. The range of choices available for individuals will greatly expand. The ultimate frontier of death will also be overcome. New technologies will liberate human beings from biology and corporeality, extending the life span, cure ageing, and make humans virtually immortal. The individual can finally obtain full mastery of his or her body. The ideal of progress, however, is not a neutral program or statement. It goes together with a reductionist and naturalist ideology. Human beings are regarded as mechanisms that can be repaired and improved. The human future will be determined by technical expertise, computer sciences, artificial intelligence, and biotechnology. Another implication of this belief in progress is that the past, history, and tradition are irrelevant. They cannot provide moral guidance for the continuously changing present. Since life is an individual accomplishment within a particular constellation of time and space, it can be disconnected from prior experiences.

## Detached concern

> The doctor said that so-and-so indicated that there was so-and-so inside the patient, but if the investigation of so-and-so did not confirm this, then he must assume that and that. If he assumed that and that, then . . . and so on. To Ivan Ilyich only one question was important: was his case serious or not? But the doctor ignored that inappropriate question. From his point of view, it was not the one under consideration, the real question was to decide between a floating kidney, chronic catarrh, or appendicitis. It was a question the doctor solved brilliantly, as it seemed to Ivan Ilyich, in favour of the appendix, with the reservation that should an examination of the urine give fresh indications the matter would be reconsidered . . . From the doctor's summing up Ivan Ilyich concluded that things were bad, but that for the doctor, and perhaps for everybody else, it was a matter of indifference. [103]

This passage from Tolstoy's *The death of Ivan Ilyich* illustrates another powerful image in present-day healthcare. Although Tolstoy presents a caricature, it is the image of the physician as an expert with detached concern.

Declarations that the soul has disappeared from medicine and healthcare are often associated with the idea that the belief in technology and medication has eliminated subjective experiences from the realm of medicine. These experiences alter, and often distort, the way in which complaints are presented. Within the dominant materialistic and naturalistic world view of medical science, the mind and thus subjectivity are not especially relevant. Emotions and feelings such as empathy and compassion should not play a role in the proceedings of medical practice. The image of the competent professional is detached concern. Doctors should not become emotionally involved. They should maintain some distance in order to safeguard their objectivity. At the same time, it is acknowledged that interpersonal relations and empathic understanding are important. Doctors cannot merely be detached rational agents. But detachment is an important ethical value, and that is what they learn in medical school. The ideal is that they are neutral moral agents who do not allow emotions to interfere with their scientific approach.

Detachment is justified with several arguments. It is a way to protect oneself from burnout. Practitioners have to concentrate on painful procedures and they can only execute them when they are not too much involved in the patient's personal circumstances. It is also necessary to care for patients in an impartial way. Professionals cannot let their emotions and feelings determine how they will act. Emotions are subjective and can easily interfere with objective and rational judgment. Professionals should be free from bias and prejudice. [104]

The image of the detached healthcare provider is connected to other images discussed earlier. One of the implications of the image of the body as mechanism is that the physician is primarily concerned with the diseased body of the patient. He or she should not enter the subjective world of the patient. In fact, the physician must operate as a mechanic. The image of *homo economicus* emphasizes rational decision-making. The supposition is that people make decisions on the basis of adequate information so that they can develop a rational judgment and can provide reasons for decisions. Healthcare providers therefore should provide reliable and objective information so that patients can weigh the benefits and harms of possible interventions. Emotions and imagination should not interfere. Finally, detached concern is the best approach in the context of individualism. It respects the autonomy of the patient and does not unduly influence the individual's decisions.

Traditionally, sympathy and compassion have always been regarded as crucial for medical practice, and especially for contributing to healing. In medicine, it is impossible to ignore the needs of patients for emotional interactions with physicians and other care providers. Attending to the subjective experiences of patients not only will deliver important information but also will engage physicians in more effective communication. It will build trust with patients and will improve the effectiveness of medical treatment. The concept of relational autonomy is helpful in this regard. It is essential for patient-centered care because it focuses attention to the patient as a whole person within his or her social context. It also enhances shared decision-making, communication, and partnership, supporting the autonomous capacities of the patient. [105]

The image of detached concern therefore is unsatisfactory. Empathy should supplement objective knowledge. George Engel, in his critique of the biomedical model, denounces the model as cold and impersonal. It is unsatisfying not only for patients but also for physicians. If they are insensitive to the personal problems of patients and their families, they experience disenchantment and feel that they neglect their patients. [106] The negative effects of such disenchantment are increasingly recognized nowadays. A recent Editorial in *The Lancet* signals a global crisis of physician burnout. In the United States, 78% of physicians are affected by burnout, and in the United Kingdom 80%. Although exact data are not available, similar phenomena of emotional exhaustion, depersonalization, and a sense of reduced personal accomplishment are observed in many other countries. It is not only a tragedy for individual physicians but also threatening healthcare systems and patients' care. [107]

Feelings of negativism and cynicism are not sufficiently addressed during medical education. It is a common finding since a long time that empathy is declining in medical school and residency. It is estimated that 75% of medical students become more cynical about the medical profession, especially in the first 4 years of their education. [108] This education emphasizes emotional detachment, affective distance, and clinical neutrality. Reasons for decline of empathy and idealism are not clear. It may be a manifestation of distress because of mistreatment by superiors and mentors, negative role models, failure to deal with anxieties concerning illness and suffering, vulnerability, social support problems, emphasis on financial regulations, and high workload. Anyway, the result is that students identify "with a cold and uncaring role model." [109] This is a reason for concern since empathy and compassionate care are generally regarded as essential for good relationships between patient and physician. The learning environment is usually blamed. There is an absence of specific educational programs to cultivate humanistic qualities. There is need for systematic training of such qualities in medical schools. But most probably more will be needed to nurture empathy. [110] We will address the role of education in Chapter 7.

## Consumer and client

The modern citizen is regarded as consumer rather than producer. He or she is a choosing self, a responsible subject making his or her choices among a large variety of options, according to his or her own preferences and values. The image of patients as consumers and clients has been introduced in healthcare since the 1960s and 1970s. [111] Especially in the United States, healthcare came to be regarded as a business. Patients are addressed as active, self-empowered health consumers with individual choice and personal responsibility as main values. Consumerism is attractive because it promises to liberate people from paternalism. In bioethics, the principle of respect for individual autonomy includes the same promise against medical paternalism. In healthcare policies, the ethical point of view could be easily aligned with the dominant market ideology. Policies suppose that citizens will be active consumers who not only will search and check the available information relevant for their health, but also are interested in a healthy lifestyle and will demonstrate responsible conduct in the decisions they make. The assumption is that real empowerment as consumers and clients will lead to the right choices. [112] Another assumption is that consumerism requires the introduction of competition, and that competitiveness will constrain costs and optimize quality of care. Patients will shop for their insurance plans, doctors, hospitals, tests, and treatments, and they purchase what is best for them. These ideas fit very well with the concept of the neoliberal subject (also articulated in the images of the *homo economicus* and lone ranger) that is focused on the proper government of life. The burden of maintaining health is on the individual. The ideal subject is the responsible consumer who actively seeks information and produces health as the outcome of choices. What is needed is correct information and proper education. Health knowledge is like capital; it should grow and expand. This is an attractive view because it no longer solely relies on the authority of medical experts. It also refers to the idea of scientific progress. Like in other markets, new tools and resources will be constantly available to realize healthy lifestyles. [113]

In the domain of healthcare, the consumer image is deficient. Several arguments are advanced for its inadequacy. The first argument points out that the discourse of choice is problematic.

Adequate information as the basis for choices and decisions is often lacking or does not exist or is kept private. If information is available, it is less reliable and harder to evaluate than elsewhere. The focus on economic considerations is overemphasized. Doctors and patients do not regularly discuss costs. [114] The main source of medical information for patients often is the internet but the reliability of information is questionable and difficult to assess. Whether or not they like it, patients are envisioned in current health policies as having the duty to exercise choice. [115] It is associated with responsibilization: people are responsible for the choices they make. However, not everyone is in the same position to make choices. And not all consequences of decisions are the result of individual choices. The effect of the discourse of choice is that social solidarity is regarded as less important. This point is illustrated by Margo Trappenburg. [116] In the 1960s and 1970s, care institutions for psychiatric patients and people with learning disabilities were dismantled in the Netherlands. Deinstitutionalization was guided by the ideology of giving choices to people: they could indicate whether they prefer to continue living in an institution or moving into society. Leaving the institutional setting behind, people could have more opportunities, live according to their preferences, and be included in society. In hindsight, this ideology created challenges. These patient populations are not typical consumers; they are vulnerable, weak, and disabled; they have serious disadvantages in social adaptation, employment, and networking. They have to rely more often on family members to sustain themselves outside institutions. Active solidarity is also requested from able-bodied citizens. They are asked for help and care. But not everybody will have the same sense of solidarity. Benevolent people who already provide care will have most of the burden of deinstitutionalization. Trappenburg furthermore questions the freedom of choice. She argues that the choice to leave the institution is not an isolated one. It is a collective action problem where individuals take into account what other individuals will supposedly do. When mildly disabled people choose to live outside the institution, the people remaining will be the more severely afflicted. The institutional environment will therefore change, making the choice to stay less attractive. In the end, only the frailest of the frail will remain institutionalized.

The second critique on the consumer image contends that it is based on misconceptions about human nature. People do not make decisions all the time in search of control, shopping for the best combination of cost and quality. They are not continuously busying around to satisfy their preferences. The continuous emphasis on people being consumers is annoying. Most often, they are citizens concerned with developments in their neighborhood, community or society at large. They are family members taking care for their children or disabled elders. They want to walk around and relax in a public park without being approached as consumers. Overextending the image of consumer is particularly disturbing when health and disease are at stake. Human beings do not want to be reduced to "aggregates of data," self-tracking and moving around, regularly gathering detailed health input about themselves. Wearables, health apps, and medical data can be useful but they receive a different role when they determine our daily existence and lifestyle. As Schneider and Hall comment: ". . . people have better things to do than become healthcare experts." [117] Furthermore, the human context changes when people are ill, disabled, or suffering. While consumers are driven by desires and preferences, patients are in need of care, assistance, or treatment. Ill people do not need a market with a diversity of providers and a range of offers among which they must choose. They do not wish satisfaction of wants or preferences but care that is in their own best interest. [118]

Moreover, patients, in distinction to consumers, are vulnerable. It is precisely this aspect of vulnerability that is omitted in consumer discourse.

The third critical argument concerns the language of competition and commodity that prevails when healthcare is regarded as consumption. [119] Generalized competitiveness expresses a normative logic: the subject should relate to himself as human capital. He has continuously to invest in his health by exploring and seeking the best and most effective options for the best price possible. The idea is that competition will eliminate inefficient health services. But competition in general is limited. Healthcare costs have not decreased as a result of competition. On the contrary, hospitals and insurance companies are merging in order to better control and consolidate the market. The Pittsburgh area, for example, is dominated by two large healthcare systems that are owned by insurance companies (they are considered as charities, so they do not pay any taxes to the communities in which they operate). In the United States, the two largest insurers control more than 50% of the market. In these markets, premiums are higher. Rather than competition, companies strive for monopolies. In many European countries that regard healthcare as a public service, limited competition among health insurers is introduced but at the same time strictly regulated. This approach is based on two ethical considerations: profits should not override patient's benefits, and healthcare should be equally accessible to everybody. The emphasis on competition also assumes that consumer options are relevant and valuable. This assumption is questionable since the main guiding rule for consumerism is that consumers can satisfy their preferences. These are not necessarily similar to their healthcare needs. Commercial health services are interested in creating greater demand for care. With an ageing population in many countries, demand for healthcare is indeed rapidly growing. But demand can also be induced by offering non-essential services and promoting unnecessary medication. [120] Another type of critique focusses on the language of commodity. Health is presented as a product that can be enhanced by rational decisions and responsible conduct. But, as will be argued in Chapter 6, health is not a product like cars and televisions. Healthcare is a set of healing practices. Efficiency is not the most important value. [121]

Another critical argument against consumerism is that it has a negative impact on cooperation. As discussed earlier, humans have evolved because they have the capacity for social learning. Medical problems are often related to social issues beyond the individual level. Addressing them properly will require cooperation of many concerned actors. The question is raised whether in modern societies, human beings are losing cooperative skills. Inequalities are growing. They increase the social distance among people; they make it harder to feel mutual sympathy. The image of consumer and client does not disregard cooperation, but interprets it as an instrumental tool. It is useful if it enhances the outcomes for everybody involved, or within the perspective of the *homo economicus*, primarily when it maximizes the interests of the person engaging in cooperation. Sharing and solidarity are useful when they deliver specific outcomes. Cooperation is not valuable as an end in itself. In a market system governed by efficiency and profitability, it will not be very beneficial to cooperate with people who cannot effectively contribute much to shared endeavors. Many people nowadays have become irrelevant, useless, and superfluous. Entire populations are no longer relevant for economic development. Public services to sustain their basic needs such as health, food, and water either are unnecessary or can be cut. The Polish sociologist Zygmunt Bauman has called these discarded and disposable populations "wasted lives." [122] In present-day societies, precariousness is not an exception; it has become the rule of modern life. [123]

The fifth and final criticism points out that consumerism is based on a distorted view of values. All human values are treated as options. Individuals are the only ones that should decide about values. Ludwig von Mises, one of the philosophers of neoliberalism, stated:

> In the market economy the individual is free to act within the orbit of private property and the market. His choices are final . . . Society does not tell a man what to do and what not to do. [124]

Judgments about values are therefore not appropriate: "It is not the fault of the entrepreneurs that the consumers . . . prefer liquors to Bibles and detective stories to serious books, and that governments prefer guns to butter." [125] Values are thus equated to individual preferences. In Chapter 6, we will argue that values cannot be reduced to individual desires or preferences. They are associated with a wide range of emotions such as respect, honor, affection, and love. What people value is often plural and different in quality. They also differ over time depending on the context, conditions, and challenges of life. [126] That means that there are important differences between values, calling into question the assumption that values are commensurable, and that the most important ethical consideration is that values must be respected and regarded as decisive as long as they are the authentic expression of the value system of the autonomous individual. Moral emotions such as repugnance, anger, and disgust indicate that some values are more important than others. Child abuse and torture are wrong whatever value they may have for the perpetrators. Some transactions such as slavery, prostitution, and dwarf-tossing are also inappropriate as affronts to human dignity, even if they satisfy the preferences of individuals. [127] Values therefore are not merely important and worthy of respect since they refer to what people prefer and desire, but more importantly, they disclose what kind of person an individual wants to be, what kind of life he intends to live, and how he engages with other people. Expressing values is not a matter of getting things and purchasing commodities but of being someone.

## Conclusion

The five images discussed in this chapter are all connected with each other. They are symbolic expressions and visualizations of the world view that currently dominates science as well as healthcare. Images are used to disseminate and reinforce the basic ideas and values of the ideology of naturalism. They frame consciousness, interpretation, and reflection, and therefore influence the ethical debate. The contemporary human being is imagined as a rational and individual decision-maker, primarily motivated by self-interest. This image of *homo economicus* pervades present-day societies. It shows how economic thinking has influenced the interpretation of human existence and social life. As a rational agent, the individual governs the human body as a mechanism. The body can be understood, examined, repaired, and enhanced with the methods of the natural sciences, especially physics, which has been enormously helpful for the growth of medical science. The body as mechanism can furthermore be incorporated in the dominant framework of the market ideology. The body and its parts are commodities like other objects in the world. They can be exchanged in the market. Decisions about the uses of the body are taken by autonomous persons who are individuals, self-reliant, and independent from other people. Individualism is a dominant image, not only in Western cultures but also particularly in mainstream bioethics discourse with its emphasis on the principle of respect for autonomy. Another common image is the detached health professional. Subjective and personal experiences are not relevant for medicine, according to the prevailing naturalist ideology. The doctor should focus on objective findings and make rational decisions. Finally, consumer discourse has vanquished healthcare. Patients are imagined as clients and consumers who select services and providers, guided by efficiency and their own preferences.

As argued in this chapter, all images have drawbacks and shortcomings. They are, often already since a long time, criticized as deficient, wrong, unjust, and one-sided. The important point, however, is that these images determine the context in which ethical discussions frequently operate. Such determination is subtle; it is usually not explicit. The images frame and shape the possible ways in which ethical challenges are addressed, how problems are formulated, and what kind of solutions are proposed and found reasonable. An example is the ASBH Code of Ethics for clinical ethics consultants. The Code requests to pay attention to disparities, discrimination, and inequities in healthcare. But the images of individualism, *homo economicus*, and rational consumer do not encourage to address issues of justice and social context. The voices of marginalized patients are not heard within medical interactions. The dominating images make it difficult to realize the requirements of the Code. [128]

To overcome the ideological context of contemporary healthcare and bioethics, it will be indispensable to widen the moral vocabulary to make room for richer ethical perspectives. The images discussed in this chapter are limited and biased. They present a reductive view of human beings and social life. The images are especially inadequate within the present global environment of bioethics. They do not inspire cooperation, partnership, and sustainable efforts to fight against ecological disasters, pandemic diseases, and planetary collapse. Many argue that a fundamental shift in values and world view is necessary. [129] New visions can be imagined since humans are the only creatures with the capacity for imagination. As *homo imaginens*, the human being can articulate alternative futures. The significance of moral imagination for bioethics will be elaborated in the next chapter.

## References


1 Thomas Nagel, *Mind and cosmos: Why the materialist Neo-Darwinian conception of nature is almost certainly false* (Oxford: Oxford University Press, 2012), 128.

2 Theodore Adorno, Else Frenkel-Brunswik, Daniel J. Levinson, and R. Newitt Sanford, *The authoritarian personality* (New York: Harper, 1950), 2.

3 John Gerring, "Ideology: A definitional analysis," *Political Research Quarterly* 50, no. 4 (1997): 3.

4 Jürgen Habermas, "Technology and science as 'ideology'," in *Toward a rational society*, Jürgen Habermas (Boston: Beacon, 1970), 81–122.

5 See, for example, Bert Baumgaertner, Juliet E. Carlisle, and Florian Justwan, "The influence of political ideology and trust on willingness to vaccinate," *PLoS One* 13, no. 1 (2018): e0191728.

6 Antara Haldar, "Intrinsic goodness," *Times Literary Supplement* (2 November 2018): 10–11; David Wilson and William Dixon, *A history of Homo Economicus. The nature of the moral in economic theory* (London and New York: Routledge, 2013).

7 Adam Smith, *An Inquiry into the Nature and Causes of the Wealth of Nations*. Edited by S. M. Soares (Amsterdam: Meta Libri Digital Library, 2007), 16.

8 John D. Bishop, "Adam Smith's invisible hand argument," *Journal of Business Ethics* 14, no. 3 (1995): 165–180.

9 Ayn Rand, *The virtue of selfishness: A new concept of egoism* (New York: Signet/Penguin, 2014).

10 Friedrich Hayek, *The road to serfdom* (Chicago and New York: University of Chicago Press, 2005).

11 Milton Friedman, "The social responsibility of business is to increase its profits," *The New York Times Magazine* (13 September 1970).

12 Samuel Bowles, and Herbert Gintis, "Social preferences, homo economicus and zoon politicon," in *The Oxford Handbook of Contextual Political Analysis*, eds. Robert E. Goodin and Charles Tilly (Oxford: Oxford University Press, 2006), 172–186.

13 Amartya K. Sen, "Rational fools: A critique of the behavioral foundations of economic theory," *Philosophy & Public Affairs* 6, no. 4 (1977): 336.

14 Joseph Henrich, Robert Boyd, Samuel Bowles, Colin Camerer, Ernst Fehr, Herbert Gintis, and Richard McElreath, "In search of homo economicus: Behavioral experiments in 15 small-scale societies," *American Economic Review* 91, no. 2 (2001): 73–84.

15 Samuel Bowles, *The moral economy. Why good incentives are no substitute for good citizens* (New Haven and London: Yale University Press, 2016). See also: Mark Granovetter, *Society and economy. Framework and principles* (Cambridge and London: The Belknap Press of Harvard University Press, 2017).

16 Herbert Gintis, "Strong reciprocity and human sociality," *Journal of Theoretical Biology* 206 (2000): 169–179.

17 Alain Cohen, Michel André Maréchal, David Tannenbaum, and Christian Lukas Zünd, "Civic honesty around the globe," *Science* 365 (2019): 70–73.

18 Herbert Gintis, *Individuality and entanglement: The moral and material bases of social life* (Princeton and Oxford: Princeton University Press, 2017), 51 ff.

19 Henk ten Have, *Global bioethics. An introduction* (London and New York: Routledge, 2016), 67–71.

20 See, for example, the work of Thomas Sowell who is concerned with disparities, discrimination and vulnerabilities but argues that humans are motivated by pay and self-interest. Thomas Sowell, *Basic economics. A common sense guide to the economy* (New York: Basic Books, 2015). See also: Wilson and Dixon, *A history of Homo Economicus*.

21 Bowles, *The moral economy*, 57–63, 75–76. See also: David Wilson and William Dixon, *A history of Homo Economicus. The nature of the moral in economic theory* (London and New York: Routledge, 2012).

22 Dorothy Nelking, and Lori Andrews, "Homo economicus. Commercialization of body tissue in the age of biotechnology," *Hastings Center Report* 28, no. 5 (1998): 30–39.

23 A human being is therefore better classified as *homo reciprocans*. Samuel Bowles, and Herbert Gintis, "Homo reciprocans," *Nature* 415, no. 6868 (2002): 125–128. "The capacity to band together to make societies is indeed a biological feature of our species . . ." And also: ". . . we humans are unusual in our ability to cooperate with unrelated individuals." Nicholas A. Christakis, *Blueprint. The evolutionary origins of a good society* (New York, Boston and London: Little, Brown Spark, 2019), 13 and 384. See furthermore, Jeremy Rifkin, *The empathic civilization* (Cambridge: Polity Press, 2009): "Empathy is the very means by which we create social life and advance civilization." (p. 10).

24 Tor Helge Holmas, Egil Kjerstad, Hilde Luras, and Odd Rune Straume, "Does monetary punishment crowd out pro-social motivation? A natural experiment on hospital length of stay," *Journal of Economic Behavior & Organization* 75 (2010): 261–267.

25 Richard M. Titmuss, *The gift relationship: From human blood to social policy* (London: Allen and Unwin, 1970).

26 David Archard, "Selling yourself: Titmuss's argument against a market in blood," *The Journal of Ethics* 6, no. 1 (2002): 87–103.

27 Alvin E. Roth, "Repugnance as a constraint on markets," *The Journal of Economic Perspectives* 21, no. 3 (2007): 37–58.

28 Charles L. Briggs, and Daniel C. Hallin, "Biocommunicability. The neoliberal subject and its contradictions in news coverage of health issues," *Social Text* 25, no. 4 (2007): 43–66.

29 Eva Illouz, *Cold intimacies: The making of emotional capitalism* (Cambridge: Polity Press, 2007).

30 Pierre Dardot, and Christian Laval, *The new way of the world. On neo-liberal society* (London and New York: Verso, 2017), 112.

31 Margaret Thatcher, Interview for the Sunday Times (7 May 1988); www.margaretthatcher.org/document/104475.

32 Sanford F. Schram, *The return of ordinary capitalism. Neoliberalism, precarity, occupy* (Oxford: Oxford University Press, 2015).

33 Ten Have, *Global bioethics*, 71–74.

34 Bruce Rogers-Vaughn, *Caring for souls in a neoliberal age* (New York: Palgrave Macmillan, 2019), 223, 231.

35 Alastair V. Campbell, *The body in bioethics* (Routledge, London and New York, 2009).

36 Eduard J. Dijksterhuis, *De mechanisering van het wereldbeeld* (Amsterdam: Meulenhoff, 1950).

37 Mary Midgley, *The ethical primate: Humans, freedom and morality* (London and New York: Taylor & Francis Group, 1994), 96–97.

38 Dorothy Nelkin, "Molecular metaphors: The gene in popular discourse," *Nature Reviews: Genetics* 2, no. 7 (2001): 555–559.

39 Gerrit A. Lindeboom, *Descartes and medicine* (Amsterdam: Rodopi, 1979), 59.

40 Peter Machamer, Lindley Darden, and Carl F. Craver, "Thinking about mechanisms," *Philosophy of Science* 67, no. 1 (2000): 1–25.

41 Lori B. Andrews, "My body, my property," *Hastings Center Report* 16, no. 5 (1986): 28–38; Courtney S. Campbell, "Body, self, and the property paradigm," *Hastings*

*Center Report* 22, no. 5 (1992): 34–42; Nelkin, and Andrews, "Homo economicus," 30–39.

42 See: Campbell, *The body in bioethics*.

43 "Our bodies demonstrate, albeit silently, that we are more than just a complex version of our animal ancestors, and, conversely, that we are also more than an enlarged brain, a consciousness somehow grafted onto or trapped within a blind mechanism that knows only survival." Leon R. Kass, "Thinking about the body," *Hastings Center Report* 15, no. 1 (1985): 26. See also: Michael A. Schwartz, and Osborne P. Wiggins, "Psychosomatic medicine and the philosophy of life," *Philosophy, Ethics, and Humanities in Medicine* 5, no. 2 (2010).

44 Charles Taliaferro, "The virtues of embodiment," *Philosophy* 76, no. 295 (2001): 111–125.

45 Roger Scruton, *On human nature* (Princeton and Oxford: Princeton University Press, 2017).

46 Scruton, *On human nature*, 110.

47 Richard Swinburne, *Are we bodies or souls?* (Oxford: Oxford University Press, 2019).

48 Irene Papanicolas, et al., "Health care spending in the United States and other high-income countries," *JAMA* 318 (13 March 2018): 1024–1039.

49 See: Robert M. Kaplan, *More than medicine. The broken promise of American health* (Cambridge and London: Harvard University Press, 2019).

50 Robert M. Kaplan, and Veronica L. Irvin, "Likelihood of null effects of large NHLBI clinical trials has increased over time," *PLoS One* 10, no. 8 (2015): e0132382.

51 Jennifer Karas Montez, and Mark D. Hayward, "Cumulative childhood adversity, educational attainment, and active life expectancy among U.S. adults," *Demography* 51, no. 2 (2014): 413–435.

52 Stuart M. Butler, Davna Bowen Matthew, and Marcela Cabello, *Re-balancing medical and social spending to promote health: Increasing state flexibility to improve health through housing* (Washington: Brookings Institute, 15 February 2017).

53 Robert M. Kaplan, Suzanne Bennett Johnson, and Patricia Clem Kobor, "NIH behavioral and social sciences research support: 1980–2016," *American Psychologist* 72, no. 8 (2017): 808–821.

54 Anthony Bowen, and Arturo Casadevall, "Increasing disparities between resource inputs and outcomes, as measured by certain health deliverables, in biomedical research," *Proceedings of the National Academy of Sciences* 112, no. 36 (2015): 11335–11340.

55 Jacob Stegenga, *Medical nihilism* (Oxford: Oxford University Press, 2018); Barbara Ehrenreich, *Natural causes. An epidemic of wellness, the certainty of dying, and killing ourselves to live longer* (New York and Boston: Twelve/Hachette Book Group, 2018).

56 Margaret Jane Radin, *Contested commodities* (Cambridge and London: Harvard University Press, 2001).

57 See: Campbell, *The body in bioethics*; Joke I. de Witte, and Henk ten Have, "Ownership of genetic material and information," *Social Science & Medicine* 45, no. 1 (1997): 51–60.

58 Nelkin and Andrews, "Homo economicus."

59 David Greaves, *Mystery in Western medicine* (Aldershot: Avebury, 1996). See also: Jo Marchant, *Cure. A journey into the science of mind over body* (New York: Broadway Books, 2016).

60 See, for example, Yoichi Chida, Andrew Steptoe, and Lynda H. Powell, "Religiosity/spirituality and mortality," *Psychotherapy and Psychosomatics* 78 (2009): 81–90; Gail

Ironson, Rick Stuetzle, Dale Ironson, Elizabeth Balbin, Heidemarie Kremer, Annie George, Neil Schneiderman, and Mary Ann Fletcher, "View of God as benevolent and forgiving or punishing and judgmental predicts HIV disease progression," *Journal of Behavioral Medicine* 34 (2011): 414–425.

61 Farr A. Curlin, John D. Lantos, Chad J. Roach, Sarah A. Sellergren, and Marshal H. Chin, "Religious characteristics of U. S. Physicians. A national survey," *Journal of General Internal Medicine* 20 (2005): 629–634.

62 Sipco J. Vellenga, "Longing for health. A practice of religious healing and biomedicine compared," *Journal of Religion and Health* 47, no. 3 (2008): 326–337.

63 Meredith B. McGuire, "Religion and healing the mind/body/self," *Social Compass* 43 (1996): 101–116.

64 Anne M. McCaffrey, David M. Eisenberg, Anna T. Legedza, et al., "Prayer for health concerns: Results of a national survey on prevalence and patterns of use," *Archives of Internal Medicine* 164 (2004): 858–862.

65 Mary Ann Richardson, Tina Sanders, J. Lynn Palmer, Anthony Greisinger, and S. Eva Singletary, "Complementary/alternative medicine use in a comprehensive cancer center and the implications for oncology," *Journal of Clinical Oncology* 18, no. 13 (2000): 2505–2514; Karin Jors, Arndt Büssing, Niels Christian Hyidt, and Klaus Baumann, "Personal prayer in patients dealing with chronic illness: A review of the research literature," *Evidence-Based Complementary and Alternative Medicine* (2015): 927–973; doi: 10.1155/2015/927973.

66 Chittaranjan Andrade, and Pajiv Radhakrihnan, "Prayer and healing: A medical and scientific perspective on randomized controlled trials," *Indian Journal of Psychiatry* 51, no. 4 (2009): 247–253.

67 Marek Jantos, and Hosen Kiat, "Prayer as medicine: How much have we learned?" *Medical Journal of Australia* 186, no. 10 (2007): S51.

68 Leanne Roberts, Irshad Ahmed, and Andrew Davidson, "Intercessory prayer for the alleviation of ill health," *Cochrane Database of Systematic Reviews*, no. 2 (2009). Art. No.: CD000368; doi:10.1002/14651858.CD000368.pub3.

69 Candy Gunther Brown, *Testing prayer. Science and healing* (Boston: Harvard University Press, 2012).

70 McCaffrey, Eisenberg, Legedza, et al., "Prayer for health concerns."

71 Diane O'Leary, "Why bioethics should be concerned with medically unexplained symptoms," *The American Journal of Bioethics* 18, no. 5 (2018): 6–15.

72 Lukas van Oudenhove, and Stefan Cuypers, "The relevance of the philosophical 'mind-body problem' for the status of psychosomatic medicine: A conceptual analysis of the biopsychosocial model," *Medicine Health Care and Philosophy* 17 (2014): 201–213; Lukas van Oudenhove, and Stefan Cuypers, "The philosophical 'mind-body problem: And its relevance for the relationship between psychiatry and the neurosciences," *Perspectives in Biology and Medicine* 53, no. 4 (2010): 545–557.

73 Eben Alexander, *Proof of heaven. A neurosurgeon's journey into the afterlife* (New York: Simon & Schuster, 2012).

74 Pim van Lommel, Ruud van Wees, Vincent Meyers, and Ingrid Elfferich, "Near-death experience in survivors of cardiac arrest: A prospective study in the Netherlands," *The Lancet* 358 (2001): 2039–2045; Sam Parnia, and Peter Fenwick, "Near death experiences in cardiac arrest: Visions of a dying brain or visions of a new science of consciousness," *Resuscitation* 52 (2002): 5–11; Pim van Lommel, *Consciousness beyond life. The science of the near-death experience* (New York: HarperCollins, 2010).

75 Russell Disivestro, "The ghost in the machine is the elephant in the room: Souls, death, and harm at the end of life," *Journal of Medicine and Philosophy* 57 (2012): 480–502.
76 Jan Claassen, Kevin Doyle, Adu Matory, Caroline Couch, et al. "Detection of brain activation in unresponsive patients with acute brain injury," *New England Journal of Medicine* 380, no. 26 (2019): 2497–2505.
77 Joseph T. Giacino, Douglas I. Katz, Nicholas D. Schiff, John Whyte, et al. "Practice guideline update recommendations summary: Disorders of consciousness," *Neurology* 91, no. 10 (2018): 450–460; Joseph J. Fins, and James L. Bernat, "Ethical, palliative, and policy considerations in disorders of consciousness," *Neurology* 91, no. 10 (2018): 471–475.
78 James A. Marcum, "Reflections on humanizing biomedicine," *Perspectives in Biology and Medicine* 51, no. 3 (2008): 392–405.
79 Ralph Fevre, *Individualism and inequality. The future of work and politics* (Cheltenham and Northampton: Edward Elgar Publishing, 2017).
80 Rand, *The virtue of selfishness*; Robert Villegas, *Individualism* (Self-published, USA, 2015), 16, 53.
81 Ralph Schroeder, "'Personality' and 'inner distance': The conception of the individual in Max Weber's sociology," *History of the Human Sciences* 4, no. 1 (1991): 61–78.
82 Max Weber, *The Protestant ethics and the 'spirit' of capitalism and other writings* (New York: Penguins Books, 2002).
83 Louis Dumont, *Essays on individualism. Modern ideology in anthropological perspective* (Chicago and London: The University of Chicago Press, 1992).
84 "Secularism is Christianity's gift to the world . . ." The crux of secularism is "It is that belief in an underlying or moral equality of humans implies that there is a sphere in which each should be free to make his or her own decisions, a sphere of conscience and free action." Larry Siedentop, *Inventing the individual. The origins of Western liberalism* (Cambridge: The Belknap Press of Harvard University Press, 2014), 360, 361.
85 Siedentop, *Inventing the individual*, 225 ff. See also: Dumont, *Essays on individualism*, 23 ff.
86 Siedentop, *Inventing the individual*, 347.
87 Renée C. Fox, *The sociology of medicine: A participant observer's view* (Englewood Cliffs: Prentice Hall, 1989).
88 Michael Sandel, *Public philosophy. Essays on morality in politics* (Cambridge and London: Harvard University Press, 2005), 153.
89 Peter Callero, *The myth of individualism. How social forces shape our lives* (Lanham, Boulder, New York and London: Rowman & Littlefield, 2018).
90 Henk ten Have, *Vulnerability. Challenging bioethics* (London and New York: Routledge, 2016).
91 Jasanoff: *Can science make sense of life?*
92 Dirk Lanzerath, and Minou Friele, eds. *Concepts and values in biodiversity* (London and New York: Routledge, 2014), 6.
93 Henk ten Have, *Wounded Planet. How declining biodiversity endangers health and how bioethics can help* (Baltimore: Johns Hopkins University Press, 2019).
94 Conceição Soares, "The philosophy of individualism: A critical perspective," *International Journal of Philosophy & Social Values* 1, no. 1 (2018): 11–34; Nancy O. Miles, "The individual in the individualism/communitarianism debate: In defense of personism," *Legon Journal of the Humanities* 29, no. 2 (2018): 241–263.

95 Michael Sandel, *Liberalism and the limits of justice* (Cambridge: Cambridge University Press, 1982); Alasdair MacIntyre, *After virtue. As study in moral theory* (Notre Dame: University of Notre Dame Press, 1984).

96 Leonard Tumaini Chuwa, *African indigenous ethics in global bioethics. Interpreting Ubundu* (New York: Springer, 2014); Nico Nortjé, Willem A. Hoffmann, and Jo-Celene De Jongh, eds., *African perspectives on ethics for healthcare professionals* (New York: Springer, 2018).

97 Myles, "The individual in the individualism/communitarianism debate," 243.

98 Thomas D. Williams, and Jan Olof Bengtsson, "Personalism", in *The Stanford Encyclopedia of Philosophy*, ed. Edward N. Zalta (Winter 2018); https://plato.stanford.edu/archives/fall2018/entries/naturalism-moral; Paul Ricoeur, "Approaching the human person," *Ethical Perspectives* 6, no. 1 (1999): 45–54; Roland Breeur, "Individualism and personalism," *Ethical Perspectives* 6, no. 1 (1999): 67–81; Emmanuel Mounier, *Le personalisme* (Paris: Presses Universitaires de France, 1949); John H. Lavely, "What is personalism," *The Personalist Forum* 7, no. 2 (1991): 1–33.

99 Daniel Callahan, "Individual good and common good: A communitarian approach to bioethics," *Perspectives in Biology and Medicine* 46, no. 4 (2003): 496–507.

100 Paul Schotsmans, "Personalism in medical ethics," *Ethical Perspectives* 6, no. 1 (1999): 10–20.

101 Catriona Mackenzie, and Natalie Stoljar, eds., *Relational autonomy. Feminist perspectives on autonomy, agency, and the social self* (New York and Oxford: Oxford University Press, 2000); Edward S. Dove, Susan E. Kelly, Federica Lucivero, Mavis Machirori, Sandi Dheensa, and Barbara Prainsack, "Beyond individualism: Is there a place for relational autonomy in clinical practice and research?" *Clinical Ethics* 12, no. 3 (2017): 150–165; Jennifer K. Walter, and Lainie Friedman Ross, "Relational autonomy: Moving beyond the limits of isolated individualism," *Pediatrics* 133 (2014): S16–S23; Janet Delgado, "Re-thinking relational autonomy: Challenging the triumph of autonomy through vulnerability," *Bioethics Update* 5 (2019): 50–65. See also: Bruce Jennings, "Reconceptualizing autonomy: A relational turn in bioethics," *Hastings Center Report* 46, no. 3 (2016): 11–16.

102 The mission statement of the Precision Medicine Initiative, launched by President Obama in 2015 is: "To enable a new era of medicine through research, technology, and policies that empower patients, researchers, and providers to work together toward development of individualized care." See: https://obamawhitehouse.archives.gov/precision-medicine.

103 Leo Tolstoy, *The death of Ivan Ilyich*, chapter IV; www.classicallibrary.org/tolstoy/ivan/index.htm.

104 Jodi Halpern, *From detached concern to empathy. Humanizing medical practice* (Oxford and New York: Oxford University Press, 2010).

105 Carolyn Ells, Matthew Hunt, and Jane Chambers-Evans, "Relational autonomy as an essential component of patient-centered care," *International Journal of Feminist Approaches to Bioethics* 4, no. 2 (2011): 79–101.

106 George L. Engel, "The need for a new medical model: A challenge for biomedicine," *Science* 196, no. 4286 (1977): 134.

107 Editorial, "Physician burnout: A global crisis," *The Lancet* 394, no. 10193 (2019): 93.

108 Mohammadreza Hojat, Salvatore Mangione, Thomas J. Nasca, Susan Rattner, James B. Erdmann, Joseph S. Gonnella, and Mike Magee, "An empirical study of decline in empathy in medical school," *Medical Education* 38 (2004): 934–941; Bruce W. Newton, Laurie Barber, James Clardy, Elton Cleveland, and Patricia

O'Sullivan, "Is there a hardening of the heart during medical school?" *Academic Medicine* 83, no. 3 (2008): 244–249; Melanie Neumann, Friedrich Edelhäuser, Diethard Tauschel, Martin R. Fischer, Markus Wirtz, Christiane Woopen, Aviad Haramati, and Christian Scheffer, "Empathy decline and its reasons: A systematic review of studies with medical students and residents," *Academic Medicine* 86, no. 8 (2011): 996–1009.

109 Hojat, et al., "An empirical study of decline of empathy in medical school," 938.

110 John Spencer, "Decline in empathy in medical education: How can we stop the rot?" *Medical Education* 38 (2004): 916–918.

111 Saras Henderson, and Alan Petersen, eds., *Consuming health. The commodification of health care* (London and New York: Routledge, 2002); Alex Mold, "Repositioning the patient: Patient organizations, consumerism, and autonomy in Britain during the 1960s and 1970s," *Bulleting of the History of Medicine* 87 (2013): 225–249; Nancy Tomes, *Remaking the American patient. How Madison Avenue and modern medicine turned patients into consumers* (Chapel Hill: The University of North Carolina Press, 2016).

112 Samantha Adams, and Antoinette de Bont, "Information Rx: Prescribing good consumerism and responsible citizenship," *Health Care Analysis* 15 (2007): 273–290; Nancy S. Lee, "Framing choice: The origins and impact of consumer rhetoric in US health care debates," *Social Science & Medicine* 138 (2015): 136–143.

113 Charles L. Briggs, and Daniel C. Hallin, "Biocommunicability. The neoliberal subject and its contradictions in news coverage of health issues," *Social Text* 25, no. 4 (2007): 43–66.

114 Carl E. Schneider, and Mark A. Hall, "The patient life: Can consumers direct health care?" *American Journal of Law & Medicine* 35, no. 1 (2009): 7–65.

115 Lars Nordgren, "Mostly empty words – what the discourse of 'choice' in health care does," *Journal of Health Organization and Management* 24, no. 2 (2010): 109–126.

116 Margo J. Trappenburg, "Active solidarity and its discontents," *Health Care Analysis* 23 (2015): 207–220.

117 Schneider, and Hall, "The patient life," 41.

118 Robin Downie, "Patient and consumers," *Journal of the Royal College of Physicians of Edinburgh* 47 (2017): 261–265; David J. Hunter, "The case against choice and competition," *Health Economics, Policy and Law* 4 (2009): 489–501.

119 See, for example, Hunter, "The case against choice and competition," 489–501; Maria Goddard, "Competition in healthcare: Good, bad or ugly?" *International Journal of Health Policy and Management* 4, no. 9 (2015): 567–569.

120 Mahmoud Keyvanara, Saeed Karimi, Elahe Khorasani, and Marzie Jarfarina Jazi, "Experts' perceptions of the concept of induced demand in healthcare: A qualitative study in Isfahan, Iran," *Journal of Education & Health Promotion* 3, no. 27 (2014).

121 Robert A. Kearns, and J. Ross Barnett, "Consumerist ideology and the symbolic landscapes of private medicine," *Health & Place* 3, no. 3 (1997): 171–180.

122 Zygmunt Bauman, *Wasted lives: Moderity and its outcasts* (Cambridge, UK: Polity Press, 2004).

123 Isabell Lorey, *Die Regierung der Prekären* (Berlin: Turia + Kant, 2012).

124 Ludwig von Mises, *Human action: A treatise on economics* (Auburn: Ludwig von Mises Institute, 1998; original 1949), 720.

125 Von Mises, *Human action*, 297.

126 Elizabeth Anderson, *Value in ethics and economics* (Cambridge and London; Harvard University Press, 1993); Jonathan Baron, and Sarah Leshner, "How serious are

expressions of protected values?" *Journal of Experimental Psychology* 6, no. 3 (2000): 183–194.

127 Roth, "Repugnance as a constraint on markets," 37–58.

128 Rachel Yarmolinsky, "Ethics for ethicists? The professionalization of clinical ethics consultation," AMA *Journal of Ethics* 18, no. 5 (2016): 509.

129 Bill Plotkin, *Nature and the human soul. Cultivating wholeness and community on a fragmented world* (Novato, CA: New World Library, 2008); Phil Cousineau, ed., *Soul. An archaeology* (New York: HarperCollins Publishers, 1995). See also: Ten Have, *Wounded Planet*, 223 ff.

# 5 Moral imagination

The French poet Charles Baudelaire called human imagination the "queen of the faculties." It is imagination that has created the world. [1] Human beings are characterized by imagination. The previous chapter has discussed certain powerful images that influence how we usually view science and healthcare. They also present a common way to consider and interpret ourselves, our relations to other people, and society. Furthermore, they are associated with particular values and virtues that prearrange the normative issues that are deemed relevant and cogent.

This chapter will discuss the role of moral imagination as faculty of the soul in bioethics. We will elaborate the suggestion of Solomon Benatar that especially in the current global context of bioethics, greater moral imagination is needed to alter our outlook and actions. [2] Global health is in a deplorable state, whereas there are significant scientific and technological advances, economic growth in many countries, and substantial philanthropic aid. At the same time, the benefits of global progress are not equally distributed, with increasing disparities, exploitation, corruption, and poor governance. The major challenge for global health, according to Benatar, is lack of moral imagination. Innovative approaches are necessary on the basis of an expanded and creative imagination. A growing number of bioethicists today argue that bioethics should rethink its agenda. It should change its focus on topics arising in wealthy countries and address common global issues. Bioethics should develop into a critical discipline that examines the social, economic, and political processes that determine bioethical problems. It is too distanced from the values of ordinary people and too far from the social contexts in which problems arise. The current environment of injustice and inequality frequently denies the fruits of science and medicine to many people. [3] But what could be a different approach in bioethics? How to envision an ethical discourse that takes into account the soul?

Imagination is regarded as an antidote to analytical and abstract theories. It offers the possibility for an authentic sense of life. It recognizes that human existence is complex and irreducible, generating a sense of wonder and appreciation for the diversity of experiences and for the transcendent nature of the world. This gives imagination a subversive character; it brings us beyond the usual framing, viewing, and structuring of experiences.

The first part of this chapter will explain that imaginary visions are not just rhetorical devices. Imagery is expressed in images, but also through metaphors. Many metaphors today are mechanistic: the organism is conceived as a machine, and genes as building blocks. Metaphors do not provide explanations but furnish ways of thinking, give structure to ideas. The concept of solidarity, for example, may broaden the moral imagination of bioethics by shaping sensibility to go beyond particular acts and individual agents. [4] Another example is the notion of vulnerability. Rather than imagining vulnerable people as victims, or as weak and miserable, they can be imagined as dignified persons, as human beings with potentials since they struggle to overcome negative forces and circumstances. Imaginary visions can reflect negative as well as positive experiences: deception and trust, horror and fascination, hope and despair, disgust and admiration, and compassion and self-interest. Mary Midgley pointed out that imaginative visions of how the world is "are the necessary background of all our living. They are likely to be much more important to us, much more influential than our factual knowledge." [5] There is a close relation between how we think and how we live. We should be looking at life as a whole, and thus considering different perspectives. She argues that there are always multiple perspectives available. For example, there are two aspects of human health: the physical aspect appropriate for medicine and science, and the imaginative or sympathetic social aspect, reflecting the point of view of the patient and the subject. Philosophy suggests new ways of thinking that call for alternative ways of living.

Subsequent paragraphs will explore why imagination has played a minor role in the history of philosophy and ethics. It has often been opposed to reason and rationality, disturbing the objectivity of knowledge with the subjectivity of feeling and fantasy. The focus of the chapter will then move explicitly to moral imagination. It is regarded as a resource for ethics because it has two capabilities that are important for ethical deliberation: it allows experiencing the situation of others, and it identifies possibilities for action. In this perspective, it is interesting to take note of the contribution from neurosciences about the meaning and role of mirror neurons, the neurons that fires both when somebody acts and when somebody observes the same action performed by another. [6] The next section will discuss how these capabilities will enable the transition from normative discourse into practical changes. It will be followed by an examination of the relationship between bioethics and civilization. Moral imagination can mobilize a variety of fundamental notions such as dignity, vulnerability, respect, and recognition that can reshape and restructure human experiences beyond the usual bioethical principles of autonomy, beneficence, and non-maleficence. It may question the dominant images of naturalism, scientism, and neoliberalism. This implies challenging the standards of appropriate behavior that govern current civilization.

The last section of this chapter will argue that moral imagination is especially critical now that bioethics is transforming into a global endeavor. Growing inequality and vulnerability, environmental degradation, and several forms of injustice have made it necessary to develop a broad approach in bioethics to address these issues. Moral imagination may help overcome experiences of disrespect, injustice, and humiliation.

## Images and imaginary visions

The most common symbol of medicine is the rod of Asclepius, a snake around a staff. Many national medical organizations have chosen this image. The logo of the World Health Organization projects a staff with a snake on a picture of the globe. In the Netherlands, doctors used to put a sticker with this image on the front window of their car, hoping that they would not receive a parking ticket if they visited a patient. It is curious that this well-known international symbol of medicine used today refers to the ancient cult of Asklepios, the god of medicine and healing, and to serpents. The snake has been a symbol for healing, rebirth, and renewal since early history. It is even more remarkable that, in fact, two different symbols are in circulation. In the United States, the caduceus is used: two snakes winding around a winged staff. It refers to the Greek god Hermes, and was used by the Army Medical Corps since the 19th century. But it is based on erroneous historical research. The rod of Asclepius has more authentic claims since this god was always imagined with a staff with a single serpent. [7] This symbol also has a wider scope. The caduceus is mostly used by commercial organizations. Hermes was the Greek god of commerce and trade.

Other images of medicine are the white coat and the stethoscope. Both are modern images, presenting medicine as a science. All images express status, prestige, and authority. The white coat was initially adopted in surgery and in the laboratory around the middle of the 19th century. Physicians presented themselves as scientists with this dress. The coat conveys the idea of purity, hygiene, and cleanliness. The color white refers to life and hope in distinction to black that is associated with death and mourning. White also implies power and authority. It shows the seriousness and professionalism of the healthcare provider. Around the same time, medical care shifted from home to hospital, and in this institutional setting clothing changed. Physicians needed to access the patient's body. By leaving behind their everyday clothing, they manifested a distance with day-to-day experiences, so that physical examinations became less threatening for patients. The white coat therefore is an instrument of detachment; it signifies that the doctor is an active scientist and the patient passive material. [8] The stethoscope reflecting scientific methodology, and especially the need for careful observation in medical practice, has the same purpose of creating some distance from the patient's body.

Bioethics does not have one representative image. There is a wealth of images and logos but not one significant symbol that characterizes the discipline. Imagery often refers to the cloud concept. It shows networked elements, connecting multiple components in different locations, and highlighting flexibility and coherence. The term "cloud" is used as metaphor for the internet. An example is the logo of the ASBH. It is a square with two blue rectangles on the right and two black boxes on the left (in the form of a D). It resembles the Microsoft logo: a red, green, yellow, and blue box within one square box. The cloud concept underlines the complexity and interdisciplinarity of bioethics emphasizing the need to share resources and expertise. Another frequent imagery of bioethics presents scientific images: test tubes, microscopes, pipettes, cell structures, and the double helix. Legal images can also be found, such as a balance and a gavel. Finally, clinical images such as a stethoscope as well as doctors in white coats are used. It is remarkable that there are almost no images referring to patients or to interaction and communication with people who need care or treatment.

### *Images*

Although images are often visual, they can evoke other sensory qualities. A sound or melody can recall certain memories or arouse particular feelings. Beethoven's Ode to Joy may give rise to imagery of unity (as the Anthem of Europe) or freedom (used during protests in Chile and China, for instance). Sounds can be transformed into visual images (e.g. musical notation) but then they are no longer auditory images. Tasting food is also associated with imagery. Gustatory images are important for cooking food and testing culinary recipes. Taste also provokes memories. Eating satay reminds one of us of a visit to Indonesia, and brings back memories of the first time he met the parents of his wife. Tastes are associated with feelings and emotions. For example, a bitter taste is unpleasant. Bitterness has become a metaphor for pain, grief, anger, and resentment. Imagery therefore is a device that appeals to our senses. Images do not need to be visual. They are often used in fiction and poetry to make a text more vivid. In philosophy, images are employed to illustrate or clarify particular arguments. A famous example is the image of the cave used by Plato in his treatise *Republic*. A powerful image is presented by Hobbes in his *Leviathan*: in the natural state before social institutions, human life was solitary, short, nasty, and poor. Rousseau presented the opposite image of the noble savage.

Generally, philosophers have distrusted the imagination. [9] The images produced can be illusions, delusions, fantasies, and hallucinations, taking them for reality. Plato condemned imagining as an inferior mental activity. For him, it is opposed to reason. But this point of view is not shared by all philosophers. For Kant, the imagination is an indispensable function of the soul without which we cannot have any knowledge. [10] Imagination is primarily a mental act. Images are mental representations. Mary Warnock defines imagination as "that which creates mental images." [11] It means thinking about objects in their absence, separating the image from that of which it is the image. Imagination is easily accessible. We can imagine whatever we wish. Another characteristic is that it is almost always successfully executed. [12] Like other mental phenomena, imagining is an intentional act. A mental image is *about* or *of* something. The problem is the ontological status of imagined objects. What is the relation between the images (ideas) in our head and things that are in the outside world?

The possible false, seductive, and delusionary character of images has been the occasion for historical struggles and attacks on images. [13] The Protestant Reformation engaged in destruction of religious images and statutes because they were regarded as idolatry. Earlier, Orthodox theology rejected images. This led to a movement of iconoclasm since the 8th century in the Byzantine empire. [14] Destruction of sacred images was justified because the divine cannot be presented in material images. Defenders of icons argued that images express expectation, hope, and desire. They do not refer to persons as they are but as they shall be. Images present a "transfigured self." This is clear in the artistic rules governing the icon. The face should directly be turned to the viewer. This frontality gives the image a dialogical and relational direction. Depicting the face in profile means fragmentation in breaking communion with the viewer and makes the person absent. The eyes of the icon, as windows of the soul, should be enlarged, representing wisdom, awareness, and spiritual insight. The icon is the image of someone. The relationship with that person is enhanced, as Constas shows, by using an inverted perspective, eliminating spatial depth, and moving the image to the viewer. [15] Through this constriction of space, the world is experienced as a world of persons sharing relations, and not as a world of things that is viewed by an observer that is distanced from the image as an object observed.

The connection between images and reality is particularly relevant in the context of art. [16] Arguably, Dutch painting in the 17th century is characterized by detailed realism. It presents everyday life scenes, ordinary people and narratives of landscapes and domestic interiors. This art reflects the time in which it is painted. The realism expresses the power of the new urban middle class, Protestant ethics, and the recent acquired freedom and growing prosperity of the Low Countries. Paintings were assumed to mirror the richness of everyday existence. One of the greatest painters was Johannes Vermeer (1632–1675). He is relatively unknown (called "the Sphinx of Delft") and his output was low (only between 33 and 35 paintings are recognized as authentic). He is renowned because of his sensibility, painting things and especially ordinary persons (mostly women) as they are in real life. He is primarily known for painting the domestic world of people playing instruments, writing letters, and receiving visitors.

Nowadays, it is pointed out that the scenes he painted were careful compositions, painstakingly arranged and rearranged. [17] He did not make portraits but painted ideal types of people, picturing everyday bourgeois life, not as it was but as symbolic for another, invisible world. He most probably used a camera obscura to intensify the play of lights and shadows, as well as the brilliant colors for which he became famous. For Vermeer, the picture is not a representation but rather an allegory, using moralistic emblems and symbols. For example, his painting *The Milkmaid* shows a footwarmer and a tile of Cupid, traditionally used as symbols for female sexuality. But Vermeer gives a sense of dignity to the woman, who is probably making bread pudding and thus involved in careful cooking. He depicts honest and hard work as a domestic virtue. [18]

## *Imagination*

Paul Ricoeur has distinguished among different uses of the term imagination. [19] First is the evocation of things that are absent and exist elsewhere. Second, imagination refers to portraits, paintings, drawings, and statutes, images that have physical existence but represent persons or things. Third, imagination refers to fictions, non-existing things, and not merely absent things, for example dreams and literary narratives. Lastly, it refers to the domain of illusion. Images can be representations of absent or non-existing things but people believe in the reality of their object; these images have pseudo-presence. Images therefore are variable according to the presence or absence of their object. For Hume, the object is there but the image is a trace or lesser presence of it; imagination is reproductive (or associative). For Sartre, the object of the image is absent; the image is other-than-present, and imagination is productive (or creative). In this view, there is a radical difference between perceiving and imagining. Ricoeur argues that the attitude of the subject is also important. The subject can be fascinated by images, and lack critical awareness, thus taking the image for real. The subject can also have critical distance, and be critically aware of the difference between the imaginary and the real. This last position is taken by Husserl who considers imagination as a critique of reality.

Husserl is usually credited as the philosopher who has recovered the imagination. He rejects the idea that imagination is simply making copies of sense experiences. It is not "secondhand recreation of perception" but, on the contrary, free and creative intentionality. [20] It takes us beyond the limitations of empirical experiences. In phenomenology, the importance of the image is its direction toward an object. It is "a *way of thinking* of something." [21] Imagination therefore has a close connection to interpretation. "Imagination is our means of interpreting the world" as Warnock emphasizes. [22] It is the ability to detach ourselves from our actual situation.

### *Metaphors*

Imagination is shaped by metaphors. When images are mental pictures, they are private. They can only be described in a public language that we have to learn. We have to find the words to express what they are and mean. By means of words, we are likening one thing to another. If the human body is imagined as a mechanism, the primary subject (body) is likened or compared to a secondary subject (mechanism). A metaphor is the understanding and experiencing of one kind of things in terms of another. Metaphors are pervasive in everyday life. [23] Especially conceptual systems have a metaphorical structure. Basic cultural values are coherent with this structure. Metaphors are helping to comprehend and make sense of phenomena in the world and to conceptualize human experiences. They also facilitate communication in objective terms. The mechanism metaphor helps us to understand the human body as an efficient and operative apparatus that can be repaired and reconstructed. It is a mistake to regard metaphors as merely a matter of language, as if reality is completely external to human beings and composed of distinct objects (which is the view of naturalism). On the contrary, metaphors are the human way to conceptualize the world and to shape experiences.

It should be noted, however, that not all metaphors are beneficial. As pointed out in the previous chapter, regarding the human body as mechanism has particular consequences for disregarding the subjective experiences of patients. Another example are military metaphors that are often used in cancer. Patients are attacked by aggressive cells that invade their body systems; they have to fight and use new magic bullets in order to survive. Recent studies have found out that such metaphors are, in fact, not beneficial. They make treatment more difficult and make patients more fatalistic about the disease. [24]

Lakoff and Johnson distinguish conventional metaphors from imaginative ones. These last metaphors provide a new understanding of our experiences; they are creative, highlighting some dimensions and hiding others. [25] They constitute new realities, and thus guide future actions. Metaphors, however, are linked not only to imagination but also to reason. Our feelings, experiences, and moral practices that are presented in images are at the same time categorized and assessed on what they entail for practical use. Metaphor is thus called "imaginative rationality." [26] It communicates experiences, produces mutual understanding, and gives us the ability to modify our world views.

### *Narratives*

Imagination is connected to narratives. Images of *homo economicus* and lone ranger assume that the individual person develops and decides independent from its context. But, in fact, the self as a moral agent is historically situated and socially constituted. Ricoeur has suggested that this context of moral agency has a narrative structure. He argues that the focus should be on language rather than perception. Imagination is semantic innovation. In his view, humans are storytelling beings. [27] They interpret themselves and their actions in a narrative that provides meaning to who they are and what they do. This is a continual process of reinterpretation and revision. Narratives give coherence to our experiences; they overcome the fragmentation of social life; they synthesize them so that our actions over time become more understandable and our life makes sense. [28] The possibility of such coherent experience is provided by imaginative activity. Narrative unity is the result of imagination. A sequence of disconnected and discrete events is configured into a meaningful whole through images of purposes, motives, and goals. They turn physical events and bodily movements into human action. The emphasis on the role of narratives provides an alternative to the abstract nature of traditional ethics. It places the focus of ethics on transforming persons, assuming that moral actions do not flow from principles but from stories enlightened by the imagination. [29]

## Imagination and philosophy

In philosophy and ethics, imagination is often distrusted and neglected. In the naturalistic perspective, images as mental representations are associated with or reduced to brain states. Philosophers such as Gilbert Ryle have argued that there are no such things as images. To imagine things is to fancy or suppose that one sees or hears them. An imagined sound is not a sound at all. Ryle concludes: there is no faculty of imagination. Imagining is a special case of pretending. [30] Mary Warnock has demonstrated that this is a counterfactual position: people do, in fact, have images. Imagination is not merely reflection or creation; it is a mixture of both active creativeness and passive representation of what is given. [31] The representational view of imagination is one-sided. For Hume, we cannot imagine anything if there is not an accompanying image. He furthermore believes that images (ideas) are the product of experiences (impressions). We can only imagine things that we have experienced previously. Someone who is blind cannot imagine the color blue. Imagining is a form of perceiving but less lively and intense than sensations. The difference between ideas and impressions, in Hume's view, is vividness. However, imagining is not necessarily to have a mental picture, although the focus of discussion is usually on mental imagery. "Imagine what will be the effect when you take prednisone" does not require a mental image. Imagining here is equivalent to supposing or thinking. [32] Richard Kearny has argued that the image-making power of human beings has undergone three paradigm shifts in the history of philosophy. [33] First, the mimetic paradigm regards imagination as representational faculty, reproducing preexisting reality. Its dominant metaphor is that of the mirror. This paradigm was dominant in premodern times but continues to be influential until now. Second is the productive paradigm of modernity, regarding imagination as a creative faculty, producing new images. Its metaphor is the lamp or light. Postmodern philosophy has promoted the third, parodic paradigm with its metaphor of labyrinth or looking glass. It argues that reality cannot be separated from images; the original is replaced by its imitation. For postmodern people, fantasy is more real than reality.

A philosophy of imagination is advanced by French philosopher Gaston Bachelard (1884–1962). He celebrated imagination as a creative faculty of the mind. It is a force of transcendence, allowing human beings to surpass and escape reality as given. "Imagination is not, as its etymology would suggest, the faculty of forming images of reality; it is rather the faculty of forming images that go beyond reality, which *sing* reality." [34] Imagination therefore opens our eyes to new types of vision. Imagining is more important than the images themselves since it is active; it changes images, forming and deforming them. This is why Bachelard calls imagination "spiritual mobility"; it renews the heart and the soul. [35]

As an epistemologist and historian of science, Bachelard was working in two different domains, the scientific and the poetic one. His aim was to bring together science, philosophy, and literature, and to reconcile the search for truth with the quest for meaning. He first regarded imagination as an epistemological obstacle to the advancement of science. Striving for rationality, objectivity, and abstraction, scientific investigation must overcome imaginative seduction. Science needs to break with life-world experiences. In this sense, science is iconoclastic. But Bachelard came to re-evaluate the role of imagination. It is also a positive force. It structures and synthesizes human experiences. In scientific discourse, images are not eradicable; they are there unsaid and unseen but still effective. In geography, the image of mother Earth is pervasive and typical, and in biology, the image of monster, and in chemistry, the image of explosion. What is repressed is frequently returning in scientific theories and research. Imagination is the prior structure that organizes observations and gives meaning to them. Images are not mere obstacles but may lead to better understanding. Imagination therefore is not negative but complementary to scientific rationality, no longer a disease of scientific thinking but a potential therapy.

Bachelard argues that the imagination is arranged around the archetypes of air, water, earth, and fire. These are the "hormones of imagination." [36] For example, earth is associated with images of solidity, resistance, courage, and permanence, while fire relates to verticality, transcendence, illumination, and eternity. An important difference for Bachelard is that between dreams and reveries. Dreams appear during sleep, without consciousness. Reveries are creative daydreams; they are a relaxed and semiconscious state in which images are perceived. They relive memories in active imagination. As a kind of meditation, they have an element of choice and freedom, contrary to dreams. Reveries as the source of imagination illustrate that imagining is a spiritual force. Imagination, furthermore, has ethical implications. Since we are willing a new world in our reveries, we also have a moral responsibility for the world that we are imagining. Thus, mental activity has two poles: the daylight one of rationality, and the nocturnal one of the soul.

In view of this polarity, Bachelard is often charged with a double anthropology. He opposes diurnal man who is rational and nocturnal man who is daydreaming, a rational philosophy of science and an imaginative philosophy of reverie. But his work is basically a reflection on human knowledge and creativity. [37] He gives primacy to human creativity. Fundamentally, there is no opposition between science and poetry but imagination is the underlying dynamism of the human mind for both domains. Images are the origins of a new consciousness and not its products. [38] For Bachelard, the contemporary soul suffers from a deficiency of imagination. We need places to dream. "The imagination, more than reason, is the unifying force of the human soul." [39] It is important to develop a "phenomenology of the soul." [40]

## Imagination and ethics

In moral reasoning, the role of imagination usually is limited, if acknowledged at all. It is regarded as subjective and non-rational. Ethics is a matter of reason. It proceeds from rules and principles that have a rational basis, and that provide arguments for moral judgments and actions. Ethics also articulates impartiality and universality: rational deliberation resulting in choices and decisions that can be justified. However, this view of moral agency is too narrow. There is a preceding phase of moral perception in which situations are perceived as morally significant and relevant. [41] Ethical discourse recognizes that a gap exists between particular situations and moral rules and principles, which is bridged by moral judgment. But it does not take into account that before a moral judgment is delivered, moral perception is needed. An example is a full and packed tram; no seating places are left. A person seated notices the discomfort of an elderly person standing. Perceiving the discomfort, he acts in relinquishing his seat. The situation is seen in a particular way, and the person feels moved to deliberate. Prior to deliberation is perception. Required is moral sensibility before a moral judgment can be made and rules and principles can be applied. Such sensibility emerges from understanding the particularity of the situation but also from recognizing particular moral features such as discomfort, distress, and compassion. If someone is not sensitive to the moral features of situations, he may not perceive them. Recognizing the significance of situations as morally relevant calls for moral perception of injustice, distress, dishonesty, and indignity. Such perception is promoted by the imagination, expanding our sympathies and imaging ourselves in the situation of other people. Before moral actions are taken, there are, what Blum calls, "nonactional responses," elicited by the imagination and invoking emotions. [42]

A broader view of moral agency is elaborated by Johnson on the basis of the significance of metaphors in ethics. [43] He argues that all aspects of morality are imaginative: fundamental moral concepts, understanding of situations, and reasoning about these situations. They all have a metaphorical structure. Metaphors define moral concepts and determine how morally problematic situations are understood. The significance of metaphors is difficult to comprehend when ethics conceives of the self as an individual, rational, and ahistorical actor. Metaphors, however, as argued earlier, are embedded in conceptual structures and cultural values. Viewing human beings as socially, culturally, and historically constituted beings provides a better understanding of the role of metaphors and thus of imagination. The roles of perception and imagination ask for a revised interpretation of imagination, beyond the historical paradigms identified by Kearney. This will focus on the ethical dimension of imagination.

## Moral imagination

What exactly makes imagination a resource for ethics? Imagination presents different ways of "seeing" and interpreting the world. This is the lesson of Husserl: imagination brings us beyond the limitations of empirical experience. It generates different framings of situations. What makes it moral are two capabilities. First, imagination enlarges our horizon and expand our sympathies. It is the ability to empathize with others. It helps us to recognize situations that demand moral action. The ability to place ourselves in the shoes of other people in very different circumstances is what make the imagination a moral resource. Through imagination, I imagine myself as the other person. I become aware of values that go beyond the limits of my own experience. Second, imagination provides various possibilities for acting. It envisions possible harm and potential help, and thus how actions may be beneficial or may hurt. This is the shaping power of imagining, projecting possibilities for future change. [44] For this reason, Iris Murdoch has designated imagination as "an exercise of freedom." [45]

An example of the moral power of imagination is the emergence of human rights in the 18th century. [46] These rights were defined as natural (i.e. inherent in human beings), equal, and universal in the American *Declaration of Independence* (1776) and the French *Declaration of the Rights of Man and Citizen* (1789). These declarations were the result of cultural processes where human beings were perceived as separate individuals and free agents with feelings, convictions, and moral judgment. It was recognized that people were equal, sharing similar feelings and sentiments, and the same desire for autonomy. The popularity of novels made readers sympathetic to the fate of others and made them empathize with their condition. This process of imaginative identification, imagining others as equals, created a favorable environment for the articulation of human rights. Accounts of torture and cruel punishment had similar effects. Increasing moral sensibility made them intolerable. Public executions common throughout the 19th century have been abolished at the end of that century in Europe and North America. Imagining how the world can be different from how it is illustrates the potential of fictional narrative.

Accordingly, what makes imagination morally relevant is the capacity of shifting perspectives. It places us in the standpoint of others. It does so by combining ideas that were not expected to be combinable; it tests opposites and searches for comparable cases so that we envision a variety of moral viewpoints. Imagination thus is, in the words of Mills, a certain playfulness of mind. [47] In like manner, Dewey has labeled moral deliberation as "dramatic rehearsal." In the imagination, we try out various competing and possible lines of action. [48] Imagination allows what Charles Peirce has called abduction. This is a way of reasoning that generates and tests hypotheses. It differs from deduction, which is the explanatory phase of reasoning, and from induction, the verification phase of reasoning. Abduction is typical for the context of discovery of knowledge. It involves the play of "musement," associating ideas in a new synthesis. In a state of free speculation, the imagination plays with ideas, like in the reveries of Bachelard. Through abduction, hypotheses are then formulated and tested, connecting imagining to reasoning. [49]

## Capabilities of imagination

Philosopher John Dewey has argued that we all have the capacity to imagine. [50] As the creative ability to make the absent become present, imagination projects ideals and values, offers possibilities for thinking and acting, helps us to bring new realities into existence, and conceives alternatives to problematic situations. It also makes use of past experiences as they suggest alternative possibilities and different ways of seeing the world. Imagination involves taking in the perspectives, feelings, and interests of others. It brings people together as human beings. Like Husserl, Dewey considers imagination as the extension of experience beyond the limited world of everyday life. It is seeing the actual in light of the possible. [51] Imagination is therefore a crucial activity for ethics.

Two capabilities make imagination especially important for ethics. First of all, it provides the capability to empathize with others. Second, moral imagination identifies various possibilities for acting. The first capability is described by Edmund

Husserl, the founder of phenomenology. *Einbildungskraft* is an image-making activity. It brings new realities into existence. His disciple Edith Stein elaborated the role of imagination in our ability to empathize with others. [52] We can imagine ourselves as the other since we recognize what we share, what is essential for all human beings, and what are invariable human goods. Imagination makes us aware of values beyond the limits of our own experience. This characteristic of imagination was further developed by John Dewey. Imagination brings human beings together. It is the extension of experience beyond our limited and familiar realm of everyday life. It fosters sympathy and dialogue because it involves taking the perspective of others. Without imagination, we cannot see situations from the viewpoint of other persons and cannot understand the experiences of others. The capability to recognize the experiences of others is especially important now that bioethics is expanding into global bioethics. Processes of globalization have contributed to an emerging global consciousness. More people than ever regard themselves as citizens of the world, living on a common planet and sharing similar fundamental challenges. Global bioethics is developing on the basis of this idea of common humanity. [53] It is argued that over time, the circle of moral concern has expanded; our moral horizon has enlarged so that the perspectives of other persons have been taken into account. Siep Stuurman, who extensively studied this historical process, concludes that it is the result of cross-cultural encounters and exchanges producing a dialectic between particularism and universalism. [54] The language of common humanity emerged in critical reflection on prevailing notions of otherness and inequality. The urge to adopt a globally inclusive concept of equality mainly came from Asian, African, and Latin American countries. The discourses of otherness and inequality were ceding ground to notions of common humanity. The empathic circle gradually widened, creating a global language of universal equality and respect for human rights and dignity. Moral imagination, in the words of John Kekes, enlarges life: it broadens its possibilities and overcomes obstacles to its realization. [55]

The second capability of moral imagination is its creative power. Dewey describes several roles of the imagination in the process of inquiry. It is conceiving alternatives to problematic situations; it suggests means to reach specific ends; it evaluates these means through considering possible consequences. The imagination does not only enable us to bring to mind future possibilities; it also allows us to make use of past experiences. [56] Social imaginaries, for example, present a conception of the moral order of society. They articulate principles of sociality. How people are living together is expressed in images and stories. This shared understanding of social existence makes common practices possible. [57]

The link between imagination and creativity emphasizes that images are not mere reproductions or recombinations of prior experiences. They are synthesizing, and not merely associating, devices that go beyond the bounds of living in the actual moment, opening up an infinite horizon of possibilities. [58] An example is the confrontation with moral injustices. These are experienced as violations of intuitive notions of justice. They often imply that there is no respect for dignity, integrity, or honor. People are denied social recognition. The normative assumptions of social interaction are violated. In many cases, people will react with anger, outrage, and indignation, particularly through social media. Moral imagination locates the discussion of these ethical issues outside of the usual space of individual autonomy, directing attention to the social, economic, and political conditions in which people live, and focusing on the common good.

Imagination can help medicine and bioethics to have a value-focused logic, which encompasses and goes beyond the technological and organic aspects of health. It is essential to have a relational perspective to focus on the meaning of our life and our responsibilities – important things always at risk of eluding the eyes. In fact, paraphrasing *The Little Prince*, by A. De Saint-Exupery, "the thing that is important is the thing that is not seen." [59]

## Possibilities for change

Bioethics is not a homogeneous discourse. It comprises various discursive practices. It moves from cases and specific situations to more elaborate and abstract arguments. This can be done in multiple ways. Imaginary processes play a role in this movement so that a richer and broader conceptual and analytical apparatus may emerge, giving voice to discourses that are easily silenced. Moral imagination, as a creative faculty of the soul, is not phantasy. It activates value systems that are not dominant and provide alternative styles of thinking that can create other norms and can resist the imposition of current norms. That ideas can be powerful and have the potential to change norms is illustrated in field of "disease diplomacy." States have been redefining their interests and responsibilities in regard to emerging infectious diseases. Now that local outbreaks of diseases quickly develop into global threats, national approaches and the traditional norms of containment (quarantine and border control) are no longer sufficient. The need for collective action, sharing information and transparency to secure global health, has changed the normative behavior of states. A new set of expectations concerning responsibilities of states, a "new package of norms," has been created, based on a greater sense of global solidarity. [60]

Another example is the use of imagination in building peace. [61] Responding to conflict, producing social change, and engineering peace are not just a technique or special form of management but also a creative process. Moral imagination may give birth to something new, to conditions and predicaments that do not yet exist. As "a capacity to perceive things beyond and at a deeper level than what initially meets the eye," it changes the way we see things and can help us to break out of usual patterns and to transcend violence. [62]

These possibilities for change through broader normative discourse problematize the usual stance of bioethics as a rational and objective discourse. Bioethics identifies itself as an academic discipline that is neutral. It assumes that there are clear boundaries between academic analysis and political engagement. Bioethics provides a "detached authority" that overrides the responses of patients, parents, families, and communities that are often emotional and not well-informed, as demonstrated in the cases of Charlie Gard (2017) and Alfie Evans (2018) in the

United Kingdom. Ethical activism, in this view, will compromise the credibility of bioethics. [63] Angus Dawson and colleagues have argued that this neutrality is a myth. They are right. Mainstream bioethics is not a neutral discourse. It endorses the ideologies of neoliberalism and scientism, neglects issues of vulnerability and solidarity, and treats justice predominantly as the distribution of resources. Confronted with human rights violations, for example the inhuman treatment of asylum seekers in Australia and elsewhere, bioethicists should criticize policies that directly harm the most vulnerable people and seriously affect their health. [64]

Moral imagination is a resource that may help overcome moral differences and disagreements. In recognizing what others value, we imagine the world, as Tivnan said, on the other side of the barricade. [65] That may help us to live with disagreements and minimize the clash of values, shaping a decent society with mutual respect. Imagination clarifies the consequences of our actions for ourselves but what makes it moral is that we are at the same time able to imagine the effects of our actions on others. It breaks through denial, inhumanity, and exploitation in formulating alternative worlds and modes of life. [66] Also, in the Christian theological perspective, it is possible to encourage and realize moral imagination, concerning all humankind and focus on more vulnerable people and the perspective of happiness and justice. [67]

## Civilization and decency

Bioethical discourse is crucially related to civilization. Bioethics learns that to understand suffering and medical problems, interpretation of moral experiences is unavoidable. Imagination is important to facilitate interpretation; it generates and produces worldviews, ideals, and values to guide moral perception. Imagination is reshaping and reconstructing our experiences. However, bioethics is important not only for individual patients and healthcare providers. It also is an expression of the values of civilization. It defines how doctors and patients should respect each other, and what is appropriate and responsible behavior in a healthcare setting. It furthermore delineates conduct and interactions in everyday life when there is no disease or disability. Hygiene is an impressive example. It has been a concern for humanity since ancient times. Drainage and toilet structures have been found in many past civilizations. The Roman Empire was known for sanitation and hygiene, manifested in baths, plumbing, and adequate supply of fresh water to towns. At the end of the 18th century, hygiene became part of health routines, as one of the standards of civilization. The germ theory developed by Pasteur and Koch also provided a scientific rationale for hygienic and clean conduct. [68]

Ethics is not just a theoretical discourse that emphasizes principles and rights but it is translated into practical behavior that governs human interaction and communication, often without explicit reflection. It is civilizing the actions and attitudes of present-day citizens. Bioethics is further related to civilization in another way. This becomes apparent when the question is asked why bioethics has emerged some decades ago. Traditional medical ethics has been transformed into a new ethical approach because the concept of life became problematic. Medical technologies and interventions obscured the distinction between life and death. They also extended and enhanced human life, and created possibilities for manipulating and constructing life. These scientific and technological innovations made the concept of "bio" inherently fluid and ambiguous, raising the ethical question of how to deal with them. Bioethics therefore can be regarded as a response to the evolution of civilization, particularly as an attempt to regain or preserve the human character of civilized life.

This evolution is especially visible in Western civilization, as Max Weber has formulated it in his thesis of disenchantment. In his view, rationalization, bureaucratization, and intellectualization are typical phenomena of our times. In healthcare, the effects of this evolution are, above all, visible since the Second World War. Medicine became a powerful technological approach that increasingly dominated the relations between care receivers and care providers. Bioethics discourse was a way to articulate the dissatisfaction with this evolution and to make it more humane, more civilized. Although bioethics itself has evolved and has lost some of its critical power, it can play a significant role in addressing the repercussions of processes of globalization. Moral imagination locates us within the stories of "undesirables," "disposables," and "victims." It interrogates our relationships to other people and how they are affected by scientism and neoliberalism. It questions the rules of civilization and standards of appropriateness. The inhumane treatment of other persons threatens "society's conception of civilized life." [69] Concepts such as respect, recognition, and dignity will then be reconfigured from a moral perspective that primarily applies to individuals into a perspective that is fundamental for society. Human dignity, for example, has motivated the search for shared humanity and therefore human rights. [70] It is the basis for mutual respect in decent societies across the world.

Reading Stephan Zweig's *Die Welt von Gestern* is not simply a reminder of a nostalgic past and a warning how civilization can deteriorate. It is also, and maybe more importantly, a vision of a future that is thoroughly humane. [71] Zweig (1881–1942), facing the death of a European civilization, and living in exile in Brazil, evokes what human dignity is about. He creates an atmosphere of tolerance and world citizenship where people are respected and feel free from bias and narrow-mindedness, where they appreciate individual liberty and spiritual independence, and at same time are connected with others and the community in which they flourish – a time in which the life of the individual and society is not dominated by the military, the political, and the commercial but by the arts, sciences, and humanities. Zweig's book is a dream about the future of Europe, a cosmopolitan vision that gives hope.

Civilization, however, is precarious. Civilizations can decay, decline, and fall. Images of disease are often applied in this context. For example, Anton Chekhov's stories are plagued by disease and untimely death. His focus on disease is symbolic of a larger depraved society. His play *Three Sisters* is less concerned with the outside threat to civilized standards represented by the protagonist Natasha than with the paradoxical nature and vulnerability of civilization to weaknesses within itself. Chekhov's stories criticize lack of goal and vision. The notion of civilization is connected to the idea of progress and human perfectibility. The assumption is that the more civilized people are, the farther they are removed from barbarism. But this connection is far from clear. The more developed a civilization, the better its capacities for making war. The 20th century has been one of the bloodiest eras in human history with hundreds of millions of people killed. Contemporary Western civilization has also created the potential for nuclear catastrophes and international terrorism. [72] The major threat at the moment is climate change and loss of biodiversity. This is clearly related to the lifestyles of current civilization. This threat was the main reason for Van Rensselaer Potter to promote his notion of (global) bioethics. Civilizations may become extinct because they are concerned with short-term decisions, neglecting policies to sustain and preserve future environment. Potter insists that the fundamental question is "what kind of an environment will be most helpful in sustaining and improving the civilized world." [73] Continuing current policies and practices will jeopardize the survival of humanity and thus of the civilized world. To reverse this trend, agreement on a common value system will be necessary, determining obligations to future generations of human beings. This is the reason, Potter argues, that a broader type of bioethics is needed, moving from an individual, to a social, and ultimately to an environmental perspective. [74] Such bioethics may contribute to make civilizations more sustainable.

Civilization is not an individual affair, although it is manifested in individuals. The moral life of individual human beings is intimately linked to that of other beings and nature. Civilization is the fabric of social life, displaying how individuals are interdependent and associated, and how they manage to live together. [75] As Norbert Elias and Lynn Hunter have demonstrated, it reflects a slow and gradual process in which sensitivities of individuals change with increasing self-awareness, more subtle communication, mutual support, and better understanding of the viewpoints of other people. [76] Civilization requires sociopolitical organization and social cooperation but it has an essential ethical dimension. [77] Albert Schweitzer has highlighted this dimension:

> the essential nature of civilization "does not lie in its material achievements, but in the fact that individuals keep in mind the ideals of the perfecting of man, and the improvement of the social and political conditions of peoples, and of mankind as a whole." [78]

In his view, civilization originate when human beings consecrate themselves to the service of life and the world. Civilizations can do this in different ways. Weber described Western civilization as determined by a specific Protestant ethos providing meaning to action. It emphasized labor, controlled wealth, domestic virtues, and material achievements – qualities reflected in the paintings of Vermeer and other Dutch painters of his time. However, Weber also made comparative investigations of the civilizations of China, India, and the ancient Near East. Each civilization is characterized by specific types of rationalism but, even more so, by world views (*Weltbilder*): coherent constellations of values that guide and justify action, and provide it with meaning. [79] These world views set standards to evaluate actions, and establish an ethical framework for policies and practices. These world views again illustrate the power of imagination. *Bild* in the German language is not only image but also picture and metaphor.

The connection between ethics and civilization challenges the distinction between ethics and morality that is commonly made in ethical discourse. Morality is regarded as customs and behaviors that are related to character and conduct. Ethics is located at the level of society and community. Ethics furthermore is regarded as reflection and critical assessment of morality, as a philosophical discipline that is rational and methodical, as systematic reflection on human conduct, while morality is the result of inner conviction, habits, and education. Ethics is theoretical, while morality is practical. In reality, morality and ethics are often used interchangeably. The difference is relative. Individual conduct is frequently determined by the codes of conduct that exists in societies and communities. This morality is described, for example, by anthropologists. Ethics has another scope. It puts emphasis on explaining concepts, developing rational arguments and justifications, and articulating principles and rules. The term "ethics" is derived from the Greek word *ethos*. This word in ancient Greece has two etymological sources: έτος, which means custom and habit, and ηθος, which refers to dwelling place and habitat. The last source of ethics has disappeared over time. Both terms were translated in Latin as *mos* (*mores*), providing a common basis for ethics and morality. The loss of connection between habits and habitats has had implications. Ethics has separated human habits from the places where human beings are living. Ricardo Rossi has argued that this has impeded an ethical approach that connects human beings, culture, and nature. It does not recognize that cultivation of moral behavior and character takes places in a setting where human beings are embedded in an environmental, social, and cultural context. [80]

## Global bioethics

Globalization, as advocated by Potter, is associated with generalization of local threats and challenges as well as with growing vulnerability. It has also encouraged the use of social media that have become an important outlet for moral outrage and anger concerning injustices. One of the major sources of injustice today is environmental degradation. Rather than stimulating theoretical discourse, it has been an inspiration for social movements and global activism in specific areas of health justice, environmental justice, food justice, and water justice. The emphasis in these movements is on violations of rights, disrespect for dignity, denial of recognition, and exclusion from participation. A different and broader concept of bioethics is necessary to face these global challenges – a concept that can be generated and cultivated through moral imagination. Imagining is a creative way of knowing as well as seeing things differently. It recognizes the complexity of human experience. It corrects the analytical and mechanical approach to the world, providing resistance against dehumanizing, objectifying, and commodifying tendencies. Moral imagination helps us to overcome experiences of disrespect and humiliation. It activates experiences of what it is to be humiliated and oppressed. But it also helps us to overcome social pathologies such as an economic order that has led to moral impoverishment of the social life-world, or the process of rationalization that is transforming all phenomena into commodities, that is objects of economic possession. [81] Moral imagination in this perspective is a remedy against moral injuries that are the result of experiences of injustice and that occur because recognition is refused or withdrawn. Particularly because human beings are not primarily autonomous entities, and because human life is intersubjective, they are vulnerable so that moral injuries are possible. But, fortunately, they have the capability of moral imagination.

Every few years, the British Broadcasting Corporation (BBC) undertakes a survey among citizens of 18 countries to explore how they identify themselves. Do they regard themselves as citizens of the world in the first place or as national citizens? Remarkably, in 2016 more than 51% of the world population regarded itself as citizen of the world, up from 45% in 2001. In Nigeria, the proportion is 73%, in China 71%, in Peru 70%, and in India 67%. In emerging economies, the majority of the population identifies itself as citizen of the world. In industrialized nations, the trend is in the other direction. In the United Kingdom and the United States, a minority (40%–45%) defines itself from a global perspective. In Germany, only 30% see themselves as global citizens (down from 60% in 2002). The strongest sense of national citizenship exists in Russia; only 25% of all respondents regard themselves as citizens of the world. [82] Of course, it is not clear what exactly people understand with the notion of "citizen of the world." It can primarily focus on economic issues; there is free trade across borders and people assume they are participating in or benefiting from this trade system; especially people in developing countries can feel that they profit economically, that poverty is declining and the burden of disease diminishing. People can also relate the notion to the awareness that humanity is facing similar problems of climate change and inequality that can only be addressed by common action. Global citizenship, for many, is first of all experienced through social media and communication. One may feel a strong sense of global citizenship through being continuously connected with family, friends, and colleagues, and even total strangers. Finally, global citizenship is experienced every day through mobility. It is easy to travel everywhere without significant obstacles from borders. Foreign countries are not really foreign anymore. Many people are migrating. The other side is that refugees are a growing issue but not necessarily regarded as a problem in an era of globalization. However, the BBC survey reveals complications and changes. Western countries that have initiated the process of globalization, and have most benefitted from this process, are now engaging in activities of de-globalization. Populist movements in several countries blame the process of globalization for many troubles and problems in their countries and regions. Instead of growing cooperation and solidarity, there are an increasing number of self-interested autocratic regimes. Narcissistic leaders denigrate human rights discourse. This is not solely a Western phenomenon, but it is remarkable that the idea that we are all connected as inhabitants of our planet is now more shared by people in developing countries than in at least some parts of the developed world.

The notion of world citizenship is moral imagination at work at the global level. It is the image that human beings transcend local perspectives and it introduces another view of their place and role in the world. Being part of the philosophy of cosmopolitanism, it is not a new image. Basically, it reflects the idea that there is a global moral community. All human beings are members of that community since they share common values and responsibilities. [83] Since Stoic philosophy, it has been acknowledged that human beings are born, and therefore rooted, in a specific place; they are localized in a native community and state. They share a common origin, language, and culture with fellow national citizens. At the same time, they are inhabitants of the same planet; they are situated in a similar space. They share the dignity and equality as members of humanity. As citizen of the world, they can transcend their localization and the boundedness of culture, tradition, community, and history. Being born in a specific place and within a particular culture with its often restrictive and traditional customs, laws and morals can be overcome in cosmopolitan perspective. Cosmopolitanism is the aspiration to live beyond bounded horizons. Human beings are not defined and should not be defined by a particular location, community, culture, or religion. From this perspective, much older than the modern processes of globalization, boundaries have no moral significance; the focus should be on what human beings have in common. Cosmopolitanism expresses therefore the moral ideal of the unity of humanity. There is a universal community that includes the whole of humanity. All human beings therefore have equal moral status.

## Conclusion

The snake as the international image of healing refers to the duality of medicine. Like the animal, healthcare involves death and rejuvenation, sin and redemption, illness and therapy. The previous chapter has illustrated that scientific and economic discourse promulgate specific images that tend to prevail in healthcare and bioethics. These images determine how human beings are perceived and treated as self-interested individuals and consumers. They specifically impact how the human body is regarded and examined as a mechanism. Care providers are imagined as detached and objective observers and researchers. Other images, for example of ageing and disability, are constructed on the basis of this fundamental imagery. They present and set up a specific reality.

This chapter has discussed the significance and role of moral imagination. With the help of philosophers such as Warnock, Johnson, Ricoeur, Dewey, and Bachelard, we have argued that imagination can play a significant role in ethical discourse because it enlarges our moral horizon, making us empathize with other people, and because it provides possibilities for moral action. This role of the imagination will be further specified in the next chapter. Instead of the images and metaphors of the dominating naturalistic and neoliberal ideologies, alternative images may activate and produce different perspectives and world views that rehabilitate and reinsert the soul in bioethical reflection and debate.

## References


1 "C'est l'imagination qui a enseigné à l'homme le sens moral de la couleur, du contour, du son et du parfum. Elle a créé, au commencement du monde, l'analogie et la métaphore. Elle décompose toute la création, et, avec les matériaux amassés et disposés suivant des règles dont on ne peut trouver l'origine que dans le plus profond de l'âme, elle crée un monde nouveau, elle produit la sensation du neuf. Comme elle a créé le monde (on peut bien dire cela, je crois, même dans un sens religieux), il est juste qu'elle le gouverne. Que dit-on d'un guerrier sans imagination? Qu'il peut faire un excellent soldat, mais que, s'il commande des armées, il ne fera pas de conquêtes. Le cas peut se comparer à celui d'un poète ou d'un romancier qui enlèverait à l'imagination le commandement des facultés pour le donner, par exemple, à la connaissance de la langue ou à l'observation des faits. Que dit-on d'un diplomate sans imagination? Qu'il peut très bien connaître l'histoire des traités et des alliances dans le passé, mais qu'il ne devinera pas les traités et les alliances contenus dans l'avenir. D'un savant sans imagination? Qu'il a appris tout ce qui, ayant été enseigné, pouvait être appris, mais qu'il ne trouvera pas les lois non encore devinées. L'imagination est la reine du vrai, et le *possible* est une des provinces du vrai. Elle est positivement apparentée avec l'infini." Charles Baudelaire, "La Reine de Facultés" in *Charles Baudelaire, Curiosités esthétiques et l'art romantique*, ed. H. Lemaitre (Paris: Garnier, 1962), 321.

2 Solomon R. Benatar, "Moral imagination: The missing component in global health," *PLoS Medicine* 12, no. 2 (2005): e400.

3 Paul Farmer, and Nicole Gastineau Campos, "Rethinking medical ethics: A view from below," *Developing World Bioethics* 4 (2004): 17–41; Solomon Benatar, Abdallah Daar, and Peter Singer, "Global health challenges: The need for an expanded discourse on bioethics," *PLoS Medicine* 2, no. 7 (2005): e143.

4 Bruce Jennings, and Angus Dawson, "Solidarity in the moral imagination of bioethics," *Hastings Center Report* 45 (2015): 31–38.

5 Mary Midgley, *What is philosophy for?* (London: Bloomsbury Academic, 2018), 73.

6 Christian Keysers, "Mirror Neurons," *Current Biology* 19, no. 21 (2010): R971–973.

7 Jan Schouten, *The rod and serpent of Aesculapius: Symbol of medicine* (London: Elsevier Publishing, 1967); Rade Nicholas Pejic, "The symbol of medicine: Aesculapius or Caduceus? JAMA 275, no. 16 (1996): 1232; Stavros A. Antoniou, George A. Antoniou, Robert Learney, Frank A. Granderath, and Athanasios I. Antoniou, "The rod and the serpent: History's ultimate healing symbol," *World Journal of Surgery* 35 (2011): 217–221.

8 Dan W. Blumhagen, "The doctor's white coat. The image of the physician in modern America," *Annals of Internal Medicine* 91 (1979): 111–116.

9 J. M. Cocking, *Imagination. A study in the history of ideas* (London and New York: Routledge, 1991).

10 Edward S. Casey, *Imagining. A phenomenological study* (Bloomington and Indianapolis: Indiana University Press, 2000), 4, 17, 178–181. See also: John Rundell, "Creativity and judgement: Kant on reason and imagination," in *Rethinking imagination. Culture and creativity*, eds. Gillian Robinson and John Rundell (London and New York: Routledge, 1994), 88–117.

11 Mary Warnock, *Imagination* (Berkeley and Los Angeles: University of California Press, 1978), 10.
12 Casey, *Imagining*, 5–6.
13 W. J. T. Mitchell, *What do pictures want? The lives and loves of images* (Chicago and London: The University of Chicago Press, 2005).
14 Nicholas Constas, "Icons and the imagination," *Logos: A Journal of Catholic Thought and Culture* 1, no. 1 (1997): 114–127.
15 Constas, "Icons and the imagination," 121–124.
16 Luciana Caenazzo, Lucia Mariani, and Renzo Pegoraro, eds., *Medical Humanities. Italian Perspectives* (Padova: Cooperativa Libraria Editrice Universita di Padova, 2015).
17 Jane Jelley, *Traces of Vermeer* (Oxford: Oxford University Press, 2017).
18 Lawrence Gowing, *Vermeer* (London: Giles de la Mare Publishers Limited, 1997); Simon Schama, *Kunstzaken. Over Rembrandt, Rubens, Vermeer en vele andere schilders* (Amsterdam and Antwerpen: Uitgeverij Contact, 1997); Anthony Bailey, *A view of Delft. Vermeer then and now* (London: Chatto & Windus, 2001).
19 Paul Ricoeur, "Imagination in discourse and in action," in *Rethinking imagination. Culture and creativity*, eds. Gillian Robinson and John Rundell (London and New York: Routledge, 1994), 119–135.
20 Terrence C. Wright, "Phenomenology and the moral imagination," *Logos: A Journal of Catholic Thought and Culture* 6, no. 4 (2003): 109.
21 Warnock, *Imagination*, 162.
22 Warnock, *Imagination*, 194.
23 George Lakoff, and Mark Johnson, *Metaphors we live by* (Chicago and London: The University of Chicago Press, 2003).
24 Jing-Bao Nie, Adam Gilbertson, Malcolm de Roubaix, Ciara Staunton, Anton van Niekerk, Joseph D. Tucker, and Stuart Rennie, "Healing without waging war: Beyond military metaphors in medicine and HIV cure research," *The American Journal of Bioethics* 16, no. 10 (2016): 3–11; David J. Hauser, and Norbert Schwarz, "Medical metaphors matter: Experiments can determine the impact of metaphors on bioethical issues," *The American Journal of Bioethics* 16, no. 10 (2016): 18–19. A classic study of the negative impact of metaphors is Susan Sontag, *Illness as metaphor & Aids and its metaphors* (London: Penguin Books, 1991).
25 Lakoff and Johnson, *Metaphors we live by*, 139 ff.
26 Lakoff and Johnson, *Metaphors we live by*, 193.
27 Ricoeur, "Imagination in discourse and in action," 212.
28 Mark Johnson, *Moral imagination. Implications of cognitive science for ethics* (Chicago and London: The University of Chicago Press, 1993), 164 ff.
29 Oliver F. Williams, ed., *The moral imagination. How literature and films can stimulate ethical reflection in the business world* (Notre Dame: The University of Notre Dame Press, 1997), 125.
30 Gilbert Ryle, *The concept of mind* (Harmondsworth: Penguin Books, 1949), 232–263.
31 Warnock, *Imagination*, 33.
32 Annis Flew, "Images, supposing, and imagining," *Philosophy* 28, no. 106 (1953): 246–254.
33 Richard Kearney, *The wake of imagination. Toward a postmodern culture* (London: Routledge, 2001).
34 Gaston Bachelard, *On Poetic Imagination and Reverie* (New York, Spring Publications, 2014), 71; Gaston Bachelard, *L'eau et les rêves. Essai sur l'imagination de la matière* (Paris: Librairie José Corti, 1942), 29.

35 Bachelard, *On Poetic Imagination and Reverie*, 76.
36 Gaston Bachelard, *L'Air et les Songes. Essai sur l'imagination du movement* (Paris: Librairie José Corti, 1943), 21.
37 Colette Gaudin, "Preface," in *On Poetic Imagination and Reverie*, ed. Gaston Bachelard (New York: Spring Publications, 2014), 16. See also: Roch C. Smith, *Gaston Bachelard. Philosopher of science and imagination* (Albany: SUNY Press, 2016); Joanne H. Stroud, *Gaston Bachelard. An elemental reverie on the world's stuff* (Dallas: The Dallas Institute of Humanities and Culture, 2015).
38 Edward K. Kaplan, "Gaston Bachelard's philosophy of imagination: An introduction," *Philosophy and Phenomenological Research* 33, no. 1 (1972): 18.
39 "L'imagination, plus que la raison, est la force d'unité de l'âme humaine." Bachelard, *L'Air et les Songes*, 176.
40 Gaston Bachelard, *La Poétique de l'Espace* (Paris: Les Presses Universitaires de France, 1957), 11, 12.
41 Lawrence A. Blum, *Moral perception and particularity* (New York: Cambridge University Press, 1994).
42 Blum, *Moral perception and particularity*, 57.
43 Johnson, *Moral imagination*, 32 ff. See also: Anders Nordgren, "Ethics and imagination. Implications of cognitive semantics for medical ethics," *Theoretical Medicine and Bioethics* 19 (1998): 117–141.
44 Wright, "Phenomenology and the moral imagination," 104–121.
45 Iris Murdoch, "Ethics and the imagination," *Irish Theological Quarterly* 52, no. 1–2 (1986): 82.
46 Lynn Hunt, *Inventing human rights. A history* (New York and London: W. W. Norton & Company, 2007).
47 C. Wright Mills, *The sociological imagination* (Oxford and New York: Oxford University Press, 2000), 7.
48 John Dewey, *Human nature and conduct. An introduction to social psychology* (New York: Henry Holt & Company, 1922), 190.
49 Sara Barrena, "Reason and imagination in Charles S. Peirce," *European Journal of Pragmatism and American Philosophy* 5, no. 1 (2013): 1–15.
50 John Dewey, *A common faith* (New Haven: Yale University Press, 1934); S. Adams, P. Blokker, N. Doyle, J. Krummel, and J. Smith, "Social imaginaries in debate," *Social Imaginaries* 1 (2015): 15–52; Steven Fesmire, *John Dewey and moral imagination. Pragmatism in ethics* (Bloomington and Indianapolis: Indiana University Press, 2003).
51 Fesmire, *John Dewey and moral imagination*, 67.
52 Alasdair MacIntyre, *Edith Stein. A philosophical prologue, 1931–1922* (Lanham: Rowman & Littlefield Publishers, 2007).
53 Henk ten Have, *Global bioethics. An introduction* (London and New York: Routledge, 2016). See also: Pope Francis, *Humana Communitas, Letter to the President of the Pontifical Academy for Life* (Vatican City: Libreri Editrice Vaticana, 2019).
54 Siep Stuurman, *The invention of humanity. Equality and cultural difference in world history* (Cambridge and London: Harvard University Press, 2017).
55 John Kekes, *The enlargement of life. Moral imagination at work* (Ithaca and London: Cornell University Press, 2006).
56 J. J. Chambliss, "John Dewey's idea of imagination in philosophy and education," *The Journal of Aesthetic Education* 25 (1991): 43–49; Andrea English, "John Dewey and the role of the teacher in a globalized world: Imagination, empathy, and 'third voice'," *Educational Philosophy and Theory* 48 (2016): 1046–1064.

57 Charles Taylor, *Modern social imaginaries* (Durham and London: Duke University Press, 2004).
58 Kearney, *The wake of imagination*, 42; Casey, *Imagining*, 183 ff.
59 Massimiliano Colucci, and Renzo Pegoraro, "Towards a Medicine of the Invisible: Bioethics and Relationship in *The Little Prince*," *Medical Humanities* 43 (2017): 9–14.
60 Sara E. Davies, Adam Kamradt-Scott, and Simon Rushton, *Disease diplomacy. International norms and global health security* (Baltimore: Johns Hopkins University Press, 2015).
61 John Paul Lederach, *The moral imagination. The art and soul of building peace* (New York: Oxford University Press, 2005).
62 Lederach, *The moral imagination*, 26–27.
63 Michael A. Ashby, and Bronwen Morrell, "To the barricades or the blackboard: Bioethics activism and the 'stance of neutrality'," *Journal of Bioethical Inquiry* 15 (2018): 479.
64 Angus Dawson, Christopher F. C. Jordens, Paul Macneill, and Deborah Zion, "Bioethics and the myth of neutrality," *Journal of Bioethical Inquiry* 15 (2018): 483–486.
65 Edward Tivnan, *The moral imagination. Confronting the ethical issues of our day* (New York: Simon & Schuster, 1995), 250.
66 Walter Brueggemann, *The prophetic imagination* (Minneapolis: Fortress Press, 2018.
67 See the *Sermon on the mount* in the Gospel of Matthew 5, 1–12. Dale C. Allison, *The Sermon on the mount: Inspiring the moral imagination* (New York: Crossroad Publications, 1999).
68 Dorothy Porter, *Health, civilization and the state: A history of public health from ancient to modern times* (London and New York: Routledge, 1999).
69 John Kekes, "Disgust and moral taboos," *Philosophy* 67 (1992): 443.
70 Richard Horton, "Rediscovering human dignity," *The Lancet* 364 (2004): 1081–1085.
71 Stefan Zweig, *Die Welt von Gestern. Erinnerungen eines Europäers* (London and Stockholm: Hamish-Hamilton and Bermann-Fischer Verlag AB, 1942).
72 Brett Bowden, "The thin ice of civilization," *Alternatives: Global, Local, Political* 36, no. 2 (2011): 118–135. See also: Jonathan Glover, *Humanity. A moral history of the twentieth century* (New Haven and London: Yale University Press, 2012).
73 Van Rensselaer Potter, *Bioethics: Bridge to the future* (Englewood Cliffs: Prentice-Hall, 1971), 130.
74 Van Rensselaer Potter, *Global bioethics. Building on the Leopold legacy* (East Lansing: Michigan State University Press, 1988).
75 "Civilization flourishes only on proportion as individuals and social groups so live that they assimilate the viewpoints of one another and develop an appreciative understanding of each other's needs. Whenever a group separates itself from others and begin to develop a framework of preoccupations peculiar to its own separate way of life, the very foundation of civilization is under threat." N. P. Jacobson, "The problem of civilization," *Ethics* 63, no. 1 (1952): 19.
76 Norbert Elias, *The civilizing process. Sociogenetic and psychogenetic investigations* (Malden: Blackwell Publishing, 2017); Hunt, *Inventing human rights*.
77 Brett Bowden, *The empire of civilization: The evolution of an imperial idea* (Chicago and London: The University of Chicago Press, 2009).
78 Albert Schweitzer, *The Philosophy of Civilization. Part II. Civilization and ethics* (New York: The Macmillan Company, 1959), 86.
79 Stephen Kalberg, "Max Weber's sociology of civilizations: The five major themes," *Max Weber Studies* 14, no. 2 (2014): 205–232.

80 Ricardo Rozzi, "Biocultural ethics: Recovering the vital links between the inhabitants, their habits, and habitats," *Environmental Ethics* 34 (2012): 27–50.

81 Axel Honneth, *Disrespect. The normative foundations of critical theory* (Cambridge: Polity Press, 2007).

82 Naomi Grimley, "Identity 2016: 'Global citizenship' rising, poll suggests," *BBC News* (28 April 2016).

83 Henk ten Have, *Global bioethics. An Introduction* (New York: Routledge, 2016), 47–49, 107–109.

# 6 Recovering the soul – inspiring images

The challenge of this chapter is how the moral imagination can activate, produce, or instigate images that rehabilitate and reinsert the soul in bioethical discourse. Images present what is absent. They do not mirror the world but make the world. They embody ideals of good life.

Images stimulate the imagination. For example, the image of the lone ranger may be associated with images of a courageous individual who explores new territories and makes fascinating discoveries. It may also provoke images of loneliness and isolation, of vulnerable individuals who desperately need social support and assistance. In turn, imagination also produces images. As a creative faculty, it provides a new understanding of our experiences, highlighting some dimensions and hiding others. The imagination may therefore constitute new realities and guide future actions. Doing so, the imagination combines cognitive and emotional dimensions. The feelings, experiences, and moral practices that are presented in images are at the same time categorized and assessed on what they entail for practical use.

Bachelard has warned that we are tempted to study images as things. But they are experienced, lived. The main characteristic of imagination is mobility. It is not static but empowers action; it transcends the earth-bound context in which we live. This is also the position of Husserl who regards the imagination as a critique of reality. The human subject can be fascinated by images, and lack critical awareness, thus taking the image for real. The subject can also have critical distance, and be apprehensive of the difference between the imaginary and the real. This illustrates that images can have power. They have a particular vitality, effectiveness, and efficacy because they elicit responses such as censorship and iconoclasm. Pictures and statues in museums have been assaulted. On the other hand, images can give pleasure, consolation, and also hope and spiritual benefits. They arouse empathy and compassion; some are venerated, consecrated, and kissed. Others provoke offense, shame, and disgust. An example is the photo of Alan Kurdi, a 3-year-old boy from Syria who drowned in the Mediterranean Sea in 2015 after trying to reach Europe. Another example is the destruction of the statue of Saddam Hussein in 2003, marking the success of the American invasion of Iraq. Many people remember and are still horrified by the images of the collapse of the Twin Towers in New York in 2001. Images are powerful; they excite emotions. [1]

They are often symbols, for example, of lack of hospitality for refugees, of cruel dictatorship and terrorism, and of capitalism and globalization.

Images play a powerful role in healthcare. Throughout the history of medicine, imagination has been regarded as a potent agent in the healing process, and imagery has been used in the treatment of a wide range of disorders. Images are healing since they can be relaxing, comforting, empowering, and promoting understanding, control, and coping. [2] Images also play a much broader role. Today, the first photo of a child is a print of the ultrasound scan at 12 weeks of the pregnancy. The images of Dolly the sheep circulated widely across the world, instigating admiration as well as horror for genetic technologies. Since ancient times, health has been imagined as harmony and balance, and disease as disorder, either deficiency or excess. [3] For some diseases, metaphors and images are mixed. Tuberculosis, for example, has been regarded as degeneration and consumption but it was also associated with images of a romantic personality, superior sensitivity, and creativity with famous patients like Chopin, Paganini, Chekhov, Kafka, and Rousseau. For cancer, the story is different. It is imagined as an insidious and devastating condition that gradually but irrevocably disintegrates the bodily structures and functions. The abnormal growth that characterizes the disease is symbolic for the excessive and isolated behavior of the *homo economicus* in contemporary societies. Cancer is imagined as an invasion by a hostile agent. The patient is expected to resist and fight, although he or she may be blamed because of smoking, unhealthy diet, or lifestyle. The images and metaphors in this case are stigmatizing and punitive. Susan Sontag has argued that they therefore should be avoided. It is better to calm the imagination when it has these negative impacts. [4] However, metaphors and images cannot be avoided in human communication. A more feasible approach is to introduce new and alternative images, to redefine common metaphors. For example, instead of military language, the image of "journey" can be used to understand illnesses, using the global framework of mobility and travel as an interpretative resource. [5]

In this chapter, we propose images that present world views that remedy the one-sidedness of the dominating ideologies of naturalism, scientism, and market thinking. They produce alternative approaches that may recover the soul in present-day discourses and practices of healthcare. Not all of these images are new. Due to the progress of science and medicine, some have been repressed and others have been neglected or discarded as irrelevant. They are all reactivated nowadays as sources of inspiration to reexamine the core of healthcare.

## The warm doctor

Francis Peabody, a celebrated and compassionate professor at Harvard Medical School from 1915 to 1927, published a short article that is often cited for its conclusion: "One of the essential qualities of the clinician is interest in humanity, for the secret of the care of the patient is in caring for the patient." [6] Peabody observed that treating a disease might be an impersonal matter but caring for a patient is always completely personal. A good physician has extensive scientific skills and knowledge but he first of all needs to know his patients, creating a personal bond with time, sympathy, and understanding. A few weeks before his death, Peabody wrote an article, published in the *Journal of the American Medical Association* with the title "The soul of the clinic." [7] Peabody argues first of all that medical care should be individualized. Physicians do not treat diseased but individual human beings. Second, he points out that hospitalization often is a dehumanizing and depersonalizing experience. What he calls a "clinical picture" is not just a photograph but "an impressionistic painting of the patient surrounded by his home, his work, his relations, his friends, his joys, sorrows, hopes and fears." [8]

Peabody's publications had a profound influence since they were regarded as the embodiment of the "noblest aspirations of the medical profession." [9] Peabody is like Hippocrates, William Osler, Albert Schweitzer, and Florence Nightingale, one of the heroes or saints of healthcare. His ideas encouraged efforts to go back to the essence of healthcare and to move beyond the disease-focused biomedical model, with approaches such as patient-centered care, individualized care, relation-centered medicine, integral care, and medicine of the person. The anthropological tradition in healthcare that we discussed in Chapter 2 also fits into this pattern of responses. What these responses have in common is the assumption of antagonism between science and art in healthcare. From different perspectives, they reject the naturalist and reductionist approach of medicine, regarding the patient as a biological organism and using universal and abstract models of disease separated from the ill person. Contrarily, they advocate a focus on the whole person, on subjective experiences, and individualized methods, thus reinserting the patient in medical discourse. [10] Peabody made a slightly different distinction: he contrasted knowledge of the mechanism of disease with the practice of medicine. For him, medical practice is not merely the field of application of scientific principles but it has its own dynamics and features. The science of medicine and the art of medicine are supplementary rather than antagonistic; they are located at different levels. Like the science of aeronautics is not the same as the art of flying, medical science is necessary for practicing medicine but not sufficient. Medical practice includes the doctor–patient relationship, and is therefore a personal matter and involves the emotional life of the patient. [11]

Subsequent concepts of patient or person-centered care, in the footsteps of Peabody, have emphasized two characteristics of good healthcare: first, the relationship of care provider and patient, including a focus on respect and dialogue, and second, the importance of individualized care. However, the scope of these concepts is limited to what it implies for the medical practitioner. He should be a virtuous professional who knows how to take care of patients. Peabody's landmark paper was based on a presentation he gave a year earlier to medical students. His primary concern was how young professionals could be properly educated and develop into good physicians. Nowadays, this spotlight on the virtues of the medical professional is directed at the notion of empathy. Physicians, and in fact all healthcare providers, should be empathic. A good doctor or nurse is an empathic person. He or she understands the experiences, needs, and wishes of a patient in order to help in the best way possible. This view is expressed in the image of the warm doctor. Empathy is perceived as warmth. Patients need a care provider who combines caring, communication, and competence – one who sits down, listens, understands, explains, and is a good communicator. [12]

### *Empathy*

Empathy starts with imagination. It demands that the care provider imagines what the patient is experiencing. As discussed in the previous chapter, we can imagine ourselves as the other person; we become aware of values beyond the limits of our own experience, and recognize shared human qualities. The imagination, in fact, encourages people to put themselves in the place of other people and relive their experiences. Imagination facilitates reciprocity of perspectives. Ethical interaction requires the ability to shift from first-person perspectives to second- and third-person perspectives and back, so that perspectives are shared and exchanged. Without moral imagination, healthcare practitioners will not develop the capacity to empathize with others. They cannot be merely detached rational agents. It is impossible to ignore the needs of patients for emotional interaction with physicians. Emotions are important in the interpersonal realm; they are "crucial for understanding reality." [13] Critically using subjective sources of information, physicians will engage in more effective communication, take fuller histories, and better understand what patients experience. They are able to discern what meaning a symptom has for an individual. Empathy supplements objective knowledge. It illustrates the statement of John Henry Newman: "The heart is commonly reached not through reason, but through the imagination." [14]

An empathic and caring physician makes a difference. A doctor who is warm and reassuring improves the patient's health. For example, symptoms are relieved faster when the doctor is nice and encouraging. [15] Empathy increases patient satisfaction and adherence to therapy; it also reduces medical errors. [16] Placebo treatment has a more powerful effect if the physician is projecting warmth and competency. [17] Concern for patient well-being is expressed verbally, but non-verbal behavior is also crucial (eye contact, open body posture, smiling, and touch). [18] Some care providers (e.g. psychiatrists, pediatricians, and general practitioners) have higher empathy scores than other professionals.

Frequently, this image of the warm healthcare provider is contrasted with that of the objective, rational, and competent professional, exemplified in the image of detached concern. Instead of an empathic communicator, it is argued, we first of all want a competent expert with professional and up-to-date skills and knowledge. This contrast between competency and empathic and communicative qualities is false. It presupposes that competency is a technical ability based on scientific, primarily biological, knowledge and specific expertise in medical procedures. But competency is more than this; it is interpersonal, reflecting skills in social interaction and communication. When we undergo surgery, we expect that the surgeon is technically competent and has the skills to perform the intervention to our benefit, and with the least harm possible. But we also expect that the surgeon has interpersonal competence, and will not treat us as a bodily machine that needs reparation; that he or she will understand our preoperative anxieties and fears, and will communicate the outcomes after the intervention, and explain what it will mean for us. An opposition between competence and empathy is therefore unnecessary. In practice, there is no trade-off between competence and empathy; they are related and are reinforcing each other. Empathic behavior increases patient perceptions of competence. [19]

Prioritizing professional competence revives the ancient antagonism between science and art. It assumes that competence is based on objective science and that empathy is subjective and affective. However, as will be argued in the following, empathy is not only the ability to share the emotions of others, but also a cognitive ability to understand these emotions. The warm healthcare provider is not lacking competence; he or she is concerned but not detached as a scientific observer. In the context of healthcare, competence and empathy are both needed for patient-centered care and relationship-centered care. Empathy in healthcare is not an additional task that comes after competency is acquired and demonstrated. It is a quality of professional communication and conduct. [20]

In the 1950s and 1960s, the ideal for medical professionalism was detached concern. Since the 1990s, interest for the role of empathy in healthcare increased, and it became a subject of training in the medical curriculum. Nowadays, empathy has an ambiguous function. The Royal Dutch Medical Association in its *Manifesto on Medical Professionalism* refers to the notion in its definition of a good doctor:

> he is a medical expert, he keeps his professional know-how up-to-date, communicates in an empathic way with his patients, cooperates with colleagues, exercises his profession within the (moral) boundaries of the professional group, organizes quality in his practice and renders account. [21]

The American Board of Medical Specialties declares that medical professionalism combines competency standards and ethical values. Its statement refers to compassion, integrity, and respect for others but does not mention empathy. [22] The *Physician Charter on Medical Professionalism*, produced in 2002, translated in many languages and endorsed by numerous organizations worldwide, defines professional responsibilities to individual patients and society. It refers to three fundamental principles: primacy of patient welfare, patient autonomy, and social justice. It mentions competence, honesty, confidentiality, and integrity but not empathy. [23] The *CanMeds Physician Competency Framework* developed by the Royal College of Physician and Surgeons of Canada in 2015 sets standards for medical education. It is now used in many other countries. The framework is based on competencies: observable abilities of healthcare professionals; and it delineates milestones at certain stages demonstrated in practice. Seven roles of the physician are distinguished: medical expert, communicator, collaborator, manager, health advocate, scholar, and professional. The concept of empathy plays a very minor role in the framework. It is only mentioned in connection to the physician as communicator. In this role, physicians form relationships with patients and their families that facilitate the gathering and sharing of essential information for effective healthcare. Empathy has an instrumental function; it is an "enabling competency." The care provider as communicator is "using a patient-centered approach that encourages patient trust and autonomy and is characterized by empathy, respect, and compassion." This competency will enable physicians to accomplish the key competency of establishing professional therapeutic relationships with patients and their families. [24] The General Medical Council in the United Kingdom in its report on medical professionalism identifies as one of the key themes the compassionate doctor. Good doctors should show compassion and empathy in their work. It underlines factors that undermine compassion such as lack of time and fragmentation of care services. Forty-four percent of the surveyed physicians believe that doctors are less compassionate than 20 years ago. [25]

These different positions regarding the role of empathy highlight some problems with the image of the warm care provider. First of all, empathy is not a clear concept. It is often confused with compassion and sympathy. It is furthermore argued that empathy may require too much. It may lead to over-identification with the suffering of the patient, and this leads to burnout. Some has argued that empathy is not necessary, at least not for all care providers. Rejection of empathy may be even broader: it is not necessary nor sufficient for good care practices. Another challenge is how empathy can be realized in daily practice. How can it be learned and taught?

Jodi Halpern has introduced the concept of *clinical empathy*. As a general notion, empathy is perhaps too broad, and needs specification in the context of healthcare. In this setting, the main concerns are with illness and the need for treatment, healing, and care. Empathy here has two goals: understanding the experiences of the patient, and communication so that a good therapeutic relation can be built. In this context, Halpern argues, empathy requires cognitive curiosity and affective attunement. [26] In general discourse, the notion of empathy is often used as synonymous with sympathy and compassion. Empathy is the English translation of the German *Einfühlung*, referring to the capacity to feel into or inside the other person, and to understand what he or she is going through and how the person is feeling. The term "sympathy" has a longer history: it is extensively used by David Hume and Adam Smith. It is argued that what they called sympathy would nowadays be called empathy. One feels with another person because of shifting perspectives. One places oneself into the situation of another person by means of the imagination. [27] Compassion is regarded as a professional virtue for healthcare providers. It is an immediate emotional response to the suffering and needs of another person. Unlike empathy and sympathy, it is asymmetrical; compassion does not require a response from the other person. [28]

### *Two questions about empathy*

If we want to elucidate the notion of empathy, two questions need to be answered. What is it? How is it possible? Numerous definitions of empathy are in use. Most of them distinguish two dimensions: affective and cognitive. Empathy is an immediate experience when we are confronted with the suffering of another person. Seeing a seriously ill child, we are emotionally touched. We directly feel what he or she is going through. Our empathic response is not the conclusion of some kind of reasoning or a copy of the same suffering as the child, but we can imagine what it is experiencing. Empathy means that we emotionally identify with another person. This identification can go too far, and this is the reason why detachment is important. However, empathy has also a cognitive component. As the capacity to understand the feelings, experiences, and thoughts of other persons, it is a way of "reading" the mind of others. It is not a spontaneous feeling but projective imagination. We understand what it means to be ill because we have the ability of perspective taking: imagining what it is to be in the situation of the other person, and at the same time maintaining a certain distance. We understand the misery and pain of the other but are aware that our situation is different; it is not *our* misery and pain. Scholars such as Petra Gelhaus regard empathy primarily as a cognitive condition. She emphasizes that it is understanding what happens inside the patient. For her, empathy is "a predominantly cognitive skill of understanding the inner processes of the patient." [29] However, she recognizes that empathy requires emotional involvement of the care provider, though not full identification. This point is articulated by Kraft-Todd and colleagues, and Nortvedt: empathy combines the ability to share the emotions of patients and the ability to understand the emotions of other. Affective and cognitive capacities therefore cannot be separated. [30] The same point is made by Halpern. She emphasizes that as a joint affective and cognitive capacity, empathy requires emotional interaction. [31] This characteristic also explains why empathy is not morally neutral. The understanding that is the result of empathy is not self-directed but concerned with the other human being. The understanding produced is not neutral. It has an impact on moral motivation. This is why, the cognition is hot rather than cold. The perception and understanding of another person's condition motivate us to work on relieving it and deliver treatment and comfort. Empathy requires a particular type of response: care, concern, and engagement. It is furthermore morally relevant since it contributes to moral perception. As discussed in the previous chapter, through the imagination we recognize others as human beings like ourselves, so that we experience and understand their predicament.

A second basic question is how we have access to the minds of other people. Can we really share the feelings of others? Simulation theories postulate that understanding of other people's experiences is possible because we have similar experiences as them. For example, we know what they feel because we have experienced pain ourselves. Although their pain is not our pain, we make an analogy with our own experiences in order to understand what they endure. Imagination plays a role here; we imagine being in the situation of the other person. Thus, we can give a third-person account of their suffering. There are two risks. One is that our own perspective is imposed. The empathic person projects his own experiences on the other person. The other risk is that understanding is superficial. From a third-person perspective, it is impossible to reproduce the mental states of another person in our own mind.

Phenomenological theories advance a second-person account. [32] Empathy is not replicating the experience of another person but appreciating it as his or her experience. It is not understanding another person because one has the same type of experience but it is an other-directed attitude, not making experiences similar to one's own experience. Empathy is more like an immediate perception that develops through interaction. We can only understand another person's mind through mutual interactive engagement, thus "being-with" one another. It is a form of joint agency, requiring mutual recognition. In some cases, empathy will not be efficient or helpful because patients do not appreciate or allow empathy. [33] This point is highlighted by Edith Stein. Empathy enables us to make the experience of the other person accessible and present but at the same time the distinction between self and other should be maintained. Otherwise, difference cannot be appreciated. [34] This view of empathy is important since it addresses the critique that empathy is too demanding and will sometimes lead to burnout, professional distress, and compassion fatigue. [35] Empathic interaction should avoid over-identification with the suffering of the patient where the boundary between self and other has evaporated. The care provider should continue to be aware of his or her own subjectivity, not mistake his or her own feelings for those of the patient, and guard against too much emotional involvement. Empathy therefore does not eliminate the distance to the other. It demands, in the words of Gelhaus, "the doctor to be sensitive, open, interested, and near, but not too near, to the patient." [35] This point of view illustrates the observation made by Reidar Pedersen that in the discourse of empathy not much attention is paid to the understanding subject. Empathy is not just gaining access to and knowledge of the patient. This assumes, as simulation theories often do, that the mental states of other people are there to be discovered and revealed, and that empathy is mirroring the experiences of other persons. This assumption neglects the role and contribution of the empathizing subject. This subject is interpreting the world, and thus other people, with presuppositions and previous experiences. It is not an abstract agent but a situated subject. The care giver brings his or her judgments, expectations, experiences, and knowledge into the empathic process. [36]

Occasionally, empathy is rejected, not because it is too ambitious but because it is not necessary and even useless. Sometimes, empathy is difficult to achieve. [37] It does not guarantee good medical practice. It is argued that in practice it can be regarded more as a form of etiquette than a moral requirement. [38] The underlying argument is that a definition of empathy that is universally accepted is missing, so that the concept is elusive. This is not a strong argument since many concepts are used in healthcare without universal agreement on how to define them (famous examples are disease, disability, and suffering). Moreover, the challenge is how empathy can be realized in practice. This challenge has two aspects. Can empathy be learned and taught? Is it possible to cultivate the capacity to empathize with other people? This brings forward the issue of education that will be discussed in the last chapter. The other aspect is that empathy is a relational ability, while the primary focus usually is on the individual care giver. Consideration of the context in which empathy can be applied and flourish is often missing. This aspect of relational engagement is particularly elaborated by Edith Stein who earned her doctorate in 1917 with a dissertation on empathy under supervision of Husserl. In empathic interaction, I become aware of the feelings and experiences of another person, recognizing him as a living body, not as a mere object or subject. I simultaneously understand myself as a unified consciousness, an embodied soul, aware that I am an object of awareness of other subjects (as a physical body and object of third-person observation, *Körper*) but also as a sensitive, living body (with first-person awareness, *Leib*). Awareness of ourselves is constituted through empathic awareness of others. Our individuality and self-knowledge derive from our situatedness in relationships with others. In Stein's philosophy, individuals are social beings and not separated from other individuals. Her account of empathy underlines intersubjectivity. Entering through empathy into the mental life of another person is crucial for understanding ourselves as intersubjectively constituted. It does not mean that there is identity. [39]

### *Interpersonal connections*

This relational and intersubjective approach to empathy shifts attention from the agent to the context, from internal mental processes to interaction and communication. Empathy is more than a character trait or professional virtue. It reflects interpersonal connection. The experiences of other persons are explored through relating and interacting with them in a certain way. Without sustained interaction, understanding and appreciation of other people's experiences will not emerge. [40] This will require attentiveness and openness but also an institutional context and medical culture that create conditions that make empathic interaction possible (e.g. leaving sufficient time to interact). In fact, this interpretation of empathy brings us back to Peabody's emphasis on practice. Empathy is a process rather than merely the result of individual acts. It is embedded in modes of caring. [41] This explains why empathy is not simply an instrumental skill or tool to gather specific information about the patient. It is a quality of communication. If patients know that a care provider behaves only instrumentally, and shows empathy to elicit results such as better compliance and effective interventions, it will undermine the desired effect. Empathy should be authentic, not merely a means to other ends. [42] The empathizing subject of the care provider cannot be separated from the empathic process, the social and communicative practice in which empathy is demonstrated. [43] A warm doctor or nurse is important but not enough. The care provider should be warm but the temperature perceived by patients depends also on the medical climate.

A final challenge is whether and how empathy can be taught and learned. It is often noted that during professional education, empathy does not increase, and even is reduced. Medical students show a decline in idealism and empathy during their training. [44] Experiences with empathy teaching programs are mixed. According to Edith Stein, the capacity to feel empathy cannot be taught. However, some studies indicate that empathy training is effective in increasing empathy levels, especially in health professionals and university students. [45] This issue of education will be discussed in Chapter 7.

## Holistic care

In a popular essay, Isaiah Berlin divided scholars and writers in hedgehogs and foxes. Foxes know many things, but they are aware that their knowledge is limited. Hedgehogs know one big thing; they have a single vision, an articulate system so that they can understand the world and "the larger scheme of things." [46] In fact, Berlin distinguished different cognitive styles. On the one hand, there are generalists (foxes). They have a broad skill set and can think outside the box. They have a holistic orientation while focused on particulars. On the other hand, there are specialists (hedgehogs) who proceed from one organizing principle that explains everything. Their knowledge is not broad but deep. They try to identify the fundamental components of the universe, and focus on generalization.

Healthcare is caught between the two metaphors. As medical science, the style of the hedgehog dominates. It proceeds from the worldview of naturalism and physicalism, using in particular two organizing visions: the image of the body as biological mechanism, and the image of the lone ranger. As argued in Chapter 4, these images imply a reductive view of human beings, rejection of subjective experiences, and a specific rationality focused on diagnosis and intervention, as well as a view of the patient disconnected from the social and environmental world. As medical practice, however, the style of the fox is more appropriate. It demands that attention is directed at the particulars of the experiencing person of the patient, and at the individual as embedded in a communal and social context, so that a relational ethics is needed. Healthcare furthermore is not an individual enterprise. It requires teamwork and thus an open and collaborative mindset. The images that are associated with this cognitive style diverge. Most commonly used is holistic care or total care but also frequent references are made to the whole person or open mindedness.

### *Obstacle: philosophy of physicalism*

The current approach to diseases in healthcare is criticized because it follows the philosophy of physicalism. It regards disease as a phenomenon of nature that is independent from social behavior, and that can be explained in terms of somatic (biochemical or neurophysiological) processes. The productiveness of this approach for the development and progress of medicine has turned it into an inescapable perspective about disease. It has become a cultural imperative, a dogma, defining what is a real disease. [47] An influential criticism of this biomedical model was the publication of George Engel in 1977 who advocates the biopsychosocial model as a new approach. Engel identifies several negative implications of the biomedical model. It separates disease from illness, making a difference between human experience and medical findings. This means that an abnormality in the human body can be present while the patient is not ill. The reverse is also true. The patient feels ill but doctors cannot find a disease. Unexplained symptoms are not uncommon. One in three consultations in primary care is concluded without specific diagnosis. [48] The biomedical model promotes a specific way of working. It encourages the healthcare professional to determine the relationship between biochemical processes in the body and clinical data, so that the symptoms of the patient can be associated with a specific disease in the body. The focus of medical attention therefore is on the underlying processes in the patient's body, not on the patient's experience, social context, or healthcare system. In this way, the biomedical model determines the role of the physician and defines what is rational medical examination. At the same time, through its focus on disease, it neglects the patient. Perhaps, this is too strong an assessment since the model assumes that the best help to the patient will be to identify or at least to rule out the presence of disease. But the model instructs the physician to not pay priority attention to the personal problems of patients and their families. This leads, as Engel concludes, to "disenchantment among some physicians with an approach to disease that neglects the patient" and stimulates the need for a holistic approach. [49] This view implies that empathy will not be sufficient. Although the person of the healthcare provider is important to establish a proper relationship with the patient, there is an overriding world view and cognitive style that determines how diseases and patient experiences are interpreted and explained.

Although Engel proposed the biopsychosocial model long ago, it has not significantly impacted medical practice. [50] On the contrary, while it is often commended, it is even after decades not implemented in daily activities. Several reasons may explain its lack of impact. One possible factor is that perhaps it is not radical enough. Simply joining together relevant dimensions will not necessarily produce a new holistic vision. The biopsychosocial model still assumes that the physical body is a necessary condition for the existence of the mind, and therefore does not escape the mind–body dualism that it criticizes in the biomedical model. Care providers are encouraged to have a broader approach, and to examine besides biological determinants psychological and social conditions, but this will not demand a new approach, a different way of understanding the patient's illness and subjective experience. Another powerful image is the "health field" promoted by the Lalonde Report in 1974. [51] It visualizes that the health of individuals is determined by four factors: biology, environment, lifestyle, and healthcare organization. The report argues that the best way to promote health is a comprehensive approach, while most efforts and finances are now directed to the determinant of biology. Again, not much has changed since then. Nowadays it is renamed as "integrative care" but faces the same challenges. Even the persistent actions of the World Health Organization to focus attention of policy-makers on social determinants of health and the overwhelming evidence that social and economic conditions have more effect on health status than medical interventions and healthcare systems have not brought significant change.

### *Obstacle: processes of rationalization and bureaucratization*

A second reason might be what Weber has called the Iron Cage. The processes of rationalization and bureaucratization that determine the delivery of present-day healthcare impede more holistic approaches. Healthcare should be efficient and not too time-consuming. In many countries, resources are scarce, and the number of healthcare providers is limited. The general complaint is that the opportunities for sufficient communication are diminishing. Most physicians are dissatisfied with time pressures, and are afraid that time for communicating with patients is decreasing. [52] In 2003, a study among American primary care physicians showed that they spend 55% of the day with face-to-face patient care. The physicians worked on average 8.6 hours each day, and saw on average 20 patients a day. An average visit lasts 17.5 minutes. [53] More than a decade later, face-to-face visits in primary practice took 49% of the physician's time, [54] while clinical face time was much lower (27.0%) in a study of four ambulatory care practices. [55] Contrary to the idea that over time the duration of outpatient visits is shortening, visits have in fact become longer. Something else is happening. Doctors have to spent more time on administrative business. More than half of their time is now devoted to activities outside of the examination room. This is called "desktop medicine": reviewing the patient record, documentation, making notes, writing prescriptions, and arranging for tests. That healthcare professionals are spending more time on paperwork and the computer is blamed on the introduction of the electronic health record. [56] But it is also related to changes in medical interaction. Doctors have more online interactions with patients: responding to online requests for prescriptions and advice, ordering and reviewing tests, and communicating with other staff members and coordinating care. [57] These changes have reduced the time available for direct face-to-face communication. Although the average time of visits has not diminished and even has become longer, during more than one-third of the direct clinical face time doctors interact with the computer rather than engaging with the patient. One study concludes that for every hour of direct clinical face time with patients, physicians spent nearly an additional 2 hours on the electronic health record and desk work. [58]

The situation in the United States is favorable compared to that in many other countries. Primary care visits last less than 5 minutes for half of the global population. Average consultation time varies from 22.5 minutes in Sweden, 2 minutes in China, to 48 seconds in Bangladesh. [59] In most European countries, face-to-face time with patients is shorter than in the United States. The interesting question is not the length of time but how the time is used. American family doctors spend more time during the visit working in the electronic record. [60] Compared with communication patterns in the Netherlands, visits in the United States were 6 minutes longer but the conversation was more instrumental than affective. American physicians were more "verbally dominant" (i.e. taking more than half of dialog time) and "biomedically intensive" (i.e. focused on physical examination and medical intervention). Dutch physicians reflected a biopsychosocial communication pattern with more attention to socioemotional aspects and rapport building. [61]

The conclusion of this data is that health professionals spent substantial time on administrative and bureaucratic tasks such as documentation and data entry, at least in resource-rich Western countries. They also have more online communication with patients and colleagues. The effect is that there is less time available for direct conversation; the computer sometimes receives more attention than individual patients. This is due to changes in the context of healthcare. There is an increasing need for team work (and thus communication with colleagues and other care providers). Other factors are the demand for documentation because of the role of insurance companies and financial regulations, and the growth of online interaction. A consequence of these contextual changes is professional dissatisfaction. One of the paradoxes of today's healthcare is that physicians and other care professionals enjoy interacting with patients, while such interaction is more and more limited. However, when time for communication is diminishing, it leads to distress and frustration. The 2018 Survey of America's Physicians indicates that for almost 80% of surveyed doctors the relationship with patients is the most satisfying dimension of professional practice. The least satisfying dimension is the electronic health record (for 39.2% of the physicians). The health record has affected medical practice; for 35.8%, it has reduced the quality of care, for 56.0% efficiency, and for 65.7% patient interaction. The survey also clarifies the impact: pessimism about the future of medicine (62% of the surveyed physicians), negative professional morale (55%), and feelings of burnout (78%). Changing career paths is considered by 46% of the physicians. [62] In the European Union, many countries are facing shortages of physicians and thus excessive workload. The level of physician satisfaction is moderate: approximately 59% of doctors working in hospitals are satisfied. [63]

Another consequence of the above-mentioned changes is that more than time, the content of the communication is significant. The opportunities available for interacting can be used differently. Here, it makes a difference whether the communication pattern reflects the biomedical or the biopsychosocial model. Studies in various countries show that what patients universally expect from medical consultation is attentive listening, enough time, being taken seriously, and being treated as a person. Patient do not like to be managed as a "bundle of symptoms." [64] Doctors should know not only the medical history of patients, but also their social and cultural background. Although patients prefer a comprehensive and holistic approach, changes are occurring. For example, while general practitioners in the Netherlands used to emphasize continuous, integral, and personal care focused on understanding the patient as a whole, since the 1990s with the introduction of evidence-based medicine and clinical guidelines, communication styles have become more task-oriented: doctors are asking questions, giving advice and information, and focusing on diagnosis according to the guidelines. Psychosocial symptoms are less discussed. Affective communication has also diminished. [65] However, this is not what patients want. [66] Their perspective is holistic. They prefer personalized and humane medical care with doctors listening and showing empathy. In medical consultations, information exchange takes most of the time. For patients, however, medical information is not technical but is associated with meaning in the context of their lives. It has an emotional dimension related to hope and trust. Healthcare providers therefore should not assume that they know what patients want: information, diagnosis, and treatment, but they should listen and give room to the voice of patients. [67]

### *Obstacle: modern medicine and its specific conceptual approach*

These findings refer to a third obstacle to holistic approaches. As we discussed in Chapter 3, modern medicine is characterized by a specific conceptual and methodological approach. Michel Foucault has called this the "clinical gaze": physicians see the patient, and especially the body, in a particular way, relating symptoms to pathological facts. This entails a focus on observation, diagnosis, and intervention. A paradigmatic change in medicine has been the result. For most of its history, medicine has done more harm than good. David Wootton argues that medicine is a "misconceived project" until 1865, when Joseph Lister first applied the germ theory in antiseptic surgery. [68] Rigorous scientific thinking and new technologies transformed medicine significantly. In Chapter 4, it is explained how this transformation is related with specific images; the view of the body as mechanism, the image of the lone ranger, and the image of detached concern. The other side of these images is that they reduced the relevancy of first-person perspectives, the idea of connectedness of individuals, and the significance of emotions in healthcare. The dominant images associated with the clinical gaze are reflected in the care that patients receive. It is commonly assumed that most people want quick solutions and "magic bullets." Almost half of all Americans are on medication. Nearly 60% of adults over 65 years of age take five or more different drugs at any one time. This strong belief in biological and chemical approaches to disease is reflected in health expenditures. The United States spends more than other countries in healthcare but Americans are not healthier than citizens of other high-income countries. For three consecutive years since 2017, life expectancy in the United States has declined. [69]

The image of holistic care promotes another way of thinking. It puts a focus on the experiencing patient, not as an abstract and isolated individual but as a situated person. This focus is expressed in the biopsychosocial model but also in the concept of patient-centered care, which is nowadays widely advocated as remedy for many deficiencies of modern healthcare: limited access, poor quality of care, and dehumanizing care experiences. It is viewed as a move away from task-centered, profession-centered, technology-centered, and disease-centered care. The concept of patient-centered care emphasizes that care providers should focus on people, not diseases and management.

Nobody will seriously argue that care should not be centered on patients but it is not clear what this will imply. Although the concept of patient-centered care is open to many different interpretations, it has two basic components. First is the concern with the individual patient within his or her unique context and situation. The particular patient as a whole person should be the center of attention, not the average patient in the guidelines. Patients want an integrated understanding of their world: "their whole person, emotional needs, and life issues." [70] Establishing an empathic relationship with patients is key to the processes of healing. Second is the view that the patient should guide the care that is provided. That means the involvement of the patient in the process of defining what is the problem, as well as shared decision-making and partnership. Both components are grounded on the notion of relational autonomy. Rather than an individualistic perspective on autonomy leading to providing information that allows the patient to decide on the basis of his or her values and preferences, patient-centered care is collaborative: it emphasizes cooperation, relationship, sharing, and involvement, going beyond the image of individualism and extending to the whole person in specific social contexts. [71] Because the patient as person is central, the medical approach is not additive: focusing on the disease and then adding the psychological and social dimensions. A holistic approach is comprehensive, starting with the needs, questions, and worries of the patient. It requests diverse responses from the healthcare provider. Because the starting point differs, the issue of vulnerability is placed at the foreground. The patient who needs care is experiencing specific vulnerabilities, for example because his physiological status is compromised, his individual identity is threatening because he does not feel well or suffers. In nursing literature, it is therefore argued that the central perspective of patient-centered care is alleviating vulnerabilities. [72] Especially at the end of life, this is an important perspective. Physical care (such as relieving symptoms) is crucial but patients, families, and healthcare practitioners agree that being treated as a whole person is at least equally important. [73] This includes that attention is paid to spirituality. Such broader view is expressed in Cicely Saunders's concept of total pain that includes the physical, emotional, social, and spiritual dimensions of distress and suffering. [74] Daniel Sulmasy has therefore proposed an expanded biopsychosocial-spiritual model for healthcare based on a philosophical anthropology of the human person in relationship. [75]

## Life as story

The medical gaze that observes and assesses the patient is a powerful way to organize the concepts and methods of medicine. The challenge in the previous section is how to broaden and humanize this gaze in order to make it holistic and centered on the patient as a person. It is also argued that there are multiple gazes, for example a relatively new gaze focused on patient safety, or a gaze outside of the hospital setting in informal care. [76] The problem with these efforts to redefine or rebalance the medical gaze is that priority is given to the health professional: it is the perception and interpretation of the medical expert that is more important than the views of the patient.

An alternative approach is suggested by the image of life as a story. The basic idea is that our lives are narratable; they can be presented as stories. Human beings are storytellers; they specifically express their values through stories. Narratives play a central role in the medical context. They testify that patients are more than interesting collections of symptoms. The attractiveness of this image is that it goes beyond visual thinking articulated by the notion of medical gaze. Visual images are the dominant mode of expression, particularly in Western culture; they often replace words. As discussed in the previous chapter, images express values but also desires. Images of clones reproduce our desires; clones want to be like us, and we want copies of ourselves. At the same time, we experience the horror of simply copying. Visual images express mastery and can therefore be seductive. [77] The medical gaze makes the invisible visible. Visualization techniques reveal the structure of the body and locate pathologies. [78] Medical students early on in their training learn to look at patients and their bodies in an objective, analytical way, searching for typical symptoms and their physical manifestation. Medical textbooks usually include illustrations, for example of anatomy and pathology but also physiological and chemical processes are imagined in pictures, diagrams, and schemata. Especially in medicine, visualization is connected to cognition. Visual images are considered to be convincing; they present evidence and realistically demonstrate what has been formulated in words. [79]

However, images are not convincing by themselves; they need interpretation. There are always various possibilities. For example, when one of us underwent a brain CT scan with contrast, the physician by accident discovered an aneurysm. This is a worrying condition and further investigation was recommended. That was in the United States. But when the same images were examined in the Netherlands, the team of specialists concluded that there was no aneurysm at all. This is not surprising. Discrepancies in interpretation of images are common. It is estimated that error rates in the interpretation of radiological images are approximately 30%. These rates have not substantially changed since the first studies on this subject in 1949. Not all discrepancies in interpretation are errors (incorrect interpretation); there is also variation among observers (difference of opinion about the correct interpretation). The consequences can be serious. False-negative interpretations may incorrectly assure patients that nothing is wrong, while false-positive interpretations may inaccurately worry patients. The point is that the conviction that visual images, such as radiographs, CT and MRI images, represent reality and are therefore reliable evidence is not sustained by practical studies. [80] Visibility is the result of artificial procedures that actively reconstruct the world and require human effort and interpretation. [81]

In healthcare interactions, the ear is often more important than the eye. Cicely Saunders was known as a good listener. As nurse, social worker, and medical doctor, she paid much attention to patient narratives. [82] Listening to patient stories demonstrates that patients are not subject-less objects but persons in specific life situations. Stories are a way to undo the separation of body as mechanism and the subjective experiences of the person. They demonstrate the unity of a single life, creating coherence among events and giving temporal structure and significance to human existence. [83] Narratives are connected to a holistic perspective while articulating the particular voice of a specific patient.

In medicine, patient histories are important. Traditionally, the anamnesis played a significant role in clarifying why the patient is visiting the doctor. Anamnesis as taking the case history, what we have learned as medical students, starts with exploring the personal situation of the patient (age, family, occupation, and social milieu). It then clarifies the main complaints, followed by the special anamnesis inquiring about the present symptoms. Ultimately, a systematic inquiry follows with questions about all the organ systems. Only then, physical examination of the body will be performed (e.g. auscultation and palpation). Nowadays, the significance of anamnesis has declined. Since it introduces the subjective context of symptoms, it is often regarded as imprecise, confusing, and irrelevant. [84]

Case presentations, team conferences, medical records, and various types of ever more sophisticated images require continuous interpretation and communication. Different kinds of narratives are circulating in healthcare: narratives of heroic journey, rescue, hope, and miracle. Doctors often remember patients through stories. Stories also provide an alternative to the tendency in medicine to prioritize visualization. The emphasis on the eye as a tool of analysis creates an objectifying distance. Stories restore the voice of patients that is usually privatized and silenced. They illustrate the crucial role of language in medicine. Rather than seeing, they emphasize hearing and therefore dialogue. Auditory communication perhaps reaches out to the soul of patients more easily than visual communication. [85]

The function of stories in bioethics is twofold. First, they are used as instruments in the teaching of ethics. In mainstream bioethics, such teaching is based on principles such as respect for autonomy and beneficence. These principles are abstract and general. They need to be applied in specific contexts. Case examples are helpful to illustrate how principles can be specified and applied. Narrative therefore complements the teaching of the methodology of principlism. [86] Second, the attention to stories introduces a critical approach in bioethics. Because they express values, they exemplify what is good life for the patient and what is good medical practice, as many physician-writers elaborate in their writings. Stories demand moral reflection and motivate ethical action. Emphasizing stories therefore presents a different view of ethics: it is not simply a matter of principles and how to apply them in a rational and impartial manner, but it also demands interpretation and sensitivity for the values of individual persons. Reason and emotion cannot be separated in ethical evaluation. Ethical studies often start with case presentations and then follow up with philosophical analysis, as if cases provide the factual and realistic context for interpretation and analysis. But, in fact, case presentations are not detached from the subsequent analysis. Narratives are expressing a particular world view, and the way cases are narrated is influenced by how ethicists see the moral world through their theoretical perspective. Case presentations are the result of a discursive strategy that is driven by a particular ethical theory. [87]

Interestingly, the image of stories sheds a particular light on Weber's thesis of disenchantment. According to this thesis, the stories peculiar for Western civilization and religion have disappeared from the public realm. Indeed, postmodernists argue that the "Grand Narratives" have been dissolved. The postmodern technological world has become impersonal and fragmented; there are no commonly shared stories. Nonetheless, the growing interest in narrative ethics indicates that this diagnosis is only partially true. On the one hand, stories give priority to particular people and situations, rather than abstract principles and theories. This illustrates the shift from the public to private domains. Stories focus the ethical attention to desires, wants, and values of individual people. Understanding stories requires affective and intellectual abilities. Because of these characteristics, stories are influencing the mind of listeners and readers; they transform their imagination. This is why they are regarded as agents of ethical empathy since they make it possible to imagining ourselves in the place of the other. [88] The appeal of stories is that they express how people feel they should live, and how they can escape from technological mastery. The world is narratable and therefore a place that we can make sense of by means of stories. On the other hand, stories are intersubjective. It is typical for stories to be shared. [89] Many of our stories originate with other people. We are not the origin of all our stories; we seek meaningful stories about ourselves by others. They are produced by relationships. Stories require an interaction and communion between a teller or writer and listener or reader. Storytelling is a reciprocal activity. Telling a story also means responding to it. Stories express the soul. Stories illustrate that our basic experience of the world is gained directly from our own particular perspective. Science only provides a second-order expression. This is why first-person perspectives as expressed in narratives are important. Contrary to the disenchantment thesis, they make the world personal. First-person experiences are also the main reason for belief in the existence of the soul. The soul as the core of our subjectivity is expressing itself in the narratives of our life. But there is another side to this view. The soul is more than the articulation of the interior dimension of human beings. Human beings have first-person perspectives because they are social beings. The implication is, as pointed out by Mary Midgley, that philosophical reflection should start in the intersubjectivity of human experience. It should not assume that we are detached observers, cut off from the living world around us. It should begin in the relation between inner and outer lives, "in our experience as a whole . . . the whole living person." [90] Thus, narrative ethics rejects the Cartesian view of the disembodied soul since this ignores the process of socialization, which is essentially a narrative process. The individual self is constituted by receiving narratives of other people and responding and renarrating to others. From a hermeneutical perspective, the self is a narrative construction. [91] It is continuously evolving and realized through our projects. It is the result of organizing one's life in a specific way. But we need others to construct our self. This means that the notion of narrative self, and the notion of soul expressed through it, will help counter the radical individualism of neoliberal ideology. [92] Since narratives are driven by imagination, they will bring us to "constantly transcend the status quo of any given society towards alternatives." [93] Narrative ethics can, in this view, also relate to the interconnectedness of all living systems and so contribute to increasing awareness of global narratives of planetary health. [94]

The application of these ideas in healthcare has fostered the notion of narrative medicine. This is an ideal of care, a new frame for clinical work. Narrative medicine, defined by Rita Charon, is "medicine practiced with the narrative competence to recognize, absorb, interpret, and be moved by the stories of illness." [95] For healthcare professionals, it is important to have "narrative competence": the ability to listen to patients, to identify the meaning of narratives, and to engage in action according to the values of the patient. Stories are a source of knowledge but they also draw the healthcare provider into the story. Narratives have the power of immersion; they appeal to the sharing of experiences. Healthcare providers cannot be detached observers but they are involved in the stories. Narratives also present a broader picture of the life of patients and in that sense demonstrate a holistic approach and encourage an empathic perspective. The resulting case reports are rooted in the experiences of patients. [96] The focus is on particular people and their situations rather than on general theories or abstract rules. Defining narrativity as a central element of medicine recognizes the role of intersubjectivity. Narrative is fundamentally communicative. [97] Practicing medicine means continuous communication, interaction and interpretation, listening to multiple voices, giving attention to subjective experiences of patients, witnessing their suffering, and imagining the consequences of intervention. Finally, the image of life as story intrinsically connects ethics and medicine. [98] The image shows that reason and emotion are related, and that understanding between human beings is a relational affair, in ethics as well as medicine.

## Sacred values

Values determine what is worthwhile and what might provide meaning. The images associated with the scientific worldview dominated by naturalism are connected with specific values. The image of *homo economicus* propagates the values of rational choice and self-interest. Values in this view are primarily preferences. Values are expressed in the choices that people make. Deciding to choose what one desires is expressing one's values. Regarding the body as mechanism has instrumental value since the body locates us in the world, is a vehicle of our actions, and relates us to other people. But this image is also connected to commodification. The body has value since it can be objectified, exchanged, and traded as individual property; it has value as an economic resource. The image of the lone ranger expresses individualism with values such as self-determination, individual rights, and privacy. Detached concern is related to the values of objectivity and impartiality. Finally, the image of the patient as consumer asserts the values of individual choice and personal responsibility.

The images that dominate current science and healthcare communicate and divulge specific values. The point, as argued in Chapter 4, is that they do so by neglecting or depreciating other values such as cooperation, relationality, and social justice. Other images may therefore articulate different value commitments. Another point is that the above-mentioned images are associated with a reductive interpretation of values: they are regarded as individual preferences. This interpretation is one of the outcomes of the process of disenchantment. Values have been relocated from the public into the private domain. Since rationalization, bureaucratization, and scientific progress dominate all spheres of modern life, values can no longer play a public role. Weber does not argue that there are no values. In his view, there are certainly ultimate values but they have been removed from public life. If values play a role, it is within the private domain as individual preferences and desires. At the collective level, values are fictions and illusions. Science therefore, in Weber's view, should operate as a value-free endeavor. The process of disenchantment has also dismissed the idea that some values are sacred, that is untouchable and inviolable. The universe is no longer understood as a sacred order. Religion has lost its significance. According to Marcel Gauchet, religion implies radical and primordial dispossession. What gives meaning to our existence comes not from us but from a different being *before us*. Whatever causes and justifies the visible human sphere lies outside this sphere. The religious perspective entails sacred dependency; in the words of Gauchet:

> The underlying belief is that we owe everything we have, our way of living, our rules, our customs, and what we know, to beings of a different nature . . . everything governing our daily lives was handed down to us. [99]

Therefore, disenchantment means that there are no longer any sacred values. The consequence is not only that values have retreated in the private sphere but also that there is no essential difference between values, or at least that overriding, untouchable values do not exist. Since science is value-free, and knowledge a neutral instrument, rational action is technical action, concerned with the efficient use of means to accomplish ends. However, there is a plurality of ends because human beings will not necessarily share the same values. There is no absolute value to order these different ends.

The view that values have retreated in the private sphere has raised critical questions. Weber's assessment of this development is ambiguous. While he argues that the modern world is characterized by impersonal structures of domination, at the same time, he describes the self as autonomous. His concept of "inner distance" is used to protect the inner core of the persons against the depersonalizing forces of the world, and to maintain individuality and the power of self-expression. As a personality, the self affirms constantly some values. The modern individual adheres self-consciously to certain values and refuses to yield to circumstances in his surroundings and life world. [100]

There are two ways to criticize this view. One is that values are not simply individual desires or preferences. They are associated with a wide range of emotions such as respect, honor, affection, and love but they cannot be reduced to feelings, emotions, and interests. Typical for values is that they connect subjective and objective elements. Values are different from preferences since they evaluate our preferences as good or desirable; they express what is worth desiring or preferring. The role of moral imagination is important: the creative power of imagining values as ideals and possibilities beyond what is desired. Furthermore, values do not express the same basic attitude (desire, preference, or pleasure) that can be more or less strong, but values differ qualitatively. What people value is often plural and different in quality. Values also differ over time depending on the context, conditions, and challenges of life. The world of values is multidimensional. [101]

In the ideology of individualism, values are attached to the individual. What is valuable emerges from human experiences, for example the experiences of violence that led to the affirmation and dissemination of human rights. Increasing empathy and sensitivity to the suffering of (imaginary) others promoted a cultural shift to regard the human person and his dignity, rather than the individual, as a sacred object. [102] Emphasizing the person implies that values are social entities. Personhood is characterized by relationality and sociality. Values arise, as Hans Joas argues, in experiences of self-formation and self-transcendence as the result of social interaction. [103]

Another critique at the privatization of values is that not only the world but also the self, and particularly its intimate relations, has been rationalized. Intimate life and emotions have been made into measurable and calculable objects. The modern subject is regarded as a self-manager. He or she has to do introspection and to clarify his or her self-image in a continuous process of communication. This has implications for values; the subject has to take values as the guides to his or her life. But the process is ambivalent. It is intensifying subjective life as the expression of personal values and authenticity but simultaneously it objectifies the means to express and exchange emotions so that others will recognize the values as components of a rational lifestyle. [104] The self needs to show self-restraint and moral autonomy in order to maintain interpersonal relationships. This requires the ability to combine two sets of values: care, cooperation, and social concern; and autonomy and self-reliance. [105] Thus, the retreat of values in the private sphere does not imply that the connection with values in the public sphere has been lost.

A fundamental problem that is raised in the above-mentioned perspectives is the exact status of values. The dominant scientific world view underlines that science aims to describe and explain the real constitution of the world. It produces facts that are not contaminated by subjective experiences and interpretations that are based on particular values. In the view of ontological naturalism, values are not real entities like the objects and phenomena studied by scientific inquiry. They are not part of the natural order. However, they can be studied as first-person perspectives that may influence science but they do not have the same status as the third-person perspectives that are delivered by scientific research. Facts and values should therefore be stringently separated. In Chapter 2, it is argued that such point of view is problematic. Husserl, for example, pointed out that the world does not exist independently from the perception of a subject. Every scientific activity is preceded by encounters of the human subject with the world, and it is therefore the product of the human lifeworld. Subjective presuppositions play a necessary role in the construction of scientific knowledge. From a phenomenological perspective, facts are not given as such and available for observation; they are discovered, delineated, and described with a specific intention. Every description is already interpretation. Facts appear within the intersubjective context of language and culture. That means that values precede facts. [106] The common, naturalistic view is that it is important that facts are first noticed and documented before they can be valued. This view not only separates facts and values but also implies that value judgments cannot be deduced from factual observations. It is not recognized that facts develop from a context of values. This is clear from visual images such as paintings, photographs, or CT scans that are not mere representations or copies of reality but expressions of specific values. The paintings of Vermeer, for example, do not reflect 17th century women or the city of Delft but present values such as domestic virtue and social order (see Chapter 5). The same dialectic coherence between facts and values is noticeable in jurisprudence. The fact that a car driver caused an accident with a cyclist will be interpreted and described differently when the driver was drunk or when he was cautious and could not avoid the deadly event. The facts differ according to value judgments of responsibility and blame. Similar coherence exists in scientific inquiry; it is permeated with the ideology of naturalism and physicalism, with objectivity, instrumental rationality, and technical control as primary values. Scientific findings can only be accepted as facts when they are the result of the application of such values. In practice, these values are often compromised. Nowadays, non-naturalistic values such as integrity and honesty are regarded as essential for scientific work. They should precede the identification and description of facts because they make them worthwhile.

In healthcare, values cannot be ignored. Patients' stories demonstrate what is valued in life. Concepts of health and disease are defined in connection to values. Goals of medicine embody values such as quality of life and prolongation of life. Health policies impose particular values on the performance of medical activities such as competition and efficiency. Ethical debates emerge because values often have a different meaning and significance for different persons. Producing an ethical decision requires the careful balancing and weighting of various values. The underlying assumption is that none of the values is overriding. The most important ethical consideration is that values are decisive if they are the appropriate expression of the value system of the autonomous person. Different medical facts emerge from this value context. When patient values predominate, the person may feel ill but no facts will be found by the physician to explain this experience. On the other hand, when doctor values prevail, medical facts may be revealed that have no significance in the perspective of the patient.

Another fundamental problem with values is that within the current market discourse values are regarded as commensurable. Objects and choices can be ranked in value according to a common scale, usually money. In this discourse, value is often equated to prize. Numbers can be used to create relations between things and actions. In this way, qualitative distinctions can be transformed into quantitative ones. Campbell describes how this has happened with the human body. When the body is turned into a commodity, there is no difference between bodies, parts, cells, or tissues. They are all fungible, that is interchangeable without any loss in value. [107] Commodification is a basic component of the market discourse. Everything that people value is a commodity with a price. This market discourse is totalitarian in the sense that all aspects of human life – love, family, babies, marriage – can be subjected to market exchanges.

Commodification presents a one-dimensional world of value. It is a form of reductionism. It does not reflect the way how people, in fact, value things. In reality, there is significant incommensurability and pluralism. It may be very difficult to translate values between different groups of people and between different historical times. [108] Certain activities are regarded as inappropriate; they elicit moral outrage, disgust, and repugnance. Even if they express individual values, these should be rejected because they are an affront to human dignity as a fundamental value. If people are confronted with injustices, they are often insulted when they are offered financial compensation or material benefits; they first of all want recognition and apologies. Repugnance and moral outrage indicate that not all values are the same. Some values are sacred; they cannot be violated because they cannot be balanced with other values. As core or essential values, they cannot be negotiated or traded-off with other values. [109] They are non-fungible and have no price. They have a transcendental significance that makes any comparison or trade-off unthinkable. They cannot be calculated, measured, or compared. In fact, any comparison will be morally disturbing because it subverts these values in an overriding calculus. [110]

Sacredness is a controversial topic because of its religious associations. The Latin word *sanctitas* has two meanings: respectability and inviolability. Values can be instrumental, personal, and intrinsic. The last category of values is sacred: they are independent from their utility or what people want; they are valuable in themselves. An example is Vermeer's painting *The Milkmaid*. This portrait has instrumental value since it gives pleasure to people admiring it. It has personal value since not everybody appreciates it. But it also has intrinsic value as a work of art. The owner of this painting will be blamed if he destroys it even if it is his own property. The work needs respect and protection. Philosopher Ronald Dworkin has explained why. He distinguishes two kinds of intrinsic value. One is incremental. For example, knowledge is valuable in itself; the more knowledge we have, the better, even if the practical utility is limited. Another type of intrinsic value relates that what is valued as soon as it exists. This is what we label as sacred value. An example is human life. It demands respect as soon as it is there. It is not incrementally valuable but when it exists it should thrive and be respected. According to Dworkin, there are two processes that make such values the object of respect: association and genesis. Values can be sacred because they are associated with something else, for example divinity. Dworkin gives the example of Ancient Egypt where cats were venerated as holy animals because they were incarnations of Bastet, the goddess of joy and love. Values can also be sacred because of their origin, the way they have been produced. Destroying *The Milkmaid* is disgustful not because a painting is annihilated but a creative product is destroyed. The same argument explains why extinction of species is horrifying; they demand respect and protection since they are creations of nature and evolution. More than the product, it is the process, the genesis of values that makes them sacred. Values are intrinsic because they embody a creative process. [111]

Contrary to the theses of Weber and Gauchet, Hans Joas has argued that the notion of the sacred has not disappeared but reappeared in multiple perspectives.

Examples are the resistance against naturalistic reduction of human beings, against discrimination and stigmatization of vulnerable people, against violations of human rights. [112] The image of sacred values is an antidote to a reductionistic view of values. A consequence of the argument that values are incommensurable is that the scope of commodification should be limited and that some realms of social life should be protected against market forces. Turning public goods and social practices such as education and healthcare into commodities is degrading and thus corrupting them. [113]

In the context of medicine, debate has focused on altruism. Market transactions are crowding out altruistic giving. People who are donating blood or organs out of a sense of solidarity or obligation are transformed into traders. Market discourse changes not only the meaning of gifts but also the motivation to give. Monetization of transactions produces objectification. Setting a price for some transactions transforms them into impersonal activities. Social relations, interactions, and their meanings are changed. Social arrangements that motivate people to care for other people are destroyed. [114] There also is significant risk of exploitation, as cases of commercial surrogate motherhood and paid organ donation have illustrated.

Emile Durkheim, one of the founders of sociology and a contemporary of Max Weber, famously argued that the idea of the sacred has not vanished at all in modern societies. There is continuity between traditional and modern societies because elementary forms of religious life permeate both. The emergence and expansion of science does not involve the collapse of religion. The world continues to be divided into the sacred and the profane. Some practices, ideas, and objects are incomparable and incommensurable with others. Secular notions such as democracy, progress, the principle of free enquiry, and equality are like religious notions in traditional societies. Corresponding to religious discourse, they are related to the common good and moral community. The sacred is expressed in the collective practices of the community. The notion of the sacred has, according to Durkheim, negative as well as positive implications. It is prohibiting certain ways of acting. But the sacred is also an object of respect and thus instigates us to act in certain ways. Since sacredness arises in collective practices, it accentuates that human life means living together. It expresses collective ideals. [115] The image of sacred values therefore directs the moral imagination toward world views and approaches that differ from the dominant images that advocate self-interest, individualism, detachment, and consumerism.

## The blue marbles

A final set of images is related to processes of globalization. In July 1969, on its way to the first manned moon landing, the spacecraft Apollo 11 took photos of the earth. It was the first time that human beings could see their planet as a whole from a distance. The pictures showed earth as a beautiful planet in a vast and dark outer space. It demonstrated vividly the vulnerability of the planet as a small, isolated, and fragile globe within an infinite universe. This sense of vulnerability was further strengthened by an even more spectacular series of pictures taken by the Apollo 17, the so-called "blue marbles." [116]

The picture of the planet as a "blue marble" has much contributed to the growth of global consciousness. Before that moment, nobody has been able to see the planet that he or she inhabits in its entirety and from a distance. The images from outer space distinctly and immediately illustrated for many people two things: all human beings have a common home, and they are an endangered species if they ruin that home. Perhaps, these images motivated Van Rensselaer Potter to launch his concept of global bioethics and intensified his concerns with the possible extinction of humanity. He used one of the Apollo 11 photos on the cover of his 1971 book on bioethics. [117]

The images of Earth as a lonely globe in outer space made all people aware that they live on the same planet, that they share the future, and that they all should worry about their destiny and that of their children and grandchildren. This sense of common home, activated by the images, triggered the moral imagination. As discussed in the previous chapter, people, especially in developing countries, are redefining themselves as "citizens of the world." They are conscious that they have to transcend local perspectives and that they are members of a global moral community, sharing common values. Though rooted in a specific place, they are situated as inhabitants of the same planet, in a shared home.

Various metaphors have been used to refer to the globe. A powerful one was "Spaceship Earth" that was influential in the 1960s and 1970s. It conceived of the earth as a technological artifact, a huge interstellar machine that is controllable, requiring human ingenuity and wise use of scarce resources. [118] The metaphor suggests that it is designed and that humans are in control, although the spaceship is vulnerable. The emphasis is on togetherness and cooperation, but the metaphor is anthropocentric in the sense that it gives a central role to human beings. Another metaphor is "web." Humans are interconnected with the environment and particularly ecosystems. The web illustrates mutual coexistence and shared destiny. At the same time, it is fragile and can easily collapse through human action. The interconnected web is complex so that the metaphor invites passivity and immobility rather than activity. [119] Market discourse has promoted the metaphor of "natural capital." The earth is a resource that can be commodified and exploited. It provides renewable and non-renewable natural resources that provide benefits to human beings. An example is water that is freely available in aquifers. A difficulty is that these resources are increasingly depleted so that the metaphor suggests a more prudent use. However, most of the natural capital is in the tropical regions of the globe (such as rainforest and wetlands). A different metaphor is "Mother Earth." It is an ancient metaphor used in mythology and theology. It emphasizes nurturing, caring, and peacefulness. The earth is regarded as a living organism that creates and nourishes life. Human beings share the same planet; they should respect it as the source of life; it is not owned by anybody and should not be exploited. Nowadays, the mother image is especially advocated by indigenous populations. [120] In 2009, the United Nations has proclaimed April 22 as International Mother Earth Day, at the initiative of Bolivia. Though the metaphor stresses the personal bond between humans and the natural world, it has been criticized since it undervalues that human beings should take care for the earth, rather than acknowledging what they receive from it in terms of nurture, warmth, and care.

Metaphors shape the imagination. They express basic cultural values and facilitate communication. They can have different effects since they conceptualize the world in various ways and elicit emotions. The image of the earth as mother evokes personification; images of spaceship and web elicit mechanization; natural capital recalls commodification. [121] Some images are connected to anthropocentric views. The earth is regarded as an object of sustainable management and responsible use, being a complicated machine or storehouse of essential resources. Other images express biocentric views focusing on the interdependence of all beings. They regard the planet more like a subject that demands respect and stewardship.

The home metaphor is different again. References to the planet as the home of humankind have been used by scientists, for example in describing the various qualities of the planet as a geophysical body. [122] The metaphor is employed in policy documents such as the *Rio Declaration on Environment and Development* (1992). Its preamble states that the earth is our home. [123] The *Earth Charter*, a civil society initiative declaring principles and values for a sustainable global future, launched in 2000, repeats the same metaphor. [124] One of its promotors was Mikhail Gorbachev, former First Secretary of the Soviet Communist Party. In a speech to the Parliamentary Assembly of the Council of Europe in July 1989, Gorbachev had outlined the idea of a "common European home," arguing that a collective effort was needed to save this home from nuclear war. [125] Having found its way in scientific, policy, and popular discourses, the home metaphor is now frequently applied in connection to the global threats of climate change, biodiversity loss, and environmental degradation. A major impetus was given in the Encyclical letter *Laudato Si'* of Pope Francis in 2015 with its subtitle "On care for our common home." [126] Home is not a specialist concept. It is familiar to everyone as the place where human beings inhabit the world, where they used to be born and die, where they generally live together in a space of intimacy and privacy in social interaction with others. It is often regarded as a haven or refuge, a secure place to retreat and feel comfortable, a setting for caring relationships and conviviality. [127] The metaphor is therefore often associated with positive emotions. [128] However, this is only part of the story. Today, many people are homeless, without any shelter or place to feel comfortable. Homes can also have a dark side. They can be places of abuse, rejection, and violence.

Home is multidimensional concept. It refers to a physical structure (a dwelling such as a house) where basic needs are satisfied and that provides shelter and security. Homes are not fixed; they can change considerably over time and across cultures. Homes are related to activity; dwelling places are transformed into homes, making them into our places. Being-at-home is the result of shaping and being shaped by the world. [129] A home is located in a specific space, so that the concept refers to territory where people are rooted. It is furthermore a center of self-identity, a place where values are imbued, where people can be themselves, where they belong. Finally, a home is a social and cultural unit, providing an emotional environment in which relationships and activities can grow and flourish. [130] For Gaston Bachelard, "home" refers to everyday experience. Being-at-home is more fundamental than activities such as working. The home allows daydreaming and is therefore the abode of imagination. At home means more than residing in a specific place. [131]

Applying the metaphor of home, especially as "common home," to the planet reformulates the connotations of the concept. The earth is now the physical structure where humans live. It is where they belong and should feel safe and secure. Like a house is divided in different rooms, the world is divided but the planet as home brings humans together as inhabitants of the same dwelling. If home is an accomplishment since it depends on our action transforming this dwelling place into home, it implies the responsibility to take care and make ourselves at home in the world. [132] Being-at-home is the experience of locality but now the local is global since human beings are part of the environmental world.

The word "home" is derived from the Greek οἶκος. The terms "ecology" and "economy" share the same etymology. Connecting the metaphor of common home with the discourse of integral ecology is therefore not surprising. Metaphors frame the debate on environment, biodiversity, and climate change in particular ways. The images of the blue marbles have quickly become symbols for globalization and its associated environmental concerns. They reinforced the idea that the planet is a globe. Three-dimensional miniature models of the Earth have been manufactured since the 15th century. [133] Presenting the earth as a globe has an impact on how we see the environment. The world is an object for admiration, contemplation, and reflection, but it is out there, not here. The world can be observed and studied because humans are detached from it. The image of the globe separates human beings from the context and ambience in which they dwell. Human beings are not integrated in the world. The environment is not their lifeworld. The planet is the location on which people are at home but it is not the world within which they live. Tim Ingold has suggested that in order to overcome the separation between planet and lifeworld, humans and their environment, another metaphor will be appropriate: the sphere. [134] It imagines that instead of being distanced from the globe as a separate entity, human beings are embedded in spheres. The environment is their lifeworld; it does not surround them but they are part of it and dependent on it. The notion of sphere also presents the world as lived experience, perceived and understood from within. The human world begins in the local rather than global because the spherical view is centrifugal. Ingold also points out that sphere is not a visual but primarily an auditory image. It is a symbol of the order and harmony that characterizes the universe. In the 6th century, Roman philosopher Boethius referred to the music of the spheres. [135]

If the image of the planet as a blue marble is connected with the image of the globe, a distance is created between human beings and the planet that they inhabit. Humanity is separated from its lifeworld. The globe is outside as a territory that can be explored and occupied. Viewed from outer space, the blue marble does not show signs of human civilization. Human activity is not visible. It reveals the beauty and wholeness of the planet but at the same time hides its most important characteristic: the human horizon. [136] Contrarily, the image of the sphere integrates humanity into nature and the environment. The natural environment is no longer the context and background of human existence. The image emphasizes that the lifeworld is viewed from within. This metaphor bridges the gap between anthropocentric and biocentric perspectives, articulating that there is no separation between earth and its inhabitants. An integral ecology is needed, based on an anthropo-cosmic sense of home, recognizing the entanglement of humans and cosmos. [137]

Similar tensions between the images of globe and sphere are noticeable in the notion of globalization. Mobility and interdependency are distinguishing features of processes of globalization. Not only people but also technology, money, images, ideas, values, and biological substances and body parts are moving. Furthermore, people are increasingly connected to other people. They are embedded in networks of relatedness. The images of "web" or "network" are used to express this interconnectedness. People experience that they are interdependent, not only with other human beings but also with the environment and the biosphere. Global phenomena such as climate change and emerging infectious diseases, and the realization that we live on a fragile planet have created a sense of vulnerability. These two features warn against a view of globalization that opposes global and local. They show that in everyday practices, the global is manifested within the local and often produced at the local level. Global processes can transform local conditions but local settings often impact and contest global processes. The dialectics between global and local is important for bioethics. As Arthur Kleinman has argued long ago: ethical deliberation is always related to local context. Moral experience is about processes and activities at the local level where values are realized in everyday life. However, local knowledge and experience must be translated into translocal frameworks. [138] The dialectics also questions the current assumption that globalization will continue to increase. Solutions to global problems (related to environmental degradation, waste disposal, and resource depletion) are more local than global. They require de-globalizing and reshoring, bringing problems and solutions closer to citizens who are confronting them. [139] Such interpretations put in effect more emphasis on the relevancy of the image of sphere than that of globe.

Moreover, there is a more fundamental worry. Processes of globalization have led to a widening of our horizon. They refer to the experience that the world has expanded, but the world here is not the planet but the comprehensive world of humankind. This global world is not a physical universe but the horizon within which events and things relate to each other and have meaning for human beings. This world is not simply given, but the result of human activity. Human beings are essentially "world-open." Because they are not, like animals, naturally integrated in and adapted to the environment, and have no special instincts, they are rather defenseless against threats. For a long time since their birth, they need protection and care by other human beings. This essential vulnerability is compensated by world-openness. Precisely because they are not enclosed in their environing world, and adapted to a specific environment, they can modify and recreate this environment into their world. Humans constitute their own environing context in which they feel at home. They focus their energies on what is not present in time and space, and make the environmental conditions into the object of reflection and action, transforming nature and construct, what Arnold Gehlen has called a "second nature" or culture. [140]

Globalization therefore concerns not the globe but the world, the *mundus* (derived from the Greek κόσμος). It is the process through which the life world is incorporating the expanded world due to global interaction and cultural diffusion. In-Suk Cha has argued that a better term is *mundalization*: "the process by which one's home world has absorbed and adapted viewpoints of the broader world into their own." [141] Rather than covering more spatial and geographic dimensions, our world as our home is integrating ideas, values, and customs from people and cultures around the globe.

## Conclusion

In previous chapters, we have argued that the dominant world view of naturalism takes the world as an impersonal environment. Reality is what natural science says it is. First-person phenomena are eliminable or reducible to third-person phenomena. This world view is disseminated through images such as the rational, self-interested individual, and consumer that have wide appeal in present-day society. Dissatisfaction with this world view refers to the experience that human beings are unique in having first-person perspectives. Without these perspectives, there is no agency, moral responsibility, or personhood. Humans belong to the ontology of the world; they give the world an in-eliminable personal aspect. These perspectives not only exhibit self-consciousness but also emerge because we are social beings. The self is not an object or thing that can be studied from a third-person perspective. The self is evolving and realized through our projects. It is the product of the specific way in which we organize and give meaning to our life, and this a narrative construction. But we need others to construct ourselves. [142] We experience ourselves as whole living person. Our subjective experiences are connected to the world that we know exists around us. Human experiences are intersubjective. [143]

The naturalistic world view also pervades contemporary medicine and healthcare. Medical history is usually constructed as progression of science. Mysteries have been eradicated and medicine now is a rational activity based on objectivity and scientific evidence. However, as David Greaves argues, mysterious qualities have not disappeared. Medicine often does not follow its own rational guidelines. Healing furthermore requires engagement with the patient as a whole person. Healthcare demands understanding sick people. There always is an element of indeterminacy and uncertainty with knowledge being incomplete and ambiguous, and interventions risky and unpredictable. Medicine is a mixture of rational and mysterious qualities. [144] Dissatisfaction with medicine and healthcare has focused on critique of the biomedical model. Human behavior is explained in terms of somatic (biochemical and neurophysiological) processes. Diseases are considered as physical and biological impairments and defects, and the body is considered as a mechanism. The biomedical model is cold and impersonal. Healthcare providers are detached; they lack interest and understanding of the personal problems of patients and their families. [145]

This chapter has presented images that provide other perspectives. They can revitalize the soul in scientific and medical discourse. The basic assumption is that soul is a relational concept. The soul is always the soul *of* some body. [146] Soul and body are intrinsically connected. The human person is not a dualistic entity but a unity. Human beings furthermore exist in a web of relationships with other beings. They are world-dependent. Human life is part of the ecology of the world. As rational beings, humans undertake activities, choosing particular ways of acting since they are valuable for them, and provide reasons for acting, explain their course of action in narratives. Images such as the warm doctor, holistic care, and life as story engage the moral imagination. Metaphors such as the blue marble and sacred values shape imagination and provide different conceptual frames going beyond the gap between the actual and the possible, opening new perspectives. Imagination can therefore have healing power. [147] The emphasis on moral imagination and the images presented in this chapter have implications for the discourse of bioethics. This issue will be explored in the following chapter.

## References

1 David Freedberg, *The power of images. Studies in the history and theory of response* (Chicago and London: The University of Chicago Press, 1989).

2 See: Anees A. Sheikh, ed., *Imagination and healing* (Farmingdale, New York: Baywood Publishing Company, 1984); Anees A. Sheikh, ed., *Healing images. The role of imagination in health* (Amityville, NY: Baywood Publishing Company, 2003).

3 G. E. R. Lloyd, *In the grip of disease. Studies in the Greek imagination* (Oxford: Oxford University Press, 2003).

4 Susan Sontag, *Illness as metaphor & Aids and its metaphors* (London: Penguin Books, 1991).

5 Jing-Bao Nie, Adam Gilbertson, Malcolm de Roubaix, Ciara Staunton, Anton van Niekerk, Joseph D. Tucker, and Stuart Rennie, "Healing without waging war: Beyond military metaphors in medicine and HIV cure research," *The American Journal of Bioethics* 16, no. 10 (2016): 3–11.

6 Francis W. Peabody, "The care of the patient," *JAMA* 88 (1927): 882.

7 Francis W. Peabody, "The soul of the clinic," *JAMA* 90, no. 15 (1928): 1193–1197.

8 Peabody, "The care of the patient," 878.

9 Pauline L. Rabin, "Francis Peabody's 'The care of the patient'," *JAMA* 252 (1984): 819. See also: James C. Harris, "Towards a restorative medicine – The science of care," *JAMA* 301, no. 16 (2009): 1710–1712.

10 Jeremy A. Greene, and Joseph Loscalzo, "Putting the patient back together – Social medicine, network medicine, and the limits of reductionism," *New England Journal of Medicine* 377 (2017): 2493–2499.

11 Peabody, "The care of the patient," 882.

12 Neil J. Stone, "Critical confidence and the three C's: Caring, communicating, and competence," *The American Journal of Medicine* 119 (2006): 1–2.

13 Jodi Halpern, *From detached concern to empathy. Humanizing medical practice* (Oxford and New York: Oxford University Press, 2010), 33.

14 John Henry Newman, *Essays and Sketches* (New York, London and Toronto: Longmans, Green and Co, 1948), 2, 204.

15 Kari A. Leibowitz, Emerson J. Hardebeck, J. Parker Goyer, and Alia J. Crum, "Physician assurance reduces patient symptoms in US adults: An experimental study," *Journal of General Internal Medicine* 33, no. 12 (2018): 2051–2052.

16 Gordon T. Kraft-Todd, Diego A. Reinero, John M. Kelley, Andrea S. Heberlein, Lee Baer, and Helen Riess, "Empathic nonverbal behavior increases ratings of both warmth and competence in a medical context," *PLoS One* 12, no. 5 (2017): e0177758.

17 Lauren C. Howe, J. Parker Goyer, and Alia J. Crum, "Harnessing the placebo effect: Exploring the influence of physician characteristics on placebo response," *Health Psychology* 36, no. 11 (2017): 1074–1082; Ted J. Kaptchuk, John M. Kelley, Lisa A. Conboy, Roger B. Davis, et al., "Components of placebo effect: Randomized controlled trial in patients with irritable bowel syndrome," *British Medical Journal* 336 (2008): 999–1003.

18 Kraft-Todd et al., "Empathic nonverbal behavior increases ratings of both warmth and competence in a medical context," 3.

19 Kraft-Todd et al., "Empathic nonverbal behavior increases ratings of both warmth and competence in a medical context," 16.

20 Jodi Halpern, "From idealized clinical empathy to empathic communication in medical care," *Medicine Health Care and Philosophy* 17 (2014): 310. See also: Howard M. Spiro, Mary G. McCrea Curnen, Enid Peschel, and Deborah St. James, eds., *Empathy and the practice of medicine. Beyond pills and the scalpel* (New Haven and London: Yale University Press, 1993).

21 Royal Dutch Medical Association (KNMG), *Medical Professionalism* (Utrecht: KNMG, 2007), 7.

22 American Board of Medical Specialties, *ABMS Definition of Medical Professionalism* (Long Form) Adopted by the ABMS Board of Directors (18 January 2012); www.abms.org/media/84742/abms-definition-of-medical-professionalism.pdf.

23 The Charter has been developed by the American Board of Internal Medicine (ABIM) Foundation joined with the American College of Physicians (ACP) Foundation and the European Federation of Internal Medicine. See: ABIM Foundation, *Medical Professionalism in the New Millennium: A Physician Charter* (2002); https://abimfoundation.org/wp-content/uploads/2015/12/Medical-Professionalism-in-the-New-Millenium-A-Physician-Charter.pdf.

24 Jason R. Frank, Linda Snell, and Jonathan Sherbino, eds., *CanMEDS 2015 Physician Competency Framework* (Ottawa: Royal College of Physicians and Surgeons of Canada, 2015).

25 General Medical Council, *Medical professionalism matters. Report and recommendations* (2016); www.gmc-uk.org/-/media/documents/mpm-report_pdf-68646225.pdf.

26 Halpern defines clinical empathy as "affectively informed engaged curiosity." Halpern, "From idealized clinical empathy to empathic communication in medical care," 304.

27 Petra Gelhaus, "The desired moral attitude of the physician: (I) empathy," *Medicine Health Care and Philosophy* 15 (2012): 103–113. See also: Lauren Wispé, "The

distinction between sympathy and empathy: To call forth a concept, a word is needed," *Journal of Personality and Social Psychology* 50, no. 2 (1986): 314–321.

28 Petra Gelhaus, "The desired moral attitude of the physician: (II) compassion," *Medicine Health Care and Philosophy* 15 (2012): 397–410.

29 Gelhaus, "The desired moral attitude of the physician: (I) empathy," 108.

30 Kraft-Todd et al., "Empathic nonverbal behavior increases ratings of both warmth and competence in a medical context," 16; Per Nortvedt, "Empathy," in *Encyclopedia of Global Bioethics*, ed. Henk ten Have (Switzerland: Springer International Publishing, 2016), Vol. 2, 1105–1112. See also: David Howe, *Empathy. What it is and why it matters* (London: Palgrave Macmillan, 2013).

31 Halpern, *From detached concern to empathy*, 67 ff.

32 Dan Zahavi, and Søren Overgaard, "Empathy without isomorphism: A phenomenological account," in *Empathy. From bench to bedside*, ed. Jean Decety (Cambridge and London: The MIT Press, 2014), 3–20.

33 Jan Slaby, "Empathy's blind spot," *Medicine Health Care and Philosophy* 17 (2014): 249–258.

34 Edith Stein, *On the problem of empathy* (Washington: ICS Publications, 1989). See also: Matthew Ratcliffe, "The phenomenology of depression and the nature of empathy," *Medicine Health Care and Philosophy* 17 (2014): 269–280.

35 Charles R. Figley, "The empathic response in clinical practice: Antecedents and consequences," in *Empathy. From bench to bedside*, ed. Jean Decety (Cambridge and London: The MIT Press, 2014), 263–273.

36 Gelhaus, "The desired moral attitude of the physician: (I) empathy," 112.

37 Reidar Pedersen, "Empathy: A world in sheep's clothing?" *Medicine Health Care and Philosophy* 11 (2008): 329. See also: Richard L. Landau, ". . . And the least of these is empathy," in *Empathy and the practice of medicine. Beyond pills and the scalpel*, eds. Howard M. Spiro, Mary G. McCrea Curnen, Enid Peschel, and Deborah St. James (New Haven and London: Yale University Press, 1993), 103–109.

38 Georgina Campelia, and Tyler Tate, "Empathic practice. The struggle and virtue of empathizing with a patient's suffering," *Hastings Center Report* 49, no. 2 (2019): 17–24.

39 Anna Smajdor, Andrea Stöckl, and Charlotte Salter, "The limits of empathy: Problems in medical education and practice," *Journal of Medical Ethics* 37, no. 6 (2011): 380–383.

40 Stein, *On the problem of empathy*. See also: Alasdair MacIntyre, *Edith Stein. A philosophical prologue, 1913–1922* (Lanham: Rowman & Littlefield Publishers, 2006); Antonio Calcagno, *The philosophy of Edith Stein* (Pittsburgh: Duquesne University Press, 2007). See also: Sylvia M. Määttä, "Closeness and distance in the nurse-patient relation. The relevance of Edith Stein's concept of empathy," *Nursing Philosophy* 7 (2006): 3–10; Marian Maskulak, "Edith Stein: A proponent of human community and a voice for social change," *Logos: A Journal of Catholic Thought and Culture* 15, no. 2 (2012): 64–83.

41 "It is through certain kinds of sustained interaction that an increasingly refined perception-like appreciation of someone's experience is achieved." Ratcliffe, "The phenomenology of depression and the nature of empathy," 276.

42 Shapiro calls this "fake empathy." Johanna Shapiro, "The paradox of teaching empathy in medical education," in *Empathy. From bench to bedside*, ed. Jean Decety (Cambridge and London: The MIT Press, 2014), 279.

43 See Campelia, and Tate, "Empathic practice."

44 See, for example, John Spencer, "Decline in empathy in medical education: How can we stop the rot?" *Medical Education* 38, no. 9 (2004): 916–918.

45 Emily Teding van Berkhout, and John M. Malouff, "The efficacy of empathy training: A meta-analysis of randomized controlled trials," *Journal of Counseling Psychology* 63, no. 1 (2016): 32–41.

46 "There exists a great chasm between those, on one side, who relate everything to a single central vision, one system, less or more coherent or articulate, in terms of which they understand, think and feel – a single, universal, organising principle in terms of which alone all that they are and say has significance – and, on the other side, those who pursue many ends, often unrelated and even contradictory, connected, if at all, only in some de facto way, for some psychological or physiological cause, related to no moral or aesthetic principle." Isaiah Berlin, *The hedgehog and the fox. An essay on Tolstoy's view of history* (London: Weidenfeld & Nicolson, 1953), 56.

47 George L. Engel, "The need for a new medical model: A challenge for biomedicine," *Science* 196, no. 4286 (1977): 129–136.

48 Marianne Rosendal, Tim C. Olde Hartman, Aase Aamland, Henriette van der Horst, Peter Lucassen, Anna Budtz-Lilly, and Christopher Burton, "'Medically unexplained' symptoms and symptom disorders in primary care: Prognosis-based recognition and classification," *BMC Family Practice* 18, no. 18 (2017).

49 Engel, "The need for a new medical model," 134.

50 Francesc Borrell-Carrió, Anthony L. Suchman, and Ronald M. Epstein, "The biopsychosocial model 25 years later: Principles, practice, and scientific inquiry," *Annals of Family Medicine* 2, no. 6 (2004): 576–582.

51 Marc Lalonde, *A new perspective on the health of Canadians. A working document* (Ottawa, 1974); www.phac-aspc.gc.ca/ph-sp/pdf/perspect-eng.pdf.

52 David Mechanic, "Physician discontent. Challenges and opportunities," *JAMA* 290, no. 7 (2003): 941–946.

53 Andrew Gottschalk, and Susan A. Flocke, "Time spent in face-to-face patient care and work outside the examination room," *Annals of Family Medicine* 3 (2005): 488–493.

54 Ming Tai-Seale, Cliff W. Olson, Jinnan Li, Albert S. Chan, Criss Morikawa, Meg Durbin, Wei Wang, and Harold S. Luft, "Electronic health record logs indicate that physicians split time evenly between seeing patients and desktop medicine," *Health Affairs* 36, no. 4 (2017): 655–662.

55 Christine Sinsky, Lacey Colligan, Ling Li, Mirela Prgomet, San Reynolds, Lindsey Goders, Johanna Westbrook, Michael Tutti, and George Blike, "Allocation of physician time in ambulatory practice: A time and motion study in 4 specialties," *Annals of Internal Medicine* 165 (2016): 753–760.

56 Richard A. Young, Sandra K. Burge, Kaparaboyna A. Kumar, Jocelyn M. Wilson, and Daniela F. Ortiz, "A time-motion study of primary care physicians' work in the electronic record era," *Family Medicine* 50, no. 2 (2018): 91–99.

57 Tai-Seale, et al. "Electronic health record logs indicate that physicians split time evenly between seeing patients and desktop medicine," 659.

58 Sinsky, et al., "Allocation of physician time in ambulatory practice: A time and motion study in 4 specialties," 758.

59 Greg Irving, Ana Luisa Neves, Hajira Dambha-Miller, Ai Oishi, Hiroko Tagashira, Anistasiya Verho, and John Holden, "International variations in primary care physician consultation time: A systematic review of 67 countries," *BMJ Open* 7 (2017): e017902.

60 Young, et al., "A time-motion study of primary care physicians' work in the electronic record era," 98.

61 Jozien M. Bensing, Debra L. Roter, and Robert L. Hulsman, "Communication patterns of primary care physicians in the United States and The Netherlands," *Journal of General Internal Medicine* 18 (2003): 335–342.

62 The Physicians Foundation, *2018 Survey of America's Physicians. Practice Patterns & Perspectives* (Merritt: Hawkins, September 2018).

63 Alicja Domagala, Malgorzata M. Bala, Juan Nicolas-Sanchez, Dawid Storman, Mateusz J. Schwierz, Mateusz Kaczmarczyk, and Monika Storman, "Satisfaction of physicians working in hospitals within the European Union: State of the evidence based on systematic review," *European Journal of Public Health* 29, no. 2 (2018): 232–241.

64 Maria Angela Mazzi, Michela Rimondini, Wienke G. W. Boerma, Christa Zimmerman, and Jozien M. Bensing, "How patient would like to improve medical consultations: Insights from a multicenter European study," *Patient Education and Counseling* 99 (2016): 53; Jozien Bensing, Myrian Deveugele, Francesca Moretti, Ian Fletcher, Liesbeth van Vliet, Marjolein Van Bogaert, and Michela Rimondini, "How to make the medical consultation more successful from a patient's perspective? Tips for doctors and patients from lay people in the United Kingdom, Italy, Belgium and the Netherlands," *Patient Education and Counseling* 84 (2011): 287–293.

65 Ligaya Butalid, Jozien M. Bensing, and Peter F. M. Verhaak, "Talking about psychosocial problems: An observational study on changes in doctor-patient communication in general practice between 1977 and 2008," *Patient Education and Counseling* 94 (2014): 314–321.

66 Paul Little, Hazel Everitt, Ian Williamson, Greg Warner, Michael Moore, Clare Gould, Kate Ferrier, and Sheila Payne, "Observational study of the effect of patient centredness and positive approach on outcomes of general practice consultations," *British Medical Journal* 323, no. 7318 (2001): 908–911; Andrew Miles, and Juan E. Mezzich, "The care of the patient and the soul of the clinic: Person-centered medicine as an emergent model of modern clinical practice," *The International Journal of Person Centered Medicine* 1, no. 2 (2011): 207–222.

67 Jozien Bensing, Michela Rimondini, and Adriaan Visser, "What patients want," *Patient Education and Counseling* 90 (2013): 287–290.

68 David Wootton, *Bad medicine. Doctors doing harm since Hippocrates* (Oxford: Oxford University Press, 2007), 13.

69 Robert M. Kaplan, *More than medicine. The broken promise of American health* (Cambridge and London: Harvard University Press, 2019), 16; Irene Papanicolas et al., "Health care spending in the United States and other high-income countries," *JAMA* 318 (2018): 1024–1039.

70 Moira Stewart, "Towards a global definition of patient centred care: The patient should be the judge of patient centred care," *British Medical Journal* 322, no. 7284 (2001): 445.

71 Carolyn Ellis, Matthew R. Hunt, and Jane Chambers-Evans, "Relational autonomy as an essential component of patient-centered care," *International Journal of Feminist Approaches to Bioethics* 4, no. 2 (2011): 79–101.

72 Jennifer Lynn Hobbs, "A dimensional analysis of patient-centered care," *Nursing Research* 58, no. 1 (2009): 52–62.

73 Karen E. Steinhauser, Nicholas A. Christakis, Elizabeth C. Clipp, Maya McNeilly, Lauren McIntyre, and James A. Tulsky, "Factors considered important at the end

of life by patient, family, physicians, and other care providers," *JAMA* 284, no. 19 (2000): 2476–2482.

74 Caroline Richmond, "Dame Cicely Saunders. Founder of the modern hospice movement," *British Medical Journal* 331 (2005): 238.

75 Daniel P. Sulmasy, *The rebirth of the clinic. An introduction to spirituality in health care* (Washington: Georgetown University Press, 2006).

76 Peter Lachman, "Redefining the clinical gaze," *BMJ Quality and Safety* (2013): 1–3; Johanna Shapiro, "(Re)examining the clinical gaze through the prism of literature," *Families, Systems and Health* 20, no. 2 (2002): 161–170; Beverly Ann Davenport, "Witnessing and the medical gaze: How medical students learn to see at a free clinic for the homeless," *Medical Anthropology Quarterly* 14, no. 3 (2000): 310–327; Janet Heaton, "The gaze and visibility of the carer: A Foucauldian analysis of the discourse of informal care," *Sociology of Health & Illness* 21, no. 6 (1999): 759–777.

77 W. J. T. Mitchel, *What do pictures want? The lives and loves of images* (Chicago and London: The University of Chicago Press, 2005).

78 Linda S. Nye, "The minds' eye. Biomedical visualization: The most powerful tool in science," *Biochemistry and Molecular Biology Education* 32, no. 2 (2004): 123–131.

79 Bruno Latour, "Visualisation and cognition: Drawing things together," in *Knowledge and Society. Studies in the Sociology of Culture Past and Present*, eds. Elizabeth Long and Henrika Kuklick (Greenwich: Jai Press, 1986), 1–40.

80 Leonard Berlin, "Accuracy of diagnostic procedures: Has it improved over the past five decades?" *American Journal of Roentgenology* 188 (2007): 1173–1178; Elizabeth A. Krupinski, "Editorial: Medical image perception: Understanding how radiologists understand images," *Journal of Medical Imaging* 3, no. 1 (2016): 011001.

81 Michael Lynch, "Discipline and the material form of images: An analysis of scientific visibility," *Social Studies of Science* 15, no. 1 (1985): 37–66.

82 Richmond, "Dame Cicely Saunders," 238.

83 Richard Kearney, *On stories* (London and New York: Routledge, 2002).

84 C. van Tellingen, "About hearsay – or reappraisal of the role of the anamnesis as an instrument of meaningful communication," *Netherlands Heart Journal* 15, no. 10 (2007): 359–362.

85 Jo Marchant, *Cure. A journey into the science of mind over body* (New York: Broadway Books, 2016); Michael J. Balboni, and Tracy A. Balboni, "Reintegrating care for the dying, body and soul," *The Harvard Theological Review* 103 (2010): 351–364.

86 David B. Morris, "Narrative medicines: Challenge and resistance," *The Permanente Journal* 12, no. 10 (2008): 88–96; Anne Hudson Jones, "Narrative in medical ethics," *British Medical Journal* 318 (1999): 253–256.

87 Tod S. Chambers, "The bioethicist as author: The medical ethics case as a rhetorical device," *Literature and Medicine* 13, no. 1 (1994): 60–78.

88 Tony E. Adams, "A review of narrative ethics," *Qualitative Inquiry* 14, no. 2 (2008): 175–194; Johanna Shapiro, "The use of narrative in the doctor-patient encounter," *Family Systems Medicine* 11, no. 1 (1993): 47–53.

89 Arthur W. Frank, "Why study people's stories? The dialogical ethics of narrative analysis," *International Journal of Qualitative Methods* 1, no. 1 (2002): 109–117.

90 Mary Midgley, "Souls, minds, bodies, and planets," in *The resounding soul. Reflections on the metaphysics and vivacity of the human person*, eds. Eric Austin Lee and Samuel Kimbriel (Eugene: Cascade Books, 2015), 177.

91 Dan Zahavi, *Subjectivity and selfhood. Investigating the first-person perspective* (Cambridge and London: The MIT Press, 2005).

92 Bruce Rogers-Vaughn, *Caring for souls in a neoliberal age* (New York: Palgrave Macmillan, 2019).
93 Richard Kearney, and James Williams, "Narrative and ethics," *Proceedings of the Aristotelian Society, Supplementary Volumes* 70 (1996): 38.
94 Susan L. Prescott, and Alan C. Logan, "Narrative medicine meets planetary health: Mindsets matter in the Anthropocene," *Challenges* 10, no. 17 (2019).
95 Rita Charon, *Narrative medicine. Honoring the stories of illness* (New York: Oxford University Press, 2006), vii; Rita Charon, "Narrative medicine. A model for empathy, reflection, profession, and trust," *JAMA* 286 (2001): 1897–1902.
96 Brian Hurwitz, and Victoria Bates, "The roots and ramifications of narrative in modern medicine," in *The Edinburgh Companion to the Critical Medical Humanities*, eds. Anne Whitehead, Angela Woods, Sarah Atkinson, Jane Macnaughton, and Jennifer Richards (Edinburgh: Edinburgh University Press, 2016), 559–576.
97 Kearney, and Williams, "Narrative and ethics," 34. See also: Morris, "Narrative medicine," 88–96.
98 Rita Charon, and Martha Montello, eds., *Stories matter. The role of narrative in medical ethics* (New York and London: Routledge, 2002).
99 Marcel Gauchet, *The disenchantment of the world. A political history of religion* (Princeton: Princeton University Press, 1997), 23–24.
100 Ralph Schroeder, "'Personality' and 'inner distance': The conception of the individual in Max Weber's sociology," *History of the Human Sciences* 4, no. 1 (1991): 61–78.
101 Elizabeth Anderson, *Value in ethics and economics* (Cambridge and London: Harvard University Press, 1993); Jonathan Baron, and Sarah Leshner, "How serious are expressions of protected values?" *Journal of Experimental Psychology* 6, no. 3 (2000): 183–194.
102 Hans Joas, *The sacredness of the person. A new genealogy of human rights* (Washington: Georgetown University Press, 2013), 49; Hans Joas, *Sind die Menschenrechte westlich?* (München: Kösel Verlag, 2015).
103 Hans Joas, *The genesis of values* (Cambridge: Polity Press, 2000).
104 Eva Illouz, *Cold intimacies: The making of emotional capitalism* (Cambridge: Polity Press, 2007), 19, 32, 38.
105 Eva Illouz, *Saving the modern soul. Therapy, emotions, and the culture of self-help* (Los Angeles and London: University of California Press, 2008).
106 Cees A. van Peursen, *Feiten, waarden, gebeurtenissen. Een deiktische ontologie* (Kampen: J. H. Kok N.V, 1972).
107 Alastair V. Campbell, *The body in bioethics* (London and New York: Routledge, 2009).
108 Margaret Jane Radin, *Contested commodities* (Cambridge and London: Harvard University Press, 2001).
109 Scott Atran, and Robert Axelrod, "Reframing sacred values," *Negotiation Journal* 24, no. 3 (2008): 221–246.
110 Philip E. Tetlock, "Thinking the unthinkable: Sacred values and taboo cognitions," *Trends in Cognitive Sciences* 7, no. 7 (2003): 320–324.
111 Ronald Dworkin, *Life's dominion. An argument about abortion and euthanasia* (London: Harper & Collins Publishers, 1993).
112 Hans Joas, *Die Macht des Heiligen. Eine Alternative zur Geschichte von der Entzauberung* (Berlin: Suhrkamp Verlag, 2017).
113 Michael J. Sandel, *What money can't buy. The moral limits of markets* (London: Allen Lane, 2012).

114 Alvin E. Roth, "Repugnance as a constraint on markets," *The Journal of Economic Perspectives* 21, no. 3 (2007): 37–58.

115 Durkheim famously stated that the idea of society is the soul of religion. Émile Durkheim, *The elementary forms of religious life* (Oxford: Oxford University Press, 2001), 314.

116 Gregory A. Petsko, "The blue marble,"' *Genome Biology* 12 (2011): 112; Denis Cosgrove, "Contested global visions: One-world, whole-earth, and the Apollo space photographs," *Annals of the Association of American Geographers* 84 (1994): 270–294. See also: Wolfgang Sachs, *Planet dialectics. Explorations in environment and development* (London: Zed Books, 2015).

117 Van Rensselaer Potter, *Bioethics: Bridge to the future* (Englewood Cliffs: Prentice-Hall, 1971).

118 Richard Samuel Deese, "The artefact of nature: 'Spaceship Earth' and the dawn of global environmentalism," *Endeavour* 33, no. 2 (2009): 70–75.

119 Star A. Muir, "The web and the spaceship: Metaphors of the environment," *ETC: A Review of General Semantics* 51, no. 2 (1994): 145–152.

120 Ronald Sandler, and Phaedra C. Pezzullo, eds., *Environmental justice and environmentalism. The social justice challenge to the environmental movement* (Cambridge and London: The MIT Press, 2007), 321.

121 Paul H. Thibodeau, Cynthia McPherson Frantz, and Matias Berretta, "The earth is our home: Systemic metaphors to redefine our relationship with nature," *Climatic Change* 142, no. 1 (2017): 287–300.

122 A. M. Selâl Şengör, "Our home, the planet earth," *Diogenes* 39, no. 155 (1991): 25–51.

123 *Rio declaration on environment and development* (1992); www.unesco.org/education/pdf/RIO_E.PDF.

124 *The earth charter* (2000); https://earthcharter.org/invent/images/uploads/echarter_english.pdf.

125 Paul Chilton, and Mikhail Ilyin, "Metaphors of political discourse: The case of the 'common European house'," *Discourse & Society* 4, no. 1 (1993): 7–31.

126 ". . . our common home is like a sister with whom we share our life and a beautiful mother who opens her arms to embrace us." Pope Francis, *Encyclical letter Laudato Si' – On care for our common home* (Rome: Vatican, 2015), 7.

127 Shelley Mallet, "Understanding home: A critical review of the literature," *Sociological Review* 52, no. 1 (2004): 62–89.

128 Thibodeau, Frantz, and Berretta, "The earth is our home."

129 "Home is lived in the tension between the given and the chosen, then and now, here and there." Mallet, "Understanding home," 80.

130 Sandy G. Smith, "The essential qualities of a home," *Journal of Environmental Psychology* 14 (1994): 31–46; Jeanne Moore, "Placing *home* in context," *Journal of Environmental Psychology* 20 (2000): 207–217.

131 Gaston Bachelard, *The poetics of space* (New York: Penguin Books, 2014), 28. According to Levinas: "To exist . . . means to dwell" (Emmanuel Levinas, *Totality and Infinity: An essay on exteriority* (Dordrecht: Kluwer Academic Publishers, 1991), 156). See also: Wim Dekkers, "Dwelling, house and home: Towards a home-led perspective on dementia care," *Medicine Health Care and Philosophy* 14 (2011): 291–300.

132 Kirsten Jacobson, "A developed nature: A phenomenological account of the experience of home," *Continental Philosophy Review* 42 (2009): 355–373.

133 The first terrestrial globe was made in 1492 in Germany and called *Erdapfel* – earth apple.

134 Tom Ingold, "Globes and spheres. The topology of environmentalism," in *The perception of the environment. Essays on livelihood, dwelling and skill*, ed. Tim Ingold (London and New York: Routledge, 2000), 209–218.

135 Otto Kinkeldey, "The music of the spheres," *Bulletin of the American Musicological Society* 11/12/13 (1948): 30–32.

136 This has changed nowadays. New technologies use satellite imagery and computer programs to provide three-dimensional maps and detailed representations on earth. *Google Earth* for example makes it possible to see your own street and house, as if from outer space. But it still presents images from the outside, as objects to be examined in much more detail than the blue marbles. The gaze is external, though extremely precise. See: Solvejg Nitzke, and Nicholas Pethes, eds., *Imagining Earth. Concepts of wholeness in cultural constructions of our home planet* (Bielefeld: Transcript Verlag, 2017).

137 An integral ecology was advocated by the Brazilian theologian Leonardo Boff in 1995 (Leonardo Boff, and Virgilio Elizondo, "Ecology and poverty: Cry of the earth, cry of the poor," *Concilium: International Journal of Theology* 5 (1995): ix–x). Integral ecology is also a central notion in the Encyclical letter of Pope Francis (Pope Francis, *Encyclical letter Laudato Si'*, 2015). See also: Sam Mickey, *On the verge of a planetary civilization. A philosophy of integral ecology* (London and New York: Rowman & Littlefield, 2014). An anthropo-cosmic perspective is developed by Gaston Bachelard, *Poetics of space*, 27, 68.

138 Arthur Kleinman, "Moral experience and ethical reflection: Can ethnography reconcile them? A quandary for 'The new bioethics'," *Daedalus* 128, no. 4 (1999): 69–97.

139 Finbarr Livesey, *From global to local. The making of things and the end of globalization* (New York: Pantheon Books, 2017).

140 Arnold Gehlen, *Man. His nature and place in the world* (New York: Columbia University Press, 1988). See also: Phillip Honenberger, *Naturalism and philosophical anthropology. Nature, life, and the human between transcendental and empirical perspectives* (Houndmills: Palgrave Macmillan, 2016).

141 In-Suk Cha, *The mundalization of home in the age of globalization: Towards a transcultural ethics* (Münster: LIT Verlag, 2012), v; In-Suk Cha, *Essais sur la mondialisation de notre demeure: vers une éthique transculturelle* (Paris: L'Harmattan, 2013).

142 Dan Zahavi, *Subjectivity and selfhood. Investigating the first-person perspective* (Cambridge and London: The MIT Press, 2005).

143 Midgley, "Souls, minds, bodies, and planets," 177.

144 David Greaves, *Mystery in Western medicine* (Aldershot: Avebury, 1996).

145 Engel, "The need for a new medical model," 129–136.

146 Denys Turner, *Thomas Aquinas. A Portrait* (New Haven and London: Yale University Press, 2013), 71.

147 Stanley W. Jackson, "The imagination and psychological healing," *Journal of the History of the Behavioral Sciences* 26 (1990): 345–358; Sheihk, *Imagination and healing*.

# 7 Another bioethics

## Introduction

This chapter will ask how bioethics can rehabilitate the soul within medicine and healthcare. In the previous chapters, we discussed the reasons why the soul has been erased in these settings. We pointed out that medical writers, health practitioners, and patients regret that medicine has lost its soul. The removal of the soul from scientific and medical discourse has been interpreted as a cultural and historical phenomenon, particularly in Western civilization; rationalization and bureaucratization came to determine social life; the sense of mystery and wonder but also emotions and meaning have been displaced from the public to the private sphere. Medicine and healthcare, in particular, have been determined by the world views of naturalism and physicalism that regard the soul as an illusion. That this is an error has already been argued by Plato in his dialogue *Charmides*. A physician cannot cure illnesses of the eyes without paying attention to the head, or cure the head without the body, or the body without the soul. Parts cannot be cured without the whole, Plato pointed out. Rather than separating the soul from the body, the physician should begin by curing the soul if he wants to heal the head and body to be well. Many bodily conditions can be treated but not cured. In healing, the charisma and charm of the healer are important for success. Humanistic qualities such as respect, compassion, and integrity are essential if physicians really want to heal and help patients. [1]

When it is argued that the eradication of the soul from healthcare is a loss and impoverishment for medical and healthcare practices, what will be the implications for the ethical debate about medicine, healthcare, and disease? Should bioethics rehabilitate the soul and how will it be able to do so? First of all, it should be recognized that "soul" is a fuzzy concept. It has different meanings: principle of life, immaterial substance, immortal personal entity, form principle of living beings, and core or essence of human beings. There are many different theories and interpretations of soul in religion, theology, and philosophy. In this book, we have been using the notion of soul in the last sense of the term. Soul refers to the deep structure of beings. It is connected to what fundamentally characterizes a being: its value, depth, heart, and personality. Leaving open the question what kind of beings can have souls, we assume that the soul of human beings refers to their humanity. Soul as reference to what fundamentally qualifies an entity is also used metaphorically, for example as the soul of a country or the soul of healthcare. Soul has been imagined in many different ways, most often as a substance or entity, but it is first of all, as formulated by Thomas Moore, "a quality or a dimension of experiencing life and ourselves." [2] This view regards the human body as a manifestation of the soul. It, moreover, articulates that the soul is not confined to the individual. As "activity of self-transcendence," it refers to community, other people, and the social context. It brings individuals in relation to self, but also others. [3] The departure of the soul implies loss of connections with others, society, and creation. Since humans are also part of nature and biodiversity, the soul connects humans with their environment. The human soul has always been related to a larger soul, the *anima mundi*.

Gilbert Meilaender, arguing that bioethics has lost the soul, regards the soul as "attention to the meaning of being human." [4] When the soul has disappeared from ethical discourse, fundamental issues about who we are and who we should be as human beings can no longer be addressed. The consequence is an impoverishment of bioethics. It also contradicts the initial inspiration of bioethics since this new discipline has emerged out of concerns with the humanity of healthcare, aspiring to reinsert the subject into an overwhelmingly scientific and technological practice. Retrieving the soul therefore requires, according to Meilaender, that bioethics goes back to "its earlier self." [5] To do that, the work of the imagination will be vital: mobilizing visions, images, models, and perspectives to elaborate what soul means in ethical discourse. A significant implication of this view is that the role of bioethics will change. It will resemble an imaginative, prophetic activity, proposing what is worthwhile and valuable. This is not how bioethics is perceived today. The role of bioethics is commonly connected to rational argumentation and justification. It addresses the query: what must be done and what should be allowed? How can particular interventions be justified from a moral point of view? How can different ethical principles be balanced and how can arguments be provided for a specific decision? Ethics is first of all an abstract system that provides rules for conduct and decision-making, especially when applied in the context of healthcare. It is practical since it assists care professionals in making decisions that follow discrete events, particularly individual cases and problems. In such context, it is attractive to view ethics as a human technology that facilitates the application of medical science and technology. New approaches can be added to make it more attractive, for example narrative ethics or the biopsychosocial model. However, these additions will not change the basic nature of bioethics if they do not reach out to the soul. That will require a different conception of ethics.

In order to focus on subjective patient experiences and a new ideal of empathic care, several considerations should be taken into account. First, ethics is a lifelong project, a way of life. It is not a succession of discrete events but the result of a continuous nurturing of moral sensibilities, emotions, and empathy. Ethics is influenced by biology and also social and cultural factors but not really determined in the sense that it is an epiphenomenon of brain states or genes, or cultural or social conditions. Webb Keane appropriately speaks of "affordances," enabling factors that allow a certain kind of ethical life to emerge without determining that it will. [6]

Second, ethical life is shared with other people. It arises in the realm of interpersonal interactions, within the tension between interpersonal demands and individual inclinations. Ethics emerges in a succession of perspectives. A full understanding of ethical life cannot be provided by the third-person point of view. A crucial feature of ethics is the capacity to move back and forth between perspectives: the first-person individual concerns, the second-person stance of mutual engagement, and the third-person perspective of detached onlooker. It is necessary, as Keane points out, to have an "orientation away from the self." [7] Such orientation is fundamentally what has been suggested in the ethical tradition as the moral point of view. Since our sympathies are limited, we are encouraged to take the point of view of other persons. It also relates to what is called the expanding circle of moral concern. The scope of ethics is widening and more beings are taken into account as morally relevant.

A third consideration, following from this, is that ethics is a social enterprise. Social interactions are not simply communications between autonomous individuals. They are intersubjective and reciprocal. They involve the sharing and exchanging of perspectives. Ethics as social ethics designates not only a different field but also a different frame for thinking and acting. The main purpose is to widen the scope of ethical considerations from individual to social, environmental, cultural, and economic concerns. This means that a wider field of concerns will be addressed. The starting point for bioethical analysis will be different. Instead of focusing on individual clinical encounters, it will focus attention to social dynamics. Injustices hurt individual people but they usually take place in specific social contexts. Bioethics should therefore start in communities of marginalized and vulnerable people where social injustices are experienced. [8] Furthermore, it is important to be aware that "the world is not flat to all people." [9] Globalization is associated with rampant inequality. Neoliberal policies have created multiple and novel sources of suffering and vulnerability. They have marginalized entire populations and disseminated widespread corruption. These policies have redefined who we are and how we relate to each other. Due to these policies, globalization has established the primacy of the economic and political over the social and ethical; it has removed the soul from ethical and cultural discourse. However, neoliberal policies are often implicitly accepted and not explicitly criticized. The dominance of the market and technocracy over society, culture, and interpersonal relationships is commonly not regarded as a fundamental ethical problem. [10] Social ethics furthermore has a distinct frame. It engages different concepts in moral analyses and debates. Examples are vulnerability, solidarity, respect, and recognition. Another example is cooperation. Humans have evolved because they have a capacity for cooperation and social learning. But in a neoliberal context the social distance between people is increasing. It is harder to feel mutual sympathy. The model of *homo economicus* implies that self-interest should be determinative, and that cooperation is only useful for instrumental purposes, not as a value in itself. Bioethics as social ethics will emphasize that cooperation itself is worthwhile. [11]

This chapter will lay out the imaginative, prophetic role of bioethics based on this broader conception of ethics. It will analyze how the images described in the previous chapter not only present alternative approaches to the dominating world view of scientism and naturalism but also entail a different approach to bioethics. Prior to that, we argue that critical reconsideration of mainstream bioethics is necessary because the contexts of ethical debate have significantly changed recently. Processes of globalization are not only increasingly criticized but strong policies of de-globalization have been initiated. The free trade market ideology is seriously in doubt. The image of *homo economicus* has few defenders nowadays. Another determinant of present-day debates is populism, creating a climate of distrust, fake news, anger, and intimidation, affecting the common values of democracy, rationality, truth, and civil deliberation. Finally, there is a sense of impending catastrophe. Global policies are unable to stop global warming and environmental destruction. The planet becomes increasingly unlivable, not in the longer run but in the very near future. Given these current contextual determinants, ethics seems futile. These cataclysmic feelings have been amplified by the Covid-19 pandemic, which demonstrated the reach of globalization and at the same time the lack of really global responses.

In the last part of the chapter, the question is raised whether ethics is perhaps too demanding. Moral theories are asking more than most of us are capable of. Can we expect health professionals to be empathic all the time, to attend to the subjective experiences of patients, and take the opportunity to listen while they function within systems that emphasize efficiency, output, and results? It seems that strict morality is not feasible in many practical circumstances. Maybe we should acknowledge that ethics has significant limitations, and that it is not an appropriate approach when faced with today's challenges. But if traditional moral theories do not provide a framework for daily life, what can be an alternative approach? Giving up on ethical reflection altogether, and accept that the world and our lives are ruled by science and economy? As argued in previous chapters, that would be a paradoxical conclusion. It entails the blind submission to the values incorporated in the world views of science and economy. It ignores that in daily life, other values, images, and ideals usually play a prominent role. Ethics, as a critical way of living, will therefore continue to be relevant for clarifying the human condition. Here, we will argue that ethics is linked to civilization. Rather than formulating abstract principles, ethics should focus on the everyday interactions between human beings that should be characterized by decency, dignity, respect, and reciprocal recognition. From this perspective, bioethics is connected to civilization, not merely because it is the expression of civil values but also because it can substantially contribute to civilized social life.

## New contexts of ethical discourse

Bioethical debates always take place within specific scientific, cultural, political, and economic circumstances. This is not a new observation, although these conditions often have not been the explicit focus of ethical analysis. Today's contexts, in our view, are significantly different from those of the recent past, with serious implications for bioethics. We distinguish three contexts: globalization and de-globalization, populism, and climate change.

### *Globalization and de-globalization*

The phenomenon of globalization is currently under severe criticism. There is an explicit return to national policies and domestic interests. This is not just a rhetorical move. Deliberate policies are undermining the existing system of economic globalization. One of the strongest global institutions, the World Trade Organization (WTO), incapacitated its dispute settlement mechanism in December 2019. The Appellate Body, established in 1995, was disabled and is no longer operative. It consists of seven judges. Some countries, especially the United States, refuse to reappoint new judges. It means that in case of trade conflicts, there is no longer any possibility of appeal. Economic relations will no longer be governed by multilateral negotiations but by power based on national interests. The idea that free trade promotes the benefit of all has gone.

Similar policies are at work to undermine international human rights discourse. Today, advocating human rights, and thus global ethics, seems more problematic than before. Heads of states, especially in autocratic regimes, publicly denounce and ridicule the discourse. Many argue that domestic laws are more important than human rights. It is also weakly defended in practice by states that used to regard themselves as champions of human rights. For instance, in the United States, traditionally priding itself on its human rights advocacy, the Obama administration downplayed human rights and freedoms in its foreign policy, while for the Trump administration human rights do not have priority at all. [12] In June 2018, the country withdrew from the UN Human Rights Council. An example of the weakness of the discourse is human trafficking, which is one of the fastest growing forms of human rights abuse. Governments are regularly accused of not doing enough against this new form of slavery. [13]

The Covid-19 pandemic has exposed a new dimension of the debate on de-globalization. It is undeniably a global event, illustrating the interconnectedness of countries and regions, transforming citizens of the world into global patients and victims. Effective responses can only be global, while the development of vaccines and medicines require cooperation and collaboration of the best research institutions across the globe. The pandemic furthermore highlights the generalized vulnerability of populations as well as the fundamental materiality of human existence. New diseases emerge since the natural balance between humans, animals, and biodiversity is disrupted by the drive for economic growth and development. At the same time, the responses to the pandemic demonstrate the policies of de-globalization that are primarily national: closing borders, restricting travel, imposing lockdowns, and quarantines. Countries are facing shortages of essential medical resources, and they are on their own, and even competing, in obtaining them. Covid-19 makes clear that globalization implies inequalities, not only in how populations are affected but also in how resources are distributed. An example is the lack of basic ingredients for tests and medicines, which are nowadays mainly produced in Asia. Rather than concluding that the pandemic signals the end of globalization, we would argue that it demands a redirection of global efforts to provide health security to all people, regardless of their nationality and domicile. Moreover, it requires stronger global institutions, particular in healthcare, to overcome the current deficiencies in cooperation and solidarity.

Covid-19 reactivated many ethical concerns related to allocation of resources, triage, end-of-life care, professional morality, human dignity, and social responsibility. In this context, we will focus on the impact on human rights. To contain the pandemic, most countries restricted the freedom of movement, the right to leave the country, the right to freedom of peaceful assembly, and sometimes the right to education. These infringements are justified by appealing to other human rights, especially the right to life and security, and by emphasizing that everyone has duties to the community, as also stated in the *Universal Declaration of Human Rights* (Article 29). However, restrictions of human rights have been varying across countries. Authoritarian regimes have adopted drastic measures, while other countries (e.g. Taiwan and Singapore) successfully implemented less intrusive policies to interrupt the chain of viral transmission. A phased strategy with sheltering in place and widespread testing not only better protected the vulnerable but also as much as possible respected human rights.

Human rights discourse is criticized as ideological and ineffective. It is claimed that human rights are not universal but an instrument of Western countries to impose their liberal values on the rest of the world. This point of view is happily endorsed by authoritarian leaders such as Duterte, Putin, and Erdogan. Questioning the legitimacy of human rights utilizes three interrelated arguments. One is that they are mainly promoted by Western countries, while the same countries no longer strongly support them nowadays. Another argument refers to ethical imperialism: human rights are representing ideas that are foreign to other cultures but imposed by powerful countries of the North. The third argument is that human rights discourse has facilitated the neoliberal policies of globalization. These arguments presuppose a specific history: they assume that human rights discourse has emerged in the global North. The point of origin can be different: the American and French revolutions in the 18th century; the 1948 adoption of the *Universal Declaration of Human Rights*; or the 1970s with explicit policies of U.S. president Carter. However, these are flawed and incomplete constructions of history. They suggest that Western countries have been the main drivers of human rights. In fact, countries such as the United States and the United Kingdom have been major obstacles to the advancement of human rights. [14] The first detailed enumeration of human rights was the *American Declaration of the Rights and Duties of Man*, mainly promoted by Latin American countries and adopted in Bogota in 1948, before the *Universal Declaration of Human Rights*. In fact, the history of human rights is much older and complicated than usually assumed. The argument that human rights are mainly promoted by Western countries is countered with the observation that oppressed people have initiated human rights struggles, as the history of de-colonization illustrates. Governments were rarely the main protagonists of human rights. It is therefore a mistake to confuse human rights movements with human rights policies of countries. Enforcement of human rights legal instruments is mostly dependent on active global civil society movements. [15]

The argument that human rights are foreign ideas imposed by the North does not recognize the diverse origins of human rights discourse in the global South as well as the North. The idea of common humanity, and thus the notion of equal rights for all human beings, emerged in many cultures across history. Famous example are the edicts of Ashoka, emperor of India in the 3rd century BCE. Human rights were promulgated by Cyrus the Great, the first Persian emperor, inaugurating policies of religious tolerance in the 6th century BCE, because humankind is one. [16] From these studies, a different history of human rights comes to light. The justification of human rights is linked to historical processes of value generalization. Human rights are cultural transformations based on universalization of the idea of human dignity. According to Hans Joas, this universalization has been at work since the axial era (800–200 BCE) in India, China, and Greece. It is the outcome of processes of sacralization of the human person, emphasizing relationality and sociality rather than individualism, in response to experiences of violence, cruelty, and suffering. The validity or rational justification of the values expressed in human rights discourse cannot be dissociated from their genesis or the formation of moral ideals. [17]

Human rights are broadly institutionalized in the global South. National courts, for example in India, South Africa, and Brazil, have articulated social-economic rights such as the right to water, food, and health. The global South has played a significant role in the development of human rights discourse. Though René Cassin from France is usually credited for the formulation of the *Universal Declaration of Human Rights* (he received the Noble Prize in 1968), contributions of representatives of developing countries have been essential (particularly Charles Malik from Lebanon, Peng-chun Chang from China, and Hansa Mehta from India, while Bertha Lutz from Brazil emphasized women's rights). [18] The extraordinary role of Latin America is now broadly recognized. The Mexican Constitution of 1917 was the first to articulate civil and political rights but also economic and social rights. In 1945, establishing the United Nations in San Francisco, human rights as one of the basic purposes of the new organization were mainly the result of efforts of developing countries (31 of the 50 participating states were from the global South). [19]

The argument that human rights discourse has made possible the neoliberal policies of globalization proceeds from an incorrect chronology. The discourse was developed and applied decades before neoliberal policies were promulgated. In practice, neoliberalism has been complicit with human rights violations, and not based on human rights ideas. Furthermore, the argument assumes that human rights are merely individual rights. The assumption is that human rights have emerged in the tradition of individualism; they are primarily individual rights and therefore cannot address the structural causes of violence and oppression. [20] This argument does not recognize that human rights are limiting self-interest and urge to take into account the needs of others. It also neglects the emergence of social, economic, and cultural rights. States should not only focus on non-interference but also protect individuals and provide services in health, education, and social security. Rather than facilitating neoliberal globalization, protection of human rights is irreconcilable with the dominant model of globalization. [21]

Critical consideration of the arguments against the legitimacy of human rights presents therefore a different and global view. Human rights have been promoted by less powerful countries to restrain the more powerful political forces. Scholars and lawmakers in Latin America, for example, regarded international human rights law as one of the "weapons of the weak" that could be used to counterbalance U.S. power. [22] The ultimate concern of human rights is the frail, vulnerable, universal human being. It requires tolerably good institutions in order to flourish. But human rights begin in small places, close to home. They have created a new norm of equal voice. [23] No wonder thus that autocrats do not like the human rights discourse. Human rights are for people, not states. They do not primarily present a grand narrative but thousands of humble stories, small everyday acts to improve the lives of ordinary people. This point of view is expressed by Payam Akhavan, who was born in Tehran but migrated with his family to Canada to escape the religious prosecution of the Baha'is. As UN prosecutor at The Hague, he was engaged in the pursuit of global justice, not because of an intellectual idea but because he was touched by human suffering. [24] Experiences of injustice motivate to imagine better worlds. This is also the message of Stephan Zweig, discussed in Chapter 5. Civilizations can deteriorate. It is therefore necessary to continuously articulate a vision of a future that is thoroughly humane. Human rights are an important tool to implement such vision, based on the notion of human dignity disseminating an atmosphere of tolerance and world citizenship. [25]

The second criticism of international human rights discourse is its lack of efficacy. The discourse is regarded as a great moral achievement with the noble intention of protecting the powerless and the vulnerable, but in reality, it is ineffective and has not improved human well-being. All major human rights treaties have been ratified by more than 150 countries, but in many countries the rights articulated in these treaties are continually violated (e.g. non-discrimination of women; prohibition of child labor). [26] Even international organizations do not take human rights seriously. Recently, for example, the UN Special Rapporteur on extreme poverty and human rights criticized the World Bank for treating "human rights more like an infectious disease than universal values and obligations." [27] They pay lip service instead of making rights operational. Furthermore, it is argued that human rights are irrelevant since they do not reduce the expanding gap between the rich and the poor. [28] We are now, as is argued, in the "endtimes of human rights." [29] It is clear that there are challenges regarding the efficacy of human rights advocacy. Measuring the frequency of rights violations is difficult. There is a tension between revealing and concealing abuses. Human rights movements bring more abuses to light even if the incidence of violations is falling. Human rights standards are not static. Increasing advocacy has expanded the scope of human rights, for example emphasizing the rights of women and LGBTQ persons.

In media reporting, abuses receive more attention than good news. Therefore, efficacy is not a straightforward notion when applied to human rights. Empirical evidence demonstrates that at least some types of human rights abuses are declining worldwide. [30] Criticism of human rights discourse is often the result of frustration because injustices continue to exist. But the fact that practices as torture, race and sex discrimination, family separation, and police brutality persist is not a reason to abandon the efforts to eradicate them or to conclude that efforts are failing. Critics do not offer more promising alternatives. For many people in precarious everyday conditions, human rights appeal to the imagination, "widening the limits of the possible." [31] There are always courageous human rights advocates in all regions of the world, although there is a need for more human rights defenders at the global level such as Nelson Mandela, Malala Yousafzai, Andrei Sakharov, and Shirin Ebadi.

During the last decades, globalization has become a commonplace word. The most outstanding place in which globalization is present is in the economy. It is the result of deliberate policies that regard the world as single market. It is this dimension of globalization that is under severe criticism nowadays. At the same time, the idea of a global ethical framework is seriously questioned, as is illustrated in the weakening and discrediting of the human rights discourse. Curiously enough, other dimensions of globalization such as communication and global travel are commonly accepted, even by the most ardent opponents of globalization. Internet, Twitter, and Facebook are global technologies used to criticize processes of globalization. News media, research organizations, and international institutions are no longer confined to boundaries and borders, and this global outreach is usually considered as enriching and beneficial. It is also significant that facing the Covid-19 pandemic, researchers and pharmaceutical industries are strongly engaging in global cooperation, while politicians only show national reflexes.

### *Populism and anger*

Another contemporary context with implications for bioethical debate is populism. It is a broad term that refers to various political approaches that appeal to ordinary people in distinction to elite groups and the establishment. It is defined as an ideology "that considers society to be ultimately separated into two homogeneous and antagonistic camps, 'the pure people' versus 'the corrupt elite'." [32] This ideology is based on normative ideas about society and human beings. The key distinction is a moral one, viz. between ordinary or common people (the "silent majority"), who do not feel represented by powerful elites, and the establishment that determines the dominant cultures and that does not take the interests and values of ordinary citizens seriously. Populism has different shapes since it usually combines with other ideologies, for example socialism, neoliberalism, and nationalism. Although populism is a recent and global phenomenon, it has existed for some time. In Latin America, for example, three waves of populism can be distinguished since the 1930s, usually combined with socialist ideas. In Europe and North America, populist movements are more conservative, rejecting government influences and bureaucratic structures as the European Union, as well as emphasizing nativism ("natives" versus "non-natives" or aliens) in response to immigration.

According to Mudde and Kaltwasser, populism is essentially a democratic phenomenon. [33] It emphasizes the general will of the people as determinative for politics, advocating better and direct representation of the interest of common people. As a relatively recent phenomenon, it is related to the global dissemination of democracy, and it can work as a corrective for authoritarian regimes. However, it may also be a threat to democracy, especially liberal democracies, which are characterized not merely by free elections, popular sovereignty, and majority rule but also by independent institutions such as courts and media to protect fundamental rights, particularly minority rights. Because populist regimes, parties, and movements criticize liberal democracies and encourage autocratic tendencies, more pessimistic views of populism point out that it introduces a new political logic that is often associated with an authoritarian art of governance, combining culture war, patronage, and mass clientelism. Populism is associated with a cult of the leader as a charismatic man of action who has a special bond with his followers, the people.

Populist regimes are frequently characterized by kleptocracy; leaders are seeking self-enrichment, buying loyalty by rewarding supporters. At the same time, non-supporters and critics are threatened. Independent judges and journalists are silenced and ridiculed, while civil society and NGOs are discredited. In some countries, we witness the rise of mafia states, using state structures and legal means for corrupt ends, controlled by "political families." [34] Populists attempt to hijack and colonize the state apparatus. [35] Some scholars therefore regard populism as an intrinsic danger to democracy. They argue that liberal democracy has indeed failed; it has eroded values and destroyed communities. [36] Democracy also has no clear answer to bureaucratic and technological power, and is unable to address environmental approaches. Citizens feel increasingly disillusioned. Calls for authoritarian approaches or a meritocracy of qualified experts ("epistocracy") are therefore attractive. [37] Democracies are not stable but can decline and end. [38] However, as we will argue later in this chapter, these pessimistic views proceed from a restricted notion of democracy. In European history, democracy is not regarded as a stable, universal political form that can be exported over the globe but has always included forms of distrust, tension, and conflict. It has taken various forms during history, as French scholar Pierre Rosanvallon has pointed out. [39] It is continuous work in action. Its institutions and manifestations have been resilient and dynamic as a permanent reorganization of social life. Its ideals can never be completely realized; it is always imperfect, indeterminate, and incomplete. Democracy is more than a political regime with institutional practices and electoral processes. It also involves forms of "counter-democracy," organized distrust. And it is a social activity of citizens, participating and interacting to reconstruct commonality. There is therefore a variety of democratic activities and experiences. Populism is not a threat but a pathology of democracy. [40]

Regarding populism first of all as a moral rather than political discourse opens up other perspectives. It is giving voice to people who do not feel represented in the present political and economic system. Social grievances are articulated that are not addressed by the current political agenda. Many people feel abandoned by the establishment that focuses on economic globalization, multiculturalism, and social integration of immigrants, and disregards the views of the common people that hardly reap the benefits of economic growth, are unemployed or have fragile jobs, diminishing pensions, and weaker social safety nets. Ordinary citizens see inequalities growing and vulnerabilities increasing, while corporations hardly pay taxes and corruption is widespread in the political system. This moral sentiment of exclusion from society and protest against elite unresponsiveness to the daily worries of most people explains the yellow vests ("gilets jaunes") movement that surfaced in France since November 2018, blocking roads and roundabouts across the country. The protests emerged spontaneously without connections to trade unions, political parties, or established institutions. The movement unites individuals with different political orientations. It appeals primarily to inhabitants of suburban and rural areas who have difficulties in making ends meet. The image of the yellow vest is important since in France every car owner is required by law to have this vest. If there is an accident or breakdown, the driver can put on the vest to ensure visibility and to avoid further accidents. To show the yellow vest means that one does not want to be run over. The protests started with a rise in gasoline taxes. But they were not a symptom of rejection of ecological measures. It was immediately clear to everybody that the tax was another measure favoring the rich at the expense of the majority of the population. Government policies have made life much more expensive especially in rural areas since jobs are usually far away and local transportation has been significantly reduced. Rural people are dependent on cars for shopping, work, and healthcare, more than people in urban areas. They also face lower salaries, pensions, and social security payments. The protest movement started with a post on Facebook. All activities were coordinated online through "groupes colères" ("angry groups") with hundreds of thousands of members. The movement is thus difficult to characterize; it has no leaders and no program. But it represents the average lower middle-class citizens who do not feel represented and even ignored by the political elites in cities such as Paris and Bordeaux. They experience that they are the victims of growing inequalities and injustices. [41] Neoliberal policies protecting the interests of the wealthy produced widespread anger and moral indignation. One of the common slogans used by the yellow vests is: "Dignity for all." It shows that it is not simply a movement of irrational anger; people feel humiliated and are acting out of a sense of social justice and human dignity. [42] Similar movements have articulated the same concerns. In 2011, popular movements called "Los indignados" ("the outraged") disturbed Spain and Greece, protesting against the austerity measures of their governments. They rejected the subjugation of politics and justice to economics. They also denounced the impotence of governments and politicians to protect citizens from injustice and hardship. Neoliberal policies are implemented by established political parties of socialists, conservatives, liberals, and Christian-democrats alike, and they subsume all values under the economic ones. In promoting the image of the occupied square in opposing the political and economic elites, the

Spanish protesters emphasized the square as a public space and global icon that represents the value of active and direct democracy. [43]

The above-mentioned examples illustrate that populism is an expression of moral outrage. It claims rhetorically that the values promulgated by the establishment and the governing elite are morally wrong. Public opinion polls indicate that more people experience feelings of anger, resentment, stress, and worry than a decade ago. [44] Moral outrage is anger because a moral standard is violated. It is a powerful emotion and a source of motivation to engage in action to reaffirm or reestablish the moral standard. Not all forms of anger are emotional responses to violations of moral transgressions. [45] Social media have transformed the expression of moral outrage. It is rare to encounter norm violations in person; only 5% of people report that in daily experiences they witness immoral acts. [46] The internet, however, exposes people to a vast range of misdeeds, corruption, trafficking, dishonesty, and fraud. Nowadays, most people learn about immoral acts online. This online content is also shared. There is evidence that immoral acts encountered online incite stronger moral outrage than immoral acts faced in person or via traditional media. [47] Digital media seem to alter the subjective experience of outrage. They make it easier to express outrage since the threshold for expressing is lower. Since there is not much chance of encountering the wrongdoer, there is little risk of physical retaliation. Anger and moral outrage can be destructive; they can elicit a desire for revenge. [48]

Anger and outrage may also have a positive meaning. They signal moral concern to others. It may enhance the reputation of those expressing them. It publicly clarifies that some behavior is socially not acceptable. Anger has always been an important human emotion. The main question is how to deal with anger and indignation. Anger can make bad situations better because people are listening, speak more honestly, and are more accommodating to complaints and grievances. Moral indignation can therefore be a force for the good. It transforms practical and economic complaints into emotional and moral issues. The protest of the yellow vests is not simply about higher taxes but about justice and equality. People do not merely want higher wages or better working conditions, but their angry movement demands to right an injustice. Moral indignation therefore locates their protest and discontent within a broader fight about rights and wrongs; it reframes complaints into moral offences. [49]

### *Climate change*

The third new context for bioethical discourse is climate change. This is not a long-term problem threatening the survival of future generations but it is a crisis happening now. Climate disasters occur every week. Tsunamis, earthquakes, wildfires, cyclones, droughts, and nuclear accidents cause immense destruction. Climate change makes the unimaginable a reality for many people across the world. Although global warming is known for at least a century (the greenhouse effect was identified in the midst of the 19th century), the Intergovernmental Panel on Climate Change (IPCC) was established in 1988, and the *United Nations Framework*

*Convention on Climate Change* was adopted in 1992, global policies have not been effective. Predicted destructive effects such as rising sea levels, violent weather, loss of biodiversity, extinction of species, desertification, oceanic dead zones, and climate refugees are no longer hypothetical but now observable everywhere. The unprecedented scale of disastrous change creates a sense of calamity. In 2018, the IPCC warned that we only have 12 years left to avoid global catastrophe. [50] This decade is therefore crucial to mitigate the effects of climate change. More and more publications are dismal, depressing, and scaring. The enormous speed of environmental destruction produces apocalyptic scenarios. The planet is rapidly becoming unlivable. Human civilization is on its way to suicide. [51] What is worse, global policies have done everything wrong, and there are no indications that they are effectively changing. Neither human rights activists nor populist movements have taken up the issue.

However, there seems to be an important divide between policy-makers and citizens. A survey in 2019 shows that for 47% of Europeans climate change is the main concern (prior to other concerns such as access to healthcare [39%], unemployment [39%], migration [32%], and terrorism [19%]). [52] Especially young people are concerned: 41% of them imagine that in the near future they have to move to another country because of global warming. They are also most hopeful, with 73% thinking that lifestyle modifications can make a difference and reverse the process of climate change. What is striking today is the activism of young people campaigning for change. Grassroots movements such as Extinction Rebellion, created in 2018, with a youth wing in 2019, engage in non-violent actions and protests. They have declared a climate emergency and demand the establishment of a Citizen's Assembly to put pressure on governments and to break the inertia of politics. [53] Environmental groups, however, have been classified, at least in some countries, as a terroristic threat and security risk, and climate activists today are met with pepper spray and police brutality, even in liberal democracies. [54]

Climate change is not a technical challenge, but primarily a moral problem. It is unlikely that technology that has caused the problem will solve it. What is required is not environmental engineering but a shift in values leading to a new lifestyle and different kind of civilization. This shift is, for example, promoted by Extinction Rebellion: from a technocratic approach focused on reducing carbon emissions to a broader perspective on equitable and just societies with special attention to the vulnerable groups of poor and indigenous people who suffer the most from the effects of global warming. At the same time, it is too easy to give up hope in view of the overwhelming magnitude of the problem. The power of non-violent activism and resistance should not be underestimated. Human beings are not only vulnerable but also resilient. They have always adapted to changed circumstances. Moreover, the human infrastructure should be made resilient, and here technologies can play a role, making housing, roads, factories, and networks for energy and water supply less vulnerable to storms, earthquakes, flooding, droughts, and extreme weather. An appropriate image here is that of bamboo: it is flexible and pliable, and therefore can adapt to the stormy winds; it is also persistent and can tolerate extreme conditions; it is strong because it has deep and interconnected roots. In traditional Chinese culture, knowing more than 400 species of bamboo, the plant symbolizes harmony between nature and human beings. Bamboo represents virtues such as integrity, modesty, loyalty, and resilience. It therefore reflects the soul and emotions of people.

## Implications for ethics

The contemporary contexts of de-globalization, populism, and climate change have moral significance since they imply normative views of human beings, community, society, and human life. First of all, they produce a demystification of dominating images. The prevailing ideology of neoliberalism, which regards the market as a self-regulating mechanism and removes constraints on free competition, has been promoted by images such as the *homo economicus*, the rational individual actor, and the consumer/client. These images may be well entrenched in public and private discourse but do no longer determine economic practices. The French economist Thomas Philippon, for example, has argued that the idea that the United States is the paragon of the free market is no longer true. Commercial sectors are dominated by monopolists and oligopolists that have eliminated effective competition. Growing company profits are not increasingly invested (as neoliberal theory would assume) but handed out as dividends to shareholders. Prices for telephone and internet subscriptions, airplane tickets, and healthcare have substantially increased. There is no stringent regulation of competition like in the European Union. Independent auditing and control are almost absent, while big companies spend large budgets on political lobbying and campaigning. [55] The field of healthcare in the United States, for instance, is characterized by mergers and oligopolistic industries that are classified as tax-exempt non-profit organizations and that reduce competition. Americans spend much more on healthcare than people in other rich countries, not because they consume more care but because the prices are higher. [56] Another example are food subsidies. Contrary to the free market ideology, governments in the United States, the European Union, and Japan provide massive subsidies to farmers. Developing countries have been forced by the WTO to deregulate: removing import restrictions and tariffs, and stopping production subsidies. Farmers in these countries are not protected against the relatively cheap, subsidized food from developed countries. This is not competition but unfair exchange between unequal parties. [57]

Although capitalism has triumphed around the world, it has significant ethical consequences. One is increased inequality and the creation of a new upper class with ideas of moral superiority, while substantial groups of people are regarded as unproductive, redundant, "undesirable," and not worthy of protection and care. The economic system has also changed values. Capitalism has created a new kind of being, prioritizing subjectivity and private experiences. [58] It has reduced social responsibility, not only for individuals but also perhaps even more so for corporations. The most profitable companies hardly pay taxes, while they benefit from the social infrastructure. The result is weakening of social cohesion, democracy, and growing plutocracy. This is exactly the point made by populism. Moreover, the insistence on continuing growth has exacerbated the processes of climate change. Several solutions are available: improve the quality of public education, introduce an inheritance tax, less taxes for the middle classes, and halt the financing of political campaigns, but politicians are not really interested in such solutions. [59]

Especially the image of *homo economicus* is under fire. It is generally accepted that it is a pathological reduction; it does not represent how most people behave in everyday interactions. In well-functioning societies, human beings cooperate and assume mutual obligations. Rather than greed and self-interest, social life is defined by friendship, cooperation, and sociality. [60] Besides, the image wrongly propagates the idea that rationality entails selfishness and non-cooperation. [61] However, in policies and practices, the image continues to prevail and to set standards for how people should behave. This leads to alienation from the discourses of globalization and politics. It is a major source of moral outrage.

Second, the new contexts have changed the role of emotions in the ethical debate. Anger has become a moral force. Injustices created by neoliberal policies produce indignation, and protest against precarity and humiliation, which is exploited by populism. In order to understand why this language of anger and outrage is more than an emotional or irrational response, it is necessary to explore the changing context of human existence. While common in present-day bioethical debates, moral outrage is often not taken seriously in bioethics. Moral outrage is a powerful moral emotion and a source of motivation for moral action, pushing for a society that is more just and sustainable. Anger can make a difference, and ethics should take up the challenge. The point is that people can provide reasons for their anger and frustration. Nowadays, globalization is regarded as exploitation of trust by an elite minority that reaps most of the benefits. The driving force of all policies seems to be the maximizing of profits. Politicians brag that it is smart to evade taxes and not contribute to the common good. Public policies no longer reflect the interests of average citizens. Social media are an important tool to mobilize people denouncing the concentration of wealth and the growth of inequality and vulnerability at the expense of the majority of the population. They also criticize practices of democracy that are not really representative. More importantly, the shared indignation motivates collective action that transforms into connective action: not focused on formal organization but on the use of digital media and sharing of personalized content through social media networks. This kind of action is more fluent and less stable. Activists and self-organizing networks are more autonomous than traditional vehicles of social change.

Third, the new contexts have impacts for deliberation and argumentation, which are the cornerstones of bioethics debate. The assumption is that rational decisions are based on empirical verifiable facts. This emphasis on rationality and facts has become problematic for at least two reasons. One is that it demarcates the public debate on ethical issues in specific ways so that it is the preferable domain of experts in bioethics, science, and policy. Ordinary citizens play a marginal role, and primarily need to be educated and better informed. Bioethics then is often considered as an elite discourse that requests qualified and enlightened participants. Yet, in practice, citizens are not apathic and powerless; they demand a voice in many public debates. Second, the connection between facts and expertise is overridden by emphasis on experience. However, experiences are viewed as subjective. Scientific experts tell us how the world really is. We may experience a beautiful sunrise but in fact the sun does not rise. Things in the world are not how they appear to be, according to the scientific world view. As discussed in Chapter 3, the process of disenchantment has stimulated the growth of subjectivism. This opposes the view that individuals are rational atomistic selves, abstracted from relationships, community, and society. The consequence is that facts have lost their determinative status in many populist debates, and are often regarded as fake and manipulated. [62] One illustration are the continuing controversies about the American healthcare system; the facts and evidence of its high costs and limited results are well known but a rational debate is impossible. Another example is the anti-vaccination movement. While, worldwide, 79% of people agree that vaccines are safe, confidence is much lower in Western Europe (59%) and Eastern Europe (40%). Distrust is highest in France where one in three people disagree that vaccines are safe. [63] "Vaccine hesitancy" is now classified by the World Health Organization as one of the ten threats to global health in 2019. [64] Skepticism about vaccine safety is often related to trust. People who have confidence in doctors and nurses also believe that vaccines are safe. Globally, 73% trust doctors and nurses, and 72% scientists. [65] Generally, in North America and Europe, people rely upon medical advice from health professionals more than government advice. While these levels of trust are high, the impression is that trust is declining. Some studies indicate that in 2016 only 39% of Americans trusted the medical system (down from 80% in 1973). [66] Levels of confidence in the healthcare system vary in Europe: 63% trust the healthcare system in Great Britain, 50% in France, and 45% in Germany. Studies on the development of trust in healthcare over time are scarce. One study in the United States concludes that between 1945 and 2000 public confidence in medicine has declined (from 73% in 1966 to 44% in 2000). [67] This decline can reflect the growing distrust of institutions, government, and policy-makers. Confidence in health professionals has remained relatively high. In the Netherlands, confidence in health professionals and institutions is stable since 1997 (90% for professionals, and 70%–80% for institutions). [68] The interpretation of this data is not straightforward. Increase of distrust in healthcare, at least in some countries, may reflect distrust in institutions, elites, and governments, as argued by populism. Studies show a highly significant positive association between voting for anti-establishment populist parties and vaccine hesitancy. [69] But respect for experts such as health professionals seems not generally declining but perhaps their authority is more in doubt now that people rely more on other sources of information (and often misinformation), and are less convinced by facts and rational arguments.

That bioethics is affected by similar phenomena, as illustrated by the Charly Gard case in the United Kingdom in 2017. Admitted to intensive care at Great Ormond Street Hospital in London when he was 2 months old, Charly was diagnosed with a rare rapidly progressing genetic disease. The hospital team recommended palliative care only. His parents searched the internet and identified an experimental treatment. They contacted the researcher who invited them to treat Charly in the United States. The hospital team in London rejected this idea. The parents thereupon started a social movement, convinced that their severely handicapped child deserved a chance to try the experimental medication. In a short time, they had several hundred thousand supporters across the world, and raised $1.67 million for possible treatment. Through mobilizing support for their case with the use of social media and the internet, the parents created a global controversy. Many people agreed with the parents because they did not trust the establishment (the doctors, hospitals, governments, courts). They were angry that families and parents were overruled, and that hope was taken away. More than 60,000 people created "Charlie's Army" on Facebook to support the parents.

Bioethics witnessed another outbreak of moral outrage at the end of November 2018 when Jiankui He, a Chinese researcher, announced that he has produced two genetically edited babies. [70] He has used the gene-editing technology of CRISPR to alter the genome and make the twin babies resistant to future HIV infection. There was a global outcry of anger and outrage, not only about what he has done but also about how he did it. He has worked outside established protocols. After his university rejected his research proposal, he went to a private hospital. Research results were not published but He used videos claiming to be the first to make edited babies. The Chinese government was embarrassed. For some time, He disappeared; his laboratory and office have been closed. In December 2019, he was sentenced to 3 years in prison. [71] However, until recently He was promoted as a star scientist in China.

The cases of Charly Gard and He Jiankui illustrate that the context of bioethical discourse has changed. First, they show the global power of social media, particularly virtual social networks. Interconnectivity and new information technologies provide people with means to share views, to denounce practices, and to mobilize for protests. Second, the cases demonstrate that in general, and bioethics in particular, debate and protest are motivated by anger and outrage. Anger seems to play a more prominent role now in contemporary societies. Healthcare professionals are confronted with angry patients, not so much directed at them as at the profession. [72]

Finally, climate change has arguably fundamental implications for bioethics. It is by far the most challenging problem today since it jeopardizes the existence of humankind. However, the magnitude of the problem is overwhelming. Daily messages and reports present a litany of plagues and horrors but no perspective on improvement. There is a general sense that it is now almost too late to stop climate change; this could have been done in the 1980s. [73] Within one generation, the planet will be seriously damaged, risking catastrophe not for our children or grandchildren but for ourselves, and the effects will persist for millennia. [74] Ethical discourse seems rather powerless. The problem simply is too big. It is multidimensional (economic, political, psychological, and cultural). Individual choices do not help much unless there is a major political and cultural change. Disaster is no longer caused by distinct decisions (e.g. about the use of nuclear weapons that are also an existential threat) or accidental events (such as the release of biological agents) but it is the outcome of processes that have been initiated long ago and are hardly influenceable today. The Covid-19 pandemic illuminates that infectious diseases are promoted by environmental degradation. Like most disasters, it is not simply a natural event but the product of human behavior, a consequence of our way of life and exploitation of the planet. Drastic measures to mitigate or reverse climate change will have effect only in the long run. Even strongly motivated individuals feel powerless. Climate fatalism, nihilism, denial, and escapism are on the rise. Against this backdrop, ethical discourse seems not only ineffectual but also futile, confronted not only with the violence from global warming, but also from populists, dividing societies, and brutal regimes ignoring human rights. [75] Nonetheless, the main solution to this greatest challenge for humankind is at first sight relatively simple: stop greenhouse gases emissions, and change to renewable energies. [76] This requires a substantial transformation in the way of life of many people. If this is true, the simple solution is not a technical one. It will call for innovative and sustained ethical efforts to prevent that the story of human civilization will come to an end.

## Bioethics dreaming

In Chapter 5, we have argued that the soul should be engaged in bioethics by appealing to the moral imagination. Gaston Bachelard advocated to "sing" reality, going beyond it and projecting other possible realities. Reality is not independent of the means of knowing. Science is not merely descriptive but first of all projective. In Bachelard's words: "The real turns out to be a particular case of the possible." [77] In his philosophy of creativity, Bachelard emphasized the connection between rationality and creativity. Reveries unleash the creative power of human beings; they put projection before reflection.

Regarding bioethics as "imaginative ethics" highlights the characteristics of moral imagination, discussed previously. The ability to imagine is more creative than representational, more productive than reproductive. [78] Imagination has transformative power. On the one hand, it enlarges the horizon of moral concern, and on the other hand, it provides possibilities for action. It interprets the actual in light of what is possible. [79] Ethics embodies the ideals in our lives. Imagination considers those ideals and anticipates the implications and consequences. Moral imagination helps us to understand "what it would be like to live according to some ideal form of life." [80] John Kekes distinguishes three modes of imagination: corrective imagination (the correction of unrealistic views of our limits and possibilities), exploratory imagination (the exploration of possibilities and what it is to live according to the possibilities we have), and disciplined imagination (aiming to make life integrated, i.e. make one's beliefs, emotions, and motives congruous). Bioethics can overcome its narrowness by employing these modes: looking backward and critically evaluating the dominating images of today; looking forward and exploring new and inspiring images; and cultivating a coherent view of human life and social existence.

## Imaginative bioethics

We have argued earlier (Chapter 5) that metaphors play a significant role in ethics. Moral concepts are metaphorical. They help us to frame particular moral situations. Moral reasoning is not merely a matter of deducing moral principles and applying them to cases but it engages the imagination. Ethics is imaginative since it envisions different framings, widens our moral sensibility and perception, and opens up alternative values and perspectives. [81] Following the modes of imagination mentioned earlier, imaginative bioethics has three dimensions.

The first is *correction*. This is the critical dimension of bioethics, reflecting on the images and metaphors that are dominating the current ethical discourse (which we have discussed in Chapter 4). As an activity of retrieval, the underlying philosophy and value perspectives of healthcare are reconsidered, accepting that basic sciences cannot define what is important in care relationships. [82]

The second dimension is *exploration*, that is the search for new images and their assessment. It highlights the creative and productive aspect of imaginative activity, transcending the real world and expanding our sympathies, as the example of the cultivation of human rights in the 18th century through the popular reading of fiction has shown. [83] This dimension releases new possibilities for action because it shifts perspectives and enlarges the moral horizon. Bioethics in this dimension is transformed into an almost prophetic and utopian exercise: it presents visions of possible futures and articulates values that are marginalized, suppressed, or overwhelmed by other value perspectives. Doing so, dominating views are criticized, for example the perception of modern economics that life is constant, endless dealing between selfish maximizers. This neoliberal dystopia assumes a fictional world that has become reality in many countries, despite overwhelming evidence that human societies are based on cooperation, learning, and love. [84] Rather than reinforcing this view by articulating images of autonomous individuals and consumers, bioethics can develop and promote alternative utopias such as the vision of universal human rights. [85] Human rights do not reflect abstract idealism; they are a mix of ethical engagement, legal formalism, and political activism. They are implemented because they inspire people at local levels and in specific circumstances to improve their daily lives. A similar utopian view is presented in the philosophy of personalism. It rejects the world view of naturalism, arguing that human beings transcend the natural order. Dualism is also rejected, arguing that there is only one existing substance, that is the human person as ensouled body. Finally, it rejects individualism, pointing out the essential interconnectedness of human life. Imagining human beings as dignified persons is utopian in the sense that it is a positive vision of future society but it is not without practical consequences. It has motivated the anthropological tradition in philosophy of medicine (see Chapter 2), emphasizing the importance of communication, holistic approaches, empathy, care, and narratives. It has also inspired the founders of the European Union. [86] Finally, the idea of globalization can, first of all, be regarded as utopian. Rather than disqualifying it as unpractical and limiting, it is a regulative and imaginative idea that embodies an ideal that considers the planet as common home, binding all living beings together with a shared destiny. Similar ideas are advanced by personalism. Articulating the interconnectedness of human beings, it promotes the notion of human community, togetherness across national borders.

These utopian views outline ideal forms of life, delineating what it means to live according to ideals of a good life. Utopias are the result of the expansion of our imagination, of dreaming of a better world. They imagine a future that is qualitatively better than the present.

Contrary to the charge that utopian visions are impractical and irrelevant, they show imagination in action. Envisioning possibilities for human life and society, they are, in fact, a precondition for doing something. [87] If there is no desire to make the world different and better than it currently is, the normative power of ethical discourse will be very limited. [88] Utopian visions resist the constraints of the technocratic and economic rationality that alienates the human being from himself. They provide opportunities to escape from Weber's Iron Cage because they reflect attempts to shape the future and open up new horizons of possibilities. [89] The utopian impulse originates from the sense that something is missing. If the soul is eliminated from ethical discourse, as we argue in this book, moral imagination as the source of utopian visions can inspire a broader vision of bioethics. Van Rensselaer Potter clarifies that global bioethics is a utopian vision directed to acceptable survival of the human species. [90] This vision is expressed in the subtitle of his book *Bioethics: Bridge to the future*. Potter was inspired by anthropologist Margaret Mead who argued that utopian visions of a possible and desirable future are of vital importance for the development of culture. [91] In order to make visions of a better world compelling and vivid, it is necessary to combine the methods of the sciences and the humanities, so that new wisdom will emerge from the combination of scientific knowledge and human values. Ethics requires an image of a better world, and in Potter's view this is the utopian vision of enlightened anthropocentrism that aims at a sustainable society and at the common good so that global survival in the long term will be achievable. [92]

The third dimension of imaginative bioethics is *integration*. This dimension combines the corrective and exploratory dimensions, is focused on the present and connecting past and future, and it integrates beliefs, emotions, and motives in order to progress toward a better life. This integration has its starting point in experiences. It is frequently argued that medicine is not sufficiently attentive to the patient's experiences of illness. As a science, it is guided by objectivity, observation, facts, and evidence. But, as we have argued in previous chapters, medicine and healthcare, in general, resist the reduction to science. They cannot neglect the significance of illness and disease for patients and their families, the quest for meaning that is provoked by the human condition, and its different predicaments of age, suffering, and death. Moreover, medicine cannot ignore the ethos of generosity and care that sustains the healing professions. [93] As imaginative ethics, bioethics recognizes the complexity of human experience. First of all, it transcends the analytic and mechanical approaches to the world that dominate scientific ideology, and scrutinizes dehumanizing and objectifying tendencies in present-day culture. It dismisses therefore abstraction and generalization, which often lead to disrespect and humiliation. Ethics starts and advances with the experiences of concrete persons. Second, persons cannot simply be reduced to individuals. They are essentially characterized by relationality. This means that ethics should do more than analyzing the connections and interactions between individuals but should take embeddedness in relational webs as its core notion. As a way of life, ethics is shared with other people. Third, bioethics is primarily a social enterprise based on reciprocity, intersubjectivity, and solidarity. Assisted by moral imagination, it can overcome social pathologies associated with neoliberal ideology and manifested in injustices, inequality, and commodification, and emphasize commonality and the common good.

- ***Back to the actual person***

Bodily experiences are the starting point for healthcare. Phenomena such as illness, suffering, disability, and dying are experienced through our bodies. As embodied persons, we live in the world and are connected to other persons. If we suffer from an illness, we encounter healthcare professionals in the hope that they would attend to our first-person experiences, and not merely investigate possible disease in our body. Experiences also play a crucial role in ethics, as we argued previously. Moral sensibility and perception help us to recognize what is relevant in situations of discomfort, distress, indignity, and injustice. Moral imagination extends our experiences and shifts our perspective to understand the experiences of others. However, the ideology of naturalism and its dominating images distract from the primacy of personal experiences. The split between description and evaluation, the separation of facts and values, locates values outside the scope of reason as subjective preferences. Reason is abstracted from its object and subject, reduced to instrumental and formal rationality. Human beings are conceived as disembodied, rational actors, divorced from their bodies, feelings, and emotions. The focus on individual behavior and choice disconnects from the social environment. Subjects are abstracted from concrete other persons, while the "others" are considered in abstract categories. Human beings are furthermore detached from the natural world. The earth is no longer our home but a resource to be exploited. Globalization is regarded as a set of general processes, abstracted from particular and local conditions. Finally, ethics is seen as an abstract system of applying general principles.

Abstraction leads to alienation and depersonalization. As illustrated in the disenchantment thesis, it produces fragmentation, opposing body and soul, humans and animals, individuals and society, reason and emotion, facts and values. It enhances the power of rationalization and bureaucracy, removing an integrated vision of self and society. Mary Midgley has criticized abstractionism since it implies a narrow conception of humanness. [94] Gabriel Marcel is another philosopher who denounced what he called "the spirit of abstraction." Abstraction is a method, a mental operation to gain clarity; it is always based on concrete conditions in the world. The risk is that abstractions do not remain abstract; they tend to take a concrete life of their own. A current example is the notion of "the people" used in populist discourses without clarifying who are the persons referred to. The spirit of abstraction is therefore different from abstraction as a method. It takes abstraction as more real, certain, and reliable than the world from which it is derived. An example is the interpretation of human reality as determined by economic facts. The "economy" then determines human life. Abstraction is a reductive operation but its results are granted more reality than the reality upon which it is based. Another example is the vision of the human being as an atomistic and self-centered individual. This operation makes the individual impersonal and without any connections to other persons. In modern culture and technology, processes of degradation are at work that produce situations in which the individual "loses touch with himself." [95] For Midgley and Marcel, philosophy as well as ethics should resist processes of abstraction that degrade the human person into a mechanism, an object assimilated to the world of things. In their search for wholeness, philosophy and ethics should bring back the person and his or her immediate experiences.

- ***Relationality***

The abstractionist conception of humanness has affected the perspective of relationships. A new approach to bioethics should articulate that human persons are essentially characterized by relationality. As integrated wholes, unities of body and soul, they are embedded within communities. Relationality is not the same as relatedness. One often thinks about relationships from the perspective of individualism. A person is continuously engaging in relations with other entities. In fact, there are two different orientations to the world. In instrumental relations, we use objects and persons for ends we want to accomplish. Interpersonal relations are different since we engage with other persons for their own sake. These last relationships are possible since we are in the same predicament as other people. In this context, the notion of relationality expresses that persons not merely connect and interact with each other but belong together and are mutually dependent, engaging, taking responsibility, and shaping their lives in sharing the world with each other. Relationships with other persons define who a person is. As argued in Chapter 4, the significance of relationality has redefined the concept of individual autonomy in bioethical discourse into "relational autonomy." One implication of this redefinition is the important role of encounter, meeting, and dialogue. The person becomes himself in meeting other persons. Authentic being is being-together. According to personalist philosophers, intersubjective connections are constitutive for humanity. The primordial experience of human beings is that they share the world with others. Gabriel Marcel uses the notion of "presence" to explain that we are not simply beings that are there and then relate to world. Encounter involves being present to each other. Consciousness of being in the world implies that we are not locked into our individuality. Human beings are conscious of existence as coexistence and they need to be recognized by other persons to integrate the self as a person. An essential characteristic of the person, in Marcel's view, is availability (*disponibilité*). [96] Being available and receptive to others is not simply openness. It means the opportunity to undergo new experiences and to enhance one's life. It is also an opportunity to break through Weber's Iron Cage. [97] The self-interested *homo economicus* is not available. The difficulty is, again according to Marcel, that the world is broken, that is the essential connection between human beings and the world is fractured as the result of processes of abstraction and objectification. The human person himself is often treated as an object like other things in the world, so that personal relationships with other persons and the world have become problematic. The ideology of the market has reduced interpersonal relationships to contractual and impersonal interactions. Societies constantly move toward depersonalization, for example by categorizing persons in abstract terms as "immigrants" or "muslims." However, in exceptional circumstances such as in confrontation with disease, disability, and death, the lived experience of being together returns. [98] During the Covid-19 pandemic, one of the most commonly used sayings refer to togetherness. All people, regardless of where they are, are in this scourge together, and even when they cannot meet, physical distancing makes them more aware of the importance of relationality, the experience of "we."

Another aspect of the notion of relationality highlights the intimate connection between body and soul. Through the body, persons are situated in space and time but are also members of the world community. [99] That human persons are situated does not mean that they are static and bounded. They are continuously in quest of themselves, not simply being but being-on-the way. Humans are situated as "travelers." Rather than spectators or detached observers of the world, they are participants. Marcel therefore uses the image of the "journey" to explain the basic human condition. But it is the soul that is the traveler, "being on the way." [100] It is peculiar for human beings to live between the possible and the actual. They want to go beyond the world of facts and events, and they have the power of hope to expand horizons. The hope and desire for a better way of being and living also situates ethics between what humans are and what they should become.

Situatedness is furthermore a precarious experience. Relationality is not an option. Human beings are necessarily related. Because the body is our positioning in the world, we are exposed to the world and other persons. That implies fundamental vulnerability. Authentic relationships are both a blessing and a wound. The other person that we encounter is a blessing since we otherwise cannot become a person ourselves and flourish as a human being. But the other may also wound us. Life in community with others (*communitas*) is ambivalent; it entails pain, harm, and injury. Social life is thus related to suffering. Neoliberal ideology is focused on the possible wounds rather than blessings: others are potential negative factors, and the emphasis should be on independency. In this ideology, a specific model of cooperation is promoted with core notions such as self-interest and contractual relations with the purpose to avoid being wounded by others. Such model attempts to provide *immunitas* instead of accepting *communitas*. [101]

- ***Common good***

However, when existence is coexistence, and bioethics a social enterprise based on reciprocity and solidarity, other perspectives arise, articulating the idea of human community, togetherness across borders, with interdependency rather than interactive relationships between separate individuals. As social beings, humans are evaluative beings; they do not have a neutral or indifferent stance toward the world. Particularly since they are vulnerable beings, they want to know how important things are because they may produce suffering or enhance well-being. In other words, they have relations of concern to the world. [102] It matters to them what happens and what is done. That explains why they are sometimes outraged and feel that their dignity is not respected. Ethical theory cannot be abstracted from the social context in which human beings live and act. This conclusion also relates to the purpose of ethical discourse: avoiding harm and promoting well-being and human flourishing. Ethics cannot be reduced to principles and norms but is pertinent to our sense of flourishing and harm, taking into account our capabilities as well as vulnerability.

As a social enterprise emphasizing the relationality and embeddedness of persons, bioethics needs the notion of the common good. The person as embodied soul and social being is more than an individual. Also, society is more than the aggregate of individuals. The purpose of society is not only the well-being of discrete individuals but the good of all its members. Examples are health, peace, and justice. These goods constitute the common good since they are desirable for society as a whole and advantageous to every citizen. They cannot be achieved by individual efforts but require collective action and the engagement of all citizens and therefore solidarity and social responsibility. All members of society benefit from this common good, although it can only be attained by mutual and communal endeavors. The common good is not just a description of what is important for societies but it is a normative concept. It refers to values, virtues, and ideals that express what it means to have a good life together within society. [103]

These characteristics of the common good are evident in the Covid-19 pandemic, exemplifying the common good of public health. Measures such as staying at home, reducing contacts with other people, and regularly washing hands not only protect individual health but also diminish the harm for society and promote the common good. Physical distancing is, in fact, a social act. It makes human interconnectedness apparent to everybody. Acting for the common good requires sacrifices from an individualistic perspective. The many health professionals who put their lives at risk to treat and take care for others are an obvious illustration of this. At the same time, physical distancing is resisted from the perspective of individualism demonstrating how this perspective has downgraded the idea of the common good. It furthermore shows the inadequacy of framing the pandemics in terms of an alien invader, coming from a foreign country and positing us against them. This framing puts the focus on individual behavior, while our behavior, in fact, protects everyone. It also singles out vulnerable groups such as the elderly and people in poverty, while, in fact, everyone can be affected. Viewing social connections as threats and individual actions as harmful to others does not point out the shared conditions that increase potential harm for all citizens.

The idea of the common good, though already advanced by Aristotle, is rehabilitated in the context of globalization. In view of increasing environmental degradation, appeals are frequently made to the common good in order to protect future generations and the survival of humankind. This appeal is used to argue that individual and collective interests should be better balanced. The common good promotes a perspective beyond individual preferences and choices. The common good, however, is not contrasted to individual goods. Its proper contrast is with particular goods. It is also different from collective or public goods such as clean air, safe water, and street lights. These goods are enjoyed by many persons individually. The common good, by contrast, is enjoyed not by individuals only but by persons in their relationships to others. It is not the aggregate of particular goods. Necessary to support human flourishing, the common good is the result of collective actions as a shared goal of all citizens. Hence, the importance of participation and communication, often expressed in symbols of togetherness. Health is an example of the connection as well as difference between individual and common good. Health is a necessary and universal condition for human flourishing. It is an individual good that allows each person to live according to his or her wishes and values. At the same time, health as a common good is only realized if certain conditions are fulfilled: sanitation, clean air and safe water, adequate food, and access to essential medicines. These conditions require common efforts.

The common good is used to redefine the market ideology, arguing that a shift is necessary away from short-term efficiency and financial gains. The neoliberal ideology has not fulfilled its promises. Rising prosperity is associated with increasing levels of unhappiness. Interpersonal interactions are reduced to contractual and impersonal relationships, making people immune to each other and destroying the feeling to belong to a community with values such as reciprocity, fraternity, and gratuitousness. [104] Restoring the notion of common good will transform the market and thus economics into "civil economy," regarding the market as a place to practice civic virtues. This change will improve the quality of human relationships and therefore subjective well-being. In the tradition of civil economy, the market is based on reciprocity, mutual assistance, and friendship, while its main concern is public happiness rather than profit and wealth. [105] Rational self-interest does not produce happiness. Since happiness is a relational good, and not an instrumental good or commodity, not simply pleasure, it cannot be produced or consumed by one individual but it needs encounters, interaction with other persons. The essential role of relationality requires a different model of cooperation. Rather than regarding it as an instrument to achieve particular ends, cooperation should be regarded as valuable for its own sake. It is not so much the product delivered or the end achieved that counts but the experience and process of cooperating. The first view assumes that cooperation is the interaction between rational and self-interested individuals. It is a means to a particular purpose. There is no value in cooperating; its value is in the results that satisfy self-interested parties. In this perspective, cooperation is always instrumental. The emphasis on relationality and common good introduces a different perspective. People share common interests, for example being healthy. They cooperate because they are concerned with health as common good. Cooperation may bring benefits to themselves, though it may also include costs and sacrifices; they work together since they are concerned for humankind, for example global health or the survival of humanity; these concerns can only be address through collective and collaborative action. As a cooperative species, humans work together for the common good since they value cooperation (and solidarity) for its own sake. [106]

The notion of common good has rehabilitated the traditional concept of "commons." [107] Fishing grounds, forests, water supplies, air, and land available for public use are considered as commons, that is domains, materials, products, resources, and services not owned by anybody but shared. Water, air, the seabed, genetic diversity, and scientific knowledge are regarded as global commons since they are important for humankind as a whole. Commons share several basic features. First, they refer to collective property, jointly owned by a group of people (as in local commons) or belonging to all persons on earth (as in global commons). Second, they are essential for human subsistence and long-term survival (since they provide water, food, shelter but also health and knowledge). Third, commons need to be protected for future generations so that sustainability is important. Commons, finally, are not simply resources; they are social practices (some advocate the use of the verb "commoning"). They express a discourse of sociality, reciprocity, sharing, and social harmony. Commons refer to togetherness ("commonwealth"), not only with people but also with nature, environment, and land. Globalization has created new commons. Examples are digital commons based on the internet, but also airspace commons (for international air transport), ether space commons (for radio and television broadcasting), weather forecasting systems, and pools of crop genetic diversity. These new commons are global; they transcend national boundaries; they are shared around technologies and user communities; they require collective actions and negotiations; they are valuable for human existence and nature. The discourse of commons does not fit into the neoliberal distinction between private and public ownership; it is situated between market and state. It has received new attention in response to the global regime of intellectual property rights that allows patenting of new drugs, genetic resources, indigenous knowledge, and all forms of biological life. This regime has facilitated global inequalities, particularly impeding access to affordable medication. With the Covid-19 pandemic, questions have emerged in regard to potential treatments and vaccines; as results of common efforts, they should be considered as commons and thus should be available to all persons who will need them. They cannot be appropriated by specific countries, companies, or research institutions. The notion of commons is used to redefine science as an open and shared activity, even when it is nowadays heavily commercialized. The idea of science commons is reflected in the movement toward open access publications. Progress of science and dissemination of knowledge require that access to scientific information is unrestricted. [108] The concept of commons illustrates the recognition that there are goods that are essential for human well-being and that can only be accomplished in a common effort.

The notion of common good can furthermore be used to rethink the notion of democracy. Basically, democracy is a way of life focused on the common good. It institutes rules and practices of engagement and participation to create a better way of life for all citizens than in other political regimes. However, as pointed out earlier, currently democracy is often subordinated to capitalism and the ideology of the market. Economic growth has not equally distributed wealth, while commodification of healthcare, education, and outsourcing of employment together with increasing surveillance have led to the collapse of social networks and impoverished the idea of common good. [109] The result is anger with technocratic and neoliberal policies manifested in the rise of populism, with people arguing that they first of all need protection rather than merely economic growth. People feel forgotten and not represented by democratic institutions. Underlying this democratic disillusionment is a restricted view of democracy. Rather than with institutions and representation, democracy has to do with social relationships. It is a regime to produce a shared social life aimed at the common good. As a characteristic of civil society, it relates first of all to questions of solidarity, equality, social welfare, and social redistribution. Democracy is defined by its works; it is permanent work in progress, indeterminate and never completed, as argued by Rosanvallon. [110] Over time, democracy has shown many faces and shapes. It is not a universal political form that can be expanded over the globe, regardless of cultures and traditions. Moreover, it has included distrust, tension, and conflict with a range of practices to exert pressure on rulers and to resist political powers. Instead of arguing that democracy is declining (with abstention of voting as an example), citizens are not passive but involved in a multitude of democratic practices interacting at all levels of society, engaging and participating in different forms of political expression, in strikes, petitions, and demonstrations. Populism is democratic pathology because it uses these forms of "counter-democracy" in a destructive way with stigmatization, accusation, and repression of otherness, disseminating "alternative facts" and conspiracy theories. The good promoted is not common but first of all shared by the "real people" with the exclusion of elites and non-natives. Democracy, however, with its focus on the common good, emphasizes that sharing values will deliver long-term benefits (e.g. health, peace, and prosperity). It also offers dignity, that is respect for all persons and their views. [111]

## A new concept of bioethics

The above-mentioned concepts and arguments give substance to a new and broader concept of bioethics. First of all, by articulating the notion of human person, human beings are not regarded as abstract and de-contextualized individual entities. They are related to each other and socially connected. This interpretation does not reject the significance of individual autonomy, but uses a broader concept of autonomy as relational and as constituted through interactions in social life. The context of personal existence (especially human vulnerability) should be taken into account when bioethical analyses are produced. Second, society is not an aggregate of individuals. It provides the conditions that make human flourishing, particularly health possible. A positive image of society articulates the importance of cooperation (rather than competition), social responsibility (rather than individual responsibility), and solidarity (rather than private interests). Third, the focus on the common good emphasizes that human beings are living together and sharing resources that are essential to all of them in order to flourish and survive. Common interest refers not to the summation of private interests. The neoliberal assumption that human beings are driven by rational self-interest is rejected; they are citizens concerned with the common good. Fourth, if human beings can only flourish within relationships, it is important to continuously change and improve the conditions in which humans exist. This requires collective action and engagement, not only at the global level (with increased cooperation and global networking) but also at the local levels (with local activism).

## The end of bioethics

The journal *Nature* recently published an article on the present state of bioethics, concluding that it has been successful but that its allure is now fading away. While today there is a sense of ethical bewilderment in view of all scientific advancements and technological innovations, bioethics is increasingly lost; it is fragmented and functioning as "a dashboard of pragmatic instruments." [112] Specialized ethical expertise is less needed, and ethical guidance is more and more provided by other experts and interdisciplinary bodies. Although the article was only focused on research ethics, it has been taken as an irreverent blow to the field of bioethics. The thesis that bioethics has come to an end reminds us of the prediction of pioneer biologist Gunther Stent. In *Science* in 1968, he concluded that molecular biology has become a "workaday field." The major discoveries were made, and scientists only need to iron out the details. [113] This was stated just before research in this field exploded, especially in new areas such as genomics. At the same time, some policy-makers decided that the war on microbes has been won and that infectious diseases were history.

Another type of arguments evokes the end of bioethics from a different angle. One version is that bioethical analysis is often too abstract and does not help us to address concrete issues. Moral decisions in real everyday practice are most of the time not guided by ethical theories. Another version, the reverse of the former one, is that bioethics has become so pragmatic that ethical expertise, in fact, is superfluous. Smart people can explain and address the relevant moral issues without any help of bioethics as an academic discipline or specific field of expertise. From both arguments, it cannot be concluded that bioethics has ended, but only that the scope and impact of bioethics as it is currently practiced is rather limited and perhaps finite. Bioethics nowadays has many shapes, and precisely in response to criticism of abstract or pragmatic approaches, it is frequently redefining itself in diverse directions. But the arguments raise the fundamental question whether bioethics, regardless of its shape and approach, is facing limitations and is perhaps too demanding. Ethical discourse formulates what we should do. It uses a special vocabulary to point out our duties, rights, and responsibilities. It specifies what is the good that we should achieve. Or it underlines the character traits that we should have in order to live a good life. But, in many circumstances, the moral requirements of deontological, consequentialist, or virtue ethics theories cannot be fulfilled. They impose impossible demands. During the Covid-19 pandemic, for example, it was argued that intensive care should only be given to patients with the best chance of survival, in order to maximize the number of lives saved. Doctors should not give priority to elderly and vulnerable persons, even if they are relatives, friends, or colleagues. On the other hand, arguing that each human life is worth saving regardless of the expected outcomes will overburden the healthcare system, will not prevent that many people die, and will give priority to those who contact health professionals immediately and in an early stage of the disease. Even when healthcare workers sacrifice themselves and provide as much care as possible, they cannot save all infected persons. Living and acting according to moral theories is asking too much. Most of us do not want to be moral villains but we cannot be moral saints or heroes either.

The thesis that ethical discourse is too demanding does not imply the end of ethics. However, it necessitates a rethinking of the force of ethics in everyday life. Two options have been developed. One is to accept that ethics can sometimes demand the impossible, that it requires us to do something that we cannot do. In some situations, moral failure is unavoidable. It is important to distinguish between two types of impossible moral requirements. One type is negotiable. An example is a moral dilemma: we are confronted with two moral requirements that cannot both be satisfied but an argument can be made that one requirement is more important than the other so that we can escape from the dilemma. Other moral conflicts are non-negotiable; the moral requirements cannot be satisfied but they remain binding. This is the case when sacred values are involved; these values cannot be balanced against other values. They cannot even be subjected to critical examination since it is unthinkable not to do what they require. In such cases, the moral conflict cannot be eliminated. The moral requirement (the "ought") continues to exist even when it is impossible to fulfill (the "ought" then does not imply the "can"). This response to the impossible demands of ethics accentuates that we sometimes face moral failure that is unavoidable. The possibility of conflict is built in the nature of human beings and in the heterogeneity of moral life. [114] This first option is perhaps theoretically awkward from the perspective of bioethics as a rational discipline, but it proceeds from the experience of moral life. It underlines that moral judgment and reasoning in many cases cannot help us to solve moral conflicts. Moral judgments are often influenced by moral intuitions, emotions, and feelings, and not the result of a reasoning process. Furthermore, in moral conflicts different kind of values are involved. There is not simply value pluralism but some values are not commensurable and cannot be included in trade-offs because they are sacred. [115]

The second option to deal with the impossible demands of ethics is to find a way out in accepting the limits of the prevalent ethical theories and formulating a more feasible morality. Instead of making moral life too difficult and appealing to everyone to be an exemplary moral person, an alternative moral framework may focus on the notion of decency. This framework accepts our moral limits and nonetheless gives guidance to the way we daily live as moral beings. Such ethics of decency has been proposed by Todd May. [116] The assumption is that most people want to live a morally decent life, rather than following traditional ethical theories because the theories demand more than people are capable of. This does not mean that people do not care about ethics, but they often are committed to projects of life, and have many other non-moral engagements making life worthwhile that they cannot sacrifice because of ethical requirements. Moral decency therefore is located between moral purity and moral depravity. Another assumption is that the core notion of ethics is preserved, that is recognition of others in the world. [117] We have encounters, interpersonal contacts, usually face to face, with family and friends. The faces of other people, even if we do not know them, instigate us to treat them more humanely and decently because we recognize them as persons like us living a life like us. Furthermore, we experience similar connectedness with others when they are distant in space or in time; we recognize that we are also citizens of the world, and that we can make a contribution to the world. This perspective of ethics articulates some of the ideas we have described in previous chapters. First, it clarifies the significance of moral experience. In our daily interactions, we experience that we live together. The experience that we share the world motivates us to recognize, in the words of May, that there are others who have lives to live. This experience relativizes individualistic perspectives and motivates us to respect the humanity of others. Second, it highlights the moral relevancy of the notions of relationality and connectedness. These notions bring us beyond the simple acknowledgement that there are other beings in the world. Ethics is not an abstract exercise but involves other persons. They remind us that human beings are "fundamentally *imaginative* moral animals." [118] Because we can imagine that others have their own engagements and projects in life, we recognize and respect them. Third, this perspective does not regard ethics as a burden but emphasizes the opportunities for solidarity with another person, not because we have obligations or duties but because we share the same world. Ethics has a prophetic role. It is not a defensive enterprise that determines what should be allowed and what can be done or not, but it is a positive effort to imagine what is worthwhile and valuable, evoking a positive sense of contributing to a better world.

The discussion about the end of bioethics does not result in the conclusion that this field of activity has come to a closure. Rather, reflecting on its end opens new possibilities. Bioethics as a prophetic activity relies on the moral imagination. It accepts that human beings are the only creatures with the capacity for imagination. As *homo imaginens*, they can conceive alternative futures. Through this capacity, they can challenge the domination by rationalistic and bureaucratic forces. Imagination enables humans to apprehend that there are "more things in the universe than are dreamed of by the rationalist epistemologies and ontologies of science." [119] Introducing new metaphors and imaginary visions, bioethics can overcome the rule of the metaphors of the market: efficiency, profit, consumption, self-interest, and competition. Imagination is indispensable when bioethics is redefined in terms of moral decency. Recognition of other people with whom we share the world depends on the imaginary capability to place ourselves in their shoes. Imagining the life situation and projects of other people expands our sympathies and enlarges our horizon. This capability allows us, as we have argued earlier, to shift perspectives from first person to second person and back, and reach a third-person perspective. Shifting perspectives are necessary because humans are social beings, continuously interacting with others and involved in shared, social practices. They operate in what personalist philosophers have called the sphere of intersubjectivity, of mutuality, in which values, hopes, expectations, and fears are shared and exchanged. Humans are not only observers and spectators but also, as participants in social life, evaluative beings. They continuously evaluate themselves, other people, and the circumstances in which they live. [120] It is the consequence of vulnerability. Human existence is precarious; human beings can flourish but also suffer and be harmed. It therefore matters to them what happens in regard to their well-being, health, work, relationships, and religious and political practices. They are concerned about the world. [121] Since the quality of relationships is essential for their well-being and happiness, human beings appraise their relations with the world and with others. Such evaluation often starts with moral emotions such as indignation, outrage, and disgust, but likewise empathy, respect, and gratitude. Emotions motivate to reflect upon the situation. They express values that are not beyond the scope of reason; we can argue about them.

As a shared way of life, and social, evaluative enterprise, ethics in general identifies what human beings have in common, while at the same time acknowledging that people are different in many dimensions. They share vulnerabilities, dependencies, and basic needs; they have the same capacity for reflexivity and narrativity. This recognition has enlarged the circle of moral concern. Not only moral sensibilities but also moral responsibility and agency have expanded, as is visible in human rights and humanitarian movements across the globe. This widening of the scope of application of ethics does not impose homogeneity and uniformity. Instead, it is associated with recognition of differences and plurality of values. Against this background, the main challenge of ethics is how we should life together. The perspective of moral decency relates ethics to civilization.

## Bioethics and civilization

Contemporary civilization is strongly characterized by science, and biotechnology in particular, and globalization. We have argued in previous chapters how these influences are noticeable in the images that dominate current discourse and that frame how human beings view themselves and the world. These images establish a repertoire of activities expected from responsible people. The emergence of biopower promoted the idea of biological citizenship. Since the body is a mechanism that can be shaped and reshaped by medical and genetic technologies, each citizen is expected to act as a rational, autonomous individual who invests in his or her biological capital and takes care for the body and bodily health through self-care and self-conduct. In this new context, bioethics is not contingent. It has emerged as the peculiar expression of the values of contemporary civilization, articulating individual respect and responsibility. Introducing a new discourse, it assisted in the reconciliation of citizens with the progress of science and medicine as well as the neoliberal policies by articulating the significance of individual autonomy. The new discipline, moreover, developed governance practices that assisted society to respond to the challenges of biotechnology. [122] However, bioethics is not only expressive but also formative. It is influencing society because it advocates decent behaviors and attitudes in regard to health, science, and interactions with health-care professionals. It advances particular values to civilize the mindset and actions of citizens, for example self-determination, respect, and responsibility.

The essence of civilization, according to Collingwood, is civility: the determination to convert occasions of non-agreement into occasions of agreement. [123] Civilization is a process directed toward the ideal of civility, which is the absence of force in relationships with others. Its aim is to create a social community, escaping the state of barbarity in which actions are focused on individual survival. To civilize is to socialize. [124] In such social community, each citizen recognizes that his or her freedom is connected to the recognition of the freedom of others. This recognition means self-respect as well as respect for fellow citizens. It entails the expectation that they treat us with similar respect as we treat them. Collingwood points out that the civilizing process has three constituents. The first concerns the relations within the community. Members of the same community show civil behavior to one another, respecting their feelings, values, and freedom, and refraining from the use of force in interpersonal relations. The precise modes of civilized conduct will differ according to historical and cultural settings. The second concerns the relations with people outside the community. They are not treated as objects in the natural world that can be exploited but as human beings entitled to the same civility as members of one's own community. The third constituent are the relations with things in the natural world. They are also entitled to civil behavior. A civilized community will use nature to produce food, clothing, and medication but will do that in an intelligent way, thus not by exploiting nature so that resources will vanish. It is clear from these constituents that the achievements of civilization are fragile. The ideal state of civility can only be approximated. There is always a mixture of civil and barbarous elements. Collingwood's constituents are not factual descriptions but refer to a process of approximation of an ideal state of civilization. They illuminate that civilization is a moral concept. This normative dimension is particularly emphasized by Albert Schweitzer. [125] Civilization, according to him, implies the development and implementation of moral standards in order to organize society in a way that is not rude, savage, or barbarous. Good manners, civil conduct, politeness, and cleanliness are surface phenomena of the basic values of mutual respect and recognition. Civilization is first of all a mental disposition, "a thing of the mind" although it is manifested in material accomplishments. [126] In Schweitzer's analysis, contemporary civilization is unbalanced since the material dimension is more developed than the ethical one. The ultimate aim of civilization, in his opinion, is the spiritual and moral perfecting of individual citizens, not external, material progress. [127]

This raises the question of moral progress. As we have discussed before, in the history of humanity the moral horizon has gradually widened. People have become concerned with the predicament of distant others and with the future of the planet. Human rights have emerged as a global standard. Cultural and religious pluralism have become more widespread. Democratic regimes are more common than before. [128] Nonetheless, these accomplishments of civilization are fragile. Especially the 20th century has presented a long history of war, violence, and cruelty. Celebrities such as Zweig and Schweitzer have denounced the moral decay and decline of civilization. In his moral history of the 20th century, Jonathan Glover argues that deterioration was due to lack of moral imagination. [129] Humans could not imagine the monsters that dwell inside them, could not envision the inhumanity and savagery from which millions of people were suffering. Moral restraints failed because they were neutralized or anesthetized, or because they were overwhelmed by tribalism and ideology. Nowadays, humans are perhaps more aware of moral resources and restraints. At least, with modern communication technology, global suffering, cruelty, racism, and injustice are hard to deny. More importantly, they show the importance of small acts that reinforce human decencies in everyday life, such as stories of sheltering a Jewish family during the last war, or current student initiatives to provide food and encouragement to elderly people who are afraid to leave their home during the Covid-19 pandemic. These acts show that moral resources are mobilized: empathy with other people and respect for their dignity. They also reinforce our moral identity as members of a community who care about each other.

The role of moral imagination reinstates the significance of the soul in ethics as well as in civilization. Imagination generates different ways of interpreting the world, bringing us beyond the realities and experiences of everyday life, not accepting the inhumanities and injustices that persist in civilization. Engaging in the reveries of Bachelard or the "musement" of Peirce is to dream other avenues and possibilities, to develop alternatives to the dystopian visions of naturalism and neoliberalism. The power of moral imagination is that it expands our sympathies and enables to empathize with others. [130] For these reasons, empathy is regarded as a crucial determinant of civilization. Understanding the feelings and experiences of other persons, makes it possible to see the world from other points of view and to recognize other perspectives. It does more than facilitating relationships but fosters cooperation and civility. [131] Ethologists argue that empathy is a universal trait of human beings, part of human evolution as an innate capacity. [132] Natural selection has fostered the human capacity for cooperation, friendship, and social learning. [133] Empathy is a condition for cooperation. Without cooperation, civilization cannot materialize; it is not an individual affair; it is formed and shaped by cooperative activities focused on the common good.

Is there progress in bioethics? It is hard to deny that as a discipline and activity, bioethics has become more sophisticated and better implemented. Scholarly publications in this field are so abundant that no person is able to cope with the literature, which is increasingly specializing and subspecializing. Bioethics is nowadays an accepted component of medical education, clinical practice, and research evaluation. Governance practices in healthcare and medical research at various levels cannot neglect to address bioethical implications. Numerous media stories refer to moral queries and bioethical experts are invited to clarify them. Bioethics has become such a familiar aspect of present-day civilization that the argument that it is fading away is understandable: being so normalized, it is less visible as a separate endeavor. Yet these observations refer to the exterior advances of bioethics as a subject, activity, discipline, and enterprise. Another question is whether there is moral progress. Has bioethics contributed to improvement of healthcare? Has it succeeded in accomplishing its aims? Answering these questions is more problematic. Bioethical discourse certainly has increased awareness of patient rights. Medical practices are more concerned with careful information and communication. Research projects take into account the concerns of patients and subjects. At the same time, as we have seen in earlier chapters, bioethics is facing a continuous challenge. Since ethics is not simply a matter of applying principles and norms but reflects a way of life, it needs continuous nurturing and practicing. Knowing that informed consent is a moral requirement does not necessarily lead to a specific communicative and dialogical practice. The significance of research integrity is emphasized in all codes of conduct for scientists. Nonetheless, conflicts of interests emerge again and again. Moral progress therefore can never be assumed but requires constant vigilance and sustenance.

The limited scope of bioethics, which we have criticized in previous chapters, is an important consideration here. If it is agreed that progress is made, it is done within a restricted playing field. Bioethics could be more impactful if it has a wider scope and a prophetic approach. Explicit use of the moral imagination as one of the powers of the soul transforms bioethics into a civilizing force. Recognizing that we share the world with many different people, bioethical discourse is not just focused on solving clinical problems but it contributes to making social interactions more decent, even outside the direct context of healthcare, resisting tendencies to dehumanize people. It expresses a sense of recognition of others, as well as solidarity with others. A decent society is one whose institutions do not humiliate people. Humiliation is injury of self-respect; humans are treated as if they were not human. Respect, on the other hand, means that appropriate weight is given to the well-being and values of people. [134] Recognition, however, is not an individual but social accomplishment. The economic order promoted by neoliberal policies has led to the moral impoverishment of the social life-world. It has multiplied experiences of injustice, especially of humiliation and disrespect. Because recognition is refused or withdrawn, moral injuries will result. Dignity, integrity, and honor are not respected. The normative assumptions of social interaction are violated, and people will react with indignation and anger. These forms of disrespect should be addressed in an ethics of decency and reciprocal recognition. [135] This broader view of ethics underlines that dignity is not only an intrinsic quality of all human beings, but also a relational quality, depending on recognition and respect, thus on how people treat each other. [136] Ethics is a continuous interactive and evaluative process within the world and with others, not a series of discrete decisions on the basis of moral beliefs and principles. These considerations release a global bioethical mindset. They acknowledge that globalization has prioritized economic and political interests at the expense of social and ethical concerns. The Covid-19 pandemic brought back to mind that interpersonal relationships and social reciprocity are more elementary than commerce and market exchanges. It also learns that it is necessary to delink globalization from neoliberalism. The pandemic is not merely a global phenomenon but, like other zoonoses, the result of exploitative violations of biodiversity and animal life. It is one of the nefarious effects of globalization, and it will most probably only reinforce processes of marginalization, injustice, and inequality.

## The role of education

Ethics education is frequently advocated as an adequate antidote to the loss of soul. It should be able to produce attentive and caring physicians by nurturing their souls. [137] Given the enormous efforts made over the past decades in expanding and intensifying ethics education, it is questionable whether it can indeed help us to achieve the dream of making medicine more humanistic and holistic, especially when it is argued that bioethics itself has lost its soul. Even when it is acknowledged that medical education is in a crisis and that the current education model has serious shortcomings, it does not imply that more emphasis on ethics will be a solution.

How can the soul of medicine be recovered? Kuczewski emphasizes the role of medical humanities. [138] They show the human aspects of care and the subjective experiences of patients as well as the importance of social interaction. What is highlighted is the contribution of moral imagination. Moral imagination is not merely an inventive power that gives us different ways of seeing the world. First of all, it provides the capability to empathize with others. It helps us to experience the situation of other human beings, to recognize situations like ours, and to notice the moral demands that others make upon us. Second, moral imagination identifies various possibilities for acting. It encourages us to envision how action might help or hurt, to anticipate possible consequences of action, and to project possibilities into the future. [139]

Some scholars argue that reflection is the best way to overcome the shortcomings of medical education. [140] Assuming that the main purpose of education is not transfer of knowledge but transformation and learning how to live, they stress that medical students should be required to visit patients at home, to communicate with them and to understand how the illness influences the patient's life. Being confronted with the subjective life-world of patients is a first step to reflect on what is the fundamental fact of medical care. Another road to reinsert the soul in medical practice is the concept of spirituality. [141] Over the past 10 years, spirituality has been the subject of substantial research output (1,516 publications in 2019 according to PubMed). It has a specific role to play in medical education and is more and more included in medical curricula. Education may be regarded as an enterprise that is specifically targeting the human soul. The first defining attribute of spirituality is: teaching with all heart and soul.

The focus on spirituality illustrates the importance of accompaniment and empathy. Medical education needs to attend to clinical cases, patients' stories, illness narratives, and subjective experiences. They require skills of interpretation and making sense of things. The pragmatic view of ethics education regards ethics teaching as a way of learning skills for analyzing and resolving the moral dilemmas that will confront health professionals in their future practices. The role of bioethics education therefore is limited. It should focus on what is practical and measurable. In this educational philosophy, it is not realistic to expect that ethics education can create morally better physicians and scientists. After all, how can a limited number of courses bring about a change in behavior or character of health professionals? The primary objective therefore is to teach skills so that it will ultimately lead to better professional decisions.

Fortunately, there is another view of ethics education that is bolder and more idealistic. In this philosophy, bioethics education is not merely focused on skills to improve decision-making but is basically a long-term effort to create better health professionals and scientists. It is aimed at character formation, integrity, and professional virtues. Rather than enhancing professional skills, it aims to improve the professional himself or herself. Only in this way can bioethics teaching contribute to enhancing the quality of patient care. This broader philosophy is motivated by the fact that bioethics education was initially introduced and promoted to counteract dehumanizing and objectifying tendencies in contemporary medicine and healthcare. It is not just there to facilitate medical decision-making, but it should contribute to making medical practice more humane. For this reason, bioethics education has a broad focus on the humanities, liberal arts, social sciences, and philosophy, so that medical activity is located within a wider human context. [142]

The philosophy of bioethics education is increasingly moving toward this broader conception. While the focus on identifying and analyzing ethical issues has been characteristic for the early stages of bioethics education, at present there is more emphasis on how to influence students' attitudes, behaviors, and characters, emphasizing that the ultimate goal of bioethics education is to produce good health professionals and scientists. Good medical practice requires more than knowledge and skills. Health professionals are expected to demonstrate good conduct and action but first of all humanistic qualities. This is what education should train and nourish. The focus of bioethics education should therefore move beyond problem-solving and applying principles. Doing so, it can respond to processes of rationalization and bureaucratization that have disenchanted the modern world. It will bring back passion and inspiration in the education of future healthcare professionals.

## Conclusion

Today, many patients and health professionals are not satisfied with the way healthcare is delivered. Patients complain about lack of empathy and compassion in healthcare interactions, while professionals denounce bureaucracy and purely commercial approaches. This variety of grievances are often expressed as the loss of soul in healthcare. In this book, we explore the connections between care, ethics, and soul. The charge that the soul has been lost in healthcare as well as in bioethics conveys the uneasiness, dissatisfaction, and disquiet that many people today experience with healthcare and also with the ethical queries that emerge in care settings. That such uneasiness is expressed in terms of loss of soul has something to do with the dominant scientific worldview that has eradicated any soul-talk and that presents an objective and technical approach to human life and its vulnerabilities. This book has analyzed how and why the soul has been lost from scientific discourses, healthcare practices, and ethical discussions. Our analysis proceeds from a broad framework that explains how medicine is dominated by a scientific world view that has eliminated the soul. This is visible in images and metaphors that currently permeate healthcare discourses and practices. We have particularly discussed the images of *homo economicus*, body machine, the lone ranger, detached concern, and consumer, promulgated by the naturalistic world-view of science, that is also pervasive in medicine and healthcare, and that is reiterated in neoliberal policies. Bioethical debate frequently assumes the same images regarding the human person as a rational, self-interested individual motivated by minimizing costs and maximizing gains for himself, while the human body is primarily viewed as a complicated mechanism and commodity that can be perfected and exchanged. We have argued that the eradication of the soul expressed in these images leads to an unsatisfactory perspective on who we are and how we relate to other beings as well as our environment. It has also impoverished ethical discourse about health and disease since human experiences are marginalized as subjective and unreliable. However, another ethical discourse is possible that takes into account the subjectivity of patients and the social conditions that determine health and well-being. The notion of moral imagination is used to reframe ethical discourse by introducing different images and metaphors, so that new perspectives may open up. We want to recover the critical, philosophical power of bioethics by arguing that it can explore new inspiring images focused on what it means to be a human being with a soul rather than merely an individual body. Moral imagination provides the capability to empathize with other people, and it proposes possibilities for action. The role of imagination is especially important now that ethical debates on health and healthcare are global. To face global challenges, a different and broad concept of bioethics will be necessary. Bioethics should transform into a critical, prophetic, and social ethics that, in our view, is needed in the current era of globalization and popularism. Using our moral imagination, several images can be activated and produced that rehabilitate and reinsert the soul in healthcare and ethical debate: first, the image of the warm doctor: a professional that is compassionate and reassuring; second, the image of holistic care that goes beyond the dominating medical model; third, the metaphor of life as a story, and the use of narratives in healthcare and ethics; fourth, the image that certain values are sacred, and not all values are the same and comparable, human dignity being an example; fifth, the image of the blue marbles (the Earth as viewed from outer space) highlighting the vulnerability of the planet as the common home of humanity; it has promoted the growth of global consciousness. In the last chapter, it is shown how a different approach to ethical challenges may emerge on the basis of these images. Losing the soul means that fundamental issues about human nature and destiny cannot be addressed. To focus on subjective patient experiences and the ideal of empathic care, it is important to consider ethics as a way of life and a lifelong project involving emotions and care. Ethical life is shared with other people, so that interpersonal interactions are crucial. Bioethics is a social enterprise; it involves sharing and exchanging of perspectives. This will shift the scope of bioethical debate from the individual to social, cultural, and economic concerns. This shift is critical since the context of bioethics is different from the past now that it is confronted with challenges of globalization and de-globalization, populism, and climate change. The final part of the chapter argues that given the overwhelming impact of these challenges, perhaps ethics is too demanding. Bioethics needs to be imaginative, that is less abstract and more focused on relationality and the common good. A feasible approach might be to emphasize notions such as decency, respect, and recognition, connecting bioethical discourse with civilization. Finally, the role of ethics education is discussed, as a possible antidote to the loss of soul and as a way to produce attentive and caring health professionals. Education should appeal to the moral imagination, sharing and articulating subjective experiences and emotions, as well as reflecting on them. It is also important to recognize the growing interest in spirituality in healthcare. It is encouraging that a broader conception of medical and ethical education is emerging so that the soul will no longer be missing in the practice of healthcare.

## References


1 Plato, *Charmides*, 156e; http://classics.mit.edu/Plato/charmides.html.

2 Thomas Moore, *Care of the soul. A guide for cultivating depth and sacredness in everyday life* (New York: HarperCollins Publishers, 1992), 5.

3 Bruce Rogers-Vaughn, *Caring for souls in a neoliberal age* (New York: Palgrave Macmillan, 2019), 5, 103, 213.

4 Gilbert C. Meilaender, *Body, soul, and bioethics* (Notre Dame: University of Notre Dame Press, 2009), x.

5 Meilaender: *Body, soul, and bioethics*, 32.

6 Webb Keane, *Ethical life. Its natural and social histories* (Princeton and Oxford: Princeton University Press, 2016), 27 ff.

7 Keane, *Ethical life*, 42.

8 M. Therese Lysaught, and Michael McCarthy, eds., *Catholic bioethics and social justice. The praxis of US health care in a globalized world* (Collegeville: Liturgical Press Academic, 2018).

9 Finbarr Livesey, *From global to local. The making of things and the end of globalization* (New York: Pantheon Books, 2017), 92.

10 John Milbank, and Adrian Pabst, *The politics of virtue. Post-liberalism and the human future* (London and New York: Rowman & Littlefield, 2016).

11 Henk ten Have, *Global bioethics. An introduction* (London and New York: Routledge, 2016), 218–220.

12 Anne R. Pierce, *A Perilous Path: The Misguided Foreign Policy of Barack Obama, Hillary Clinton & John Kerry* (New York: Post Hill Press, 2016).

13 UK Human Rights Blog, "UK not doing enough to combat human trafficking and domestic slavery" (28 November 2012).

14 For example, during the Dumberton Oak Conference in 1944, discussing the establishment of the United Nations, the US delegation was instructed not to engage in any discussion of human rights. See: Kathryn Sikkink, *Evidence for hope. Making human rights work in the 21st century* (Princeton and Oxford: Princeton University Press, 2017), 26–31, 55 ff.

15 Aryeh Neier, *The international human rights movement. A history* (Princeton and Oxford: Princeton University Press, 2012).

16 See chapter 5. Also: Siep Stuurman, *The invention of humanity. Equality and cultural difference in world history* (Cambridge and London: Harvard University Press, 2017).

17 Hans Joas, *The sacredness of the person. A new genealogy of human rights* (Washington: Georgetown University Press, 2013).

18 Hans Joas, *Sind die Menschenrechte westlich?* (München: Kösel Verlag, 2015), 72; Joas, *The sacredness of the person*, 185 ff.

19 "The language adopted was not the language of the great powers, but rather that of the Global South; it was only adopted by the great powers in response to pressure from small states and civil society." Sikkink, *Evidence for hope*, 71.

20 Tony Evans, *The politics of human rights. A global perspective* (London and Ann Arbor: Pluto Press, 2005).

21 Paul O'Connell, "On reconciling irreconcilables: Neo-liberal globalization and human rights," *Human Rights Law Review* 7, no. 3 (2007): 483–509.

22 Sikkink, *Evidence for hope*, 60. "Human rights has gone global not because it serves the interests of the powerful but primarily because it has advanced the interests of the powerless." Michael Ignatieff, "Human rights as politics and idolatry," in *Human rights as politics and idolatry*, ed. Amy Gutmann (Princeton and Oxford: Princeton University Press, 2001), 7.

23 Michael Ignatieff, *The ordinary virtues. Moral order in a divided world* (Cambridge: Harvard University Press, 2017).

24 Payam Akhavan, *In search of a better world. A human rights Odyssey* ( Toronto, Canada: Anansi, 2017).

25 Stephan Zweig, *Die Welt von Gestern. Erinnerungen eines Europäers* (London and Stockholm: Hamish-Hamilton and Bermann-Fischer Verlag AB, 1942).

26 Eric A. Posner, *The twilight of human rights law* (Oxford: Oxford University Press, 2014).

27 United Nations, General Assembly, Seventieth session. 2015. *Extreme poverty and human rights* (4 August 2015).

28 Samuel Moyn, *The last utopia. Human rights in history* (Cambridge and London: The Belknap Press of Harvard University Press, 2010); Samuel Moyn, *Not enough. Human rights in an unequal world* (Cambridge and London: The Belknap Press of Harvard University Press, 2018).

29 Stephen Hopgood, *The endtimes of human rights* (Ithaca: Cornell University Press, 2013).

30 Kathryn Sikkink mentions the dramatic decline of war-related deaths and genocide, the abolition of the death penalty (today in 140 countries, up from 16 in 1977), and the substantial increase of the percentage of girls in schools since 1979. See: Sikkink, *Evidence for hope*, 139 ff.

31 Sikkink, *Evidence for hope*, 20.
32 Cas Mudde, and Cristobal Rovira Kaltwasser, *Populism. A very short introduction* (Oxford: Oxford University Press, 2017), 6.
33 Mudde, and Kaltwasser, *Populism*, 81. See also Moffitt who rejects the opposition of populism and democracy; populism as a political style has democratic and antidemocratic tendencies (Benjamin Moffitt, *The global rise of populism. Performance, political style, and representation* (Stanford: Stanford University Press, 2016), 133–151).
34 Jan-Werner Müller, *What is populism?* (London: Penguin Books, 2017).
35 Jan-Werner Müller, "Populism and the People," *London Review of Books* (23 May 2019): 35–37.
36 See, for example, Patrick J. Deneen, *Why liberalism failed* (New Haven and London: Yale University Press, 2019).
37 Jason Brennan, *Against democracy* (Princeton and Oxford: Princeton University Press, 2016).
38 David Runciman, *How democracy ends* (London: Profile Books, 2019).
39 Pierre Rosanvallon, *De democratie denken. Werk in uitvoering* (Nijmegen: Uitgeverij Vantilt, 2019); Pierre Rosanvallon, *Counter-democracy. Politics in an age of distrust* (Cambridge: Cambridge University Press, 2008).
40 Democratic activity "extends well beyond the framework of electoral-representative institutions." "*Democracy is defined by its works*, and not simply by its institutions." (Rosanvallon, *Counter-democracy*, 249, 307).
41 That the elites are protecting the interests of the wealthy was demonstrated in the first act of the new French president (a former banker) after his election: reducing the wealth tax showing that he favors powerful corporations and rich individuals, less caring about the wellbeing of ordinary citizens.
42 Vivienne Walt, "France's yellow vests straitjacket Macron," *Time* (17 December 2018): 8; Rokhaya Diallo, "Why are the 'yellow vests' protesting in France?" *Al Jazeera* (10 December 2018); Jeremy Harding, "Among the gilets jaunes," *London Review of Books* (21 March 2019): 3–11.
43 Maria Rovisco, "The indignados social movement and the image of the occupied square: The making of a global icon," *Visual Communication* 16, no. 3 (2017): 337–359. See also: Marcos Ancelovici, Pascale Dufour and Héloïse Nez, eds., *Street politics in the age of austerity. From the Indignados to Occupy* (Amsterdam: Amsterdam University Press, 2016).
44 Niraj Chokshi, "Americans are among the most stressed people in the world, poll finds," *The New York Times* (25 April 2019).
45 Anger as moral outrage should be distinguished from personal anger (which is not a moral emotion but related to the affection of one's own interests) and empathic anger (which is also not a moral emotion but triggered because somebody else's interests are thwarted, not because a moral standard is violated). See: C. Daniel Batson, Christopher L. Kennedy, Lesly-Anne Nord et al., "Anger at unfairness: Is it moral outrage?" *European Journal of Social Psychology* 37 (2007): 1272–1285.
46 M. J. Crockett, "Moral outrage in the digital age," *Nature Human Behavior* 1 (2017): 769–771.
47 Crockett, "Moral outrage in the digital age," 769.
48 Anger and outrage can lead to the perception that offenders are less than human ('monsters') and that they lack core human qualities. See: Brock Bastian, Thomas F. Denson, and Nick Haslam, "The roles of dehumanization and moral outrage in retributive justice," *PLoS One* 8, no. 4 (2013): e61841.

49 Duhigg concludes that we "need moral outrage that motivates citizens to push for a more just society." See: Charles Duhigg, "Why are we so angry? The untold story of how all got so mad at one another," *The Atlantic* (January–February 2019): 75.
50 Intergovernmental Panel on Climate Change, *Global warming of 1.5°C* (Switzerland: IPCC, 2018).
51 David Wallace-Wells, *The uninhabitable earth. A story of the future* (London: Penguin Books, 2019). See also Bill McKibben, *Falter. Has the human game begun to play itself out?* (London: Wildfire, 2019).
52 Marie Dancer, "Le climat en tête des préoccupations des Européens," *La Croix* (25 November 2019).
53 Kate Brown, "Child's play. The global quest for a Green New Deal," *Times Literary Supplement* (7 June 2019).
54 In the United States, some environmentalists has been classified as 'extremists' alongside mass killers and white nationalists (Adam Federman, "Revealed: US listed climate activist group as 'extremists' alongside mass killers," *The Guardian* (13 January 2020)). In the United Kingdom, Extinction Rebellion is included by counter-terrorism police on a list of 'extreme ideologies' (Jamie Grierson, Vikram Dodd, and Peter Walker, "Putting Extinction Rebellion on extremist list 'completely wrong,' says Keir Starmer," *The Guardian* (13 January 2020)).
55 Thomas Philippon, *The great reversal. How America gave up on free markets* (Cambridge and London: The Belknap Press of Harvard University Press, 2019).
56 Philippon, *The great reversal*, 223–239.
57 Henk ten Have, *Wounded planet. How declining biodiversity endangers health and how bioethics can help* (Baltimore: Johns Hopkins University Press, 2019), 173.
58 See chapters 3 and 4.
59 Branko Milanovic, *Capitalism alone. The future of the system that rules the world* (Cambridge and London: The Belknap Press of Harvard University Press, 2019).
60 See chapter 5. See also: Nicholas A. Christakis, *Blueprint. The evolutionary origins of a good society* (New York, Boston and London: Little, Brown Spark, 2019). Paul Collier concludes that greed is dead, and that this will be wholesome: ". . . the death of Economic Man will be balm to the soul." See Paul Collier, "Greed is dead. The recognition that we need to rely on each other rather than ourselves," *Times Literary Supplement* (6 December 2019): 4.
61 Jonathan Aldred, *Licence to be bad. How economics corrupted us* (London: Allen Lane/Penguin Random House, 2019).
62 Thomas E. McCollough, *The moral imagination and public life. Raising the ethical question* (Chatham, NJ: Chatham House Publishers, 1991).
63 Wellcome Global Monitor 2018, *How does the world feel about science and health?* (London: Wellcome, 2019).
64 World Health Organization, "Ten threats to global health in 2019"; www.who.int/emergencies/ten-threats-to-global-health-in-2019.
65 Wellcome Global Monitor 2018, *How does the world feel about science and health?* (London: Wellcome, 2019), chapter 3: 48 ff.
66 Dhruv Khullar, "Do you trust the medical profession? A growing distrust could be dangerous to public health and safety," *The New York Times* (23 January 2018).
67 Robert J. Blendon, and John M. Benson, "American's view on health policy: A fifty-year historical perspective," *Health Affairs* 20, no. 2 (2001): 33–46.
68 NIVEL, *Nederlanders hebben nog steeds veel vertrouwen in de gezondheidszorg* (Utrecht; 27 October 2016); www.nivel.nl/nl/nieuws/nederlanders-hebben-nog-steeds-

veel-vertrouwen-de-gezondheidszorg. See also: Evelien van der Schee, *Public trust in health care. Exploring the mechanisms* (Utrecht: NIVEL, 2016).

69 Jonathan Kennedy, "Populist politics and vaccine hesitancy in Western Europe: An analysis of national-level data," *European Journal of Public Health* 29, no. 3 (2019): 512–516.

70 Arthur Caplan, "He Jankui's moral mess," *PLOS Biologue* (3 December 2018).

71 Ruipeng Lei, and Renzong Qiu, "Chinese bioethicists: He Jiankui's crime is more than illegal medical practice," *The Hastings Center* (4 January 2020).

72 Kristin L. Kirschner, "Rethinking and advocacy in bioethics," *American Journal of Bioethics* 1 (2002): 60–62.

73 Nathaniel Rich, *Losing earth. The decade we could have stopped climate change* (London: Picador, 2019).

74 The damage has accelerated during the last few decades, despite all declarations and treaties. "In fact, more than half of the carbon exhaled into the atmosphere by the burning of fossil fuels has been emitted in just the past three decades." Wallace-Wells, *The uninhabitable earth*, 4.

75 Though Wallace-Wells (*The uninhabitable earth*) has a chapter on ethics, he discusses most of all fringe responses to the climate crisis, without referring to serious works in ethics.

76 McKibben, *Falter*, 203–215.

77 Gaston Bachelard, *Le nouvel esprit scientifique* (Paris: Presses Universitaires de France, 1968), 58. See also: Roch C. Smith, *Gaston Bachelard. Philosopher of science and imagination* (Albany: State University of New York Press, 2016).

78 Richard Kearney, *The wake of imagination. Toward a postmodern culture* (London: Routledge, 2001).

79 Sara Barrena, "Reason and imagination in Charles S. Peirce," *European Journal of Pragmatism and American Philosophy* 5, no. 1 (2013): 1–15. The moral imagination is ". . . the capacity to empathize with others and to discern creative possibilities for ethical action." McCollough, *The moral imagination and public life*, 16.

80 John Kekes, *The enlargement of life. Moral imagination at work* (Ithaca and London: Cornell University Press, 2006), 18.

81 Anders Nordgren, "Ethics and imagination. Implications of cognitive semantics for medical ethics," *Theoretical Medicine and Bioethics* 19 (1998): 117–141; Mark G. Hanson, "Imaginative ethics – bringing ethical practice into sharper relief," *Medicine, Health Care and Philosophy* 5 (2002): 33–42.

82 Shawn D. Whatley, "Borrowed philosophy: Bedside physicalism and the need for a sui generis metaphysic of medicine," *Journal of Evaluation in Clinical Practice* 20 (2014): 961–964.

83 Lynn Hunt, *Inventing human rights. A history* (New York and London: W. W. Norton & Company, 2007).

84 Aldred, *Licence to be bad*; see also Christakis, *Blueprint*.

85 ". . . universal human rights represent the dominant utopianism of our era." See Richard Thompson Ford, *Universal rights down to earth* (New York and London: W. W. Norton & Company, 2011), 4. Human rights discourse in his view is not abstract idealism. It requires local institutions, movements and concerns for its implementation. Samuel Moyn has also stated that human rights present a "recognizably utopian program" with "the image of another, better world of dignity and respect . . ." See: Moyn, *The last Utopia*, 1, 4.

86 The founding fathers of the European Community, Robert Schumann, Jean Monnet and Alcide de Gasperi have all been personalist, like later personalities such as Jacques Delors and Herman Van Rompuy. See: Jonas Norgaard Mortensen, *The common good. An introduction to personalism* (Wilmington: Vernon Press, 2017), 114–115.
87 Russell Jacoby, *The end of utopia. Politics and culture in an age of apathy* (New York: Basic Books, 1999); Russell Jacoby, *Picture imperfect. Utopian thought for an anti-utopian age* (New York: Columbia University Press, 2005).
88 Ruth Levitas defines utopia as "the expression of the desire for a better way of living and of being." See: Ruth Levitas, *Utopia as method. The imaginary reconstruction of society* (Houndmills: Palgrave Macmillan, 2013), 4.
89 Martin Plattel, *Utopie en kritisch denken* (Bilthoven: Amboboeken, 1970).
90 Van Rensselaer Potter, "Moving the culture toward more vivid utopias with survival as the goal," *Global Bioethics* 14, no. 4 (2001): 20.
91 ". . . utopian visions are the stuff by which men live . . ." See: Margaret Mead, "Towards more vivid utopias," *Science* 126, no. 3280 (1957): 958.
92 Van Rensselaer Potter, *Bioethics: Bridge to the future* (Englewood Cliffs: Prentice-Hall, 1971).
93 Roberto Dell'Oro, "On the ultimate that is first: Thinking beyond bioethics," *Gregorianum* 100, no. 3 (2019): 621–647.
94 See Gregory S. McElwain, *Mary Midgley. An introduction* (London: Bloomsbury Academic, 2020).
95 Gabriel Marcel, *Man against mass society* (South Bend: St. Augustine's Press, 2008), 12.
96 Gabriel Marcel, *Homo viator. Introduction to a metaphysic of hope* (New York: Harper & Row, 1962), 23.
97 Otto Friedrich Bollnow, "Marcel's concept of availability," in *The philosophy of Gabriel Marcel*, eds. Paul A. Schilpp and Lewis E. Hahn (Open Court: La Salle, 1984), 177–199.
98 Gabriel Marcel, "Reply to John E. Smith," in *The philosophy of Gabriel Marcel*, eds. Paul A. Schilpp, and Lewis E. Hahn (Open Court: La Salle, 1984), 350–353.
99 Erwin W. Straus, and Michael A. Machado, "Gabriel Marcel's notion of incarnate being," in *The philosophy of Gabriel Marcel*, eds. Paul A. Schilpp and Lewis E. Hahn (Open Court: La Salle, 1984), 123–155.
100 Marcel, *Homo viator*, 11.
101 Luigino Bruni, *The wound and the blessing. Economics, relationships, and happiness* (Hyde Park and New York: New City Press, 2012).
102 Andrew Sayer, *Why things matter to people. Social science, values and ethical life* (Cambridge: Cambridge University Press, 2011).
103 In the words of Michael Sandel: "The common good is about how we live together in community. It's about the ethical ideals we strive for together, the benefits and burdens we share, the sacrifices we make for one another. It's about the lessons we learn from one another about how to live a good and decent life." Quoted in Thomas Friedman, "Finding the 'common good' in a pandemic," *New York Times* (24 March 2020). According to Jacques Maritain, the common good ". . . includes the sum or sociological integration of all the civic conscience, political virtues and sense of right and liberty, of all the activity, material prosperity and spiritual riches, of unconsciously operative hereditary wisdom, of moral rectitude, justice, friendship, happiness, virtue and heroism in the individual lives of its members. For these things all are, in a certain

measure, communicable and so revert to each member, helping him to perfect his life and liberty of person. They all constitute the good human life of the multitude." See: Jacques Maritain, and John T. FitzGerald, "The person and the common good," *The Review of Politics* 8, no. 4 (1946): 438.

104 Bruni, *The wound and the blessing*, 63 ff.

105 Luigino Bruno, and Stefano Zamagni, *Civil economy. Another idea of the market* (Newcastle upon Tyne: Agenda Publishing, 2016). See also: Luigino Bruni, *Reciprocity, altruism and the civil society. In praise of heterogeneity* (London and New York: Routledge, 2008).

106 Ten Have, *Global bioethics*, 218–220.

107 Benjamin Coriat, ed., *Le retour des communs. La crise de l'idéologie propriétaire* (Paris: Éditions Les Liens qui Libèrent, 2015).

108 Ten Have, *Global bioethics*, 113 ff.

109 Adam Tooze, "Democracy and its discontents," *The New York Review of Books* (6 June 2019): 52–57.

110 Rosanvallon, *Counter-democracy*, 307.

111 Runciman, *How democracy ends*, 169 ff.

112 Sarah Franklin, "Ethical research – the long and bumpy road from shirked to shared," *Nature* 574, no. 7780 (2019): 629.

113 Gunther Stent, "That was the molecular biology that was," *Science* 160, no. 3826 (1968): 390–395.

114 "But a morality that makes impossible demands, demands that we'll unavoidable fail to meet, is the only kind of morality that fits what actual human beings are like." Lisa Tessman, *When doing the right thing is impossible* (New York: Oxford University Press, 2017), 165. See also: Lisa Tessman, *Moral failure. On the impossible demands of morality* (New York: Oxford University Press, 2015).

115 See Chapter 6.

116 Todd May, *A decent life. Morality for the rest of us* (Chicago and London: The University of Chicago Press, 2019).

117 ". . . decent moral action recognizes that there are others in the world who have lives to live." (May, *A decent life*, 29).

118 Mark Johnson, *Moral imagination. Implication of cognitive science for ethics* (Chicago and London: The University of Chicago Press, 1993), 1.

119 Richard Jenkins, "Disenchantment, enchantment and re-enchantment: Max Weber at the Millennium," *Max Weber Studies* 1 (2000): 12.

120 See: Keane, *Ethical life*, 6, 171.

121 See: Sayer, *Why things matter to people*, 1–2, 98 ff.

122 Jonathan Montgomery, "Bioethics as a governance practice," *Health Care Analysis* 24 (2016): 3–23.

123 "*Being civilized* means *living, so far as possible, dialectically*, that is, in constant endeavor to convert every occasion of non-agreement into an occasion of agreement." See: R. G. Collingwood, *The new Leviathan. Or man, society, civilization and barbarism* (Oxford: Clarendon Press, 1992), 326.

124 "Civilization is the process of converting a non-social community into a society. . . *to civilize is to socialize*." See: Collingwood, *The new Leviathan*, 309.

125 Albert Schweitzer, *The philosophy of civilization* (New York: The Macmillan Company, 1959).

126 Collingwood, *The new Leviathan*, 280.

127 Schweitzer, *The philosophy of civilization*, Part II. Civilization and ethics.

128 Brett Bowden, *The empire of civilization: The evolution of an imperial idea* (Chicago and London: The University of Chicago Press, 2009).

129 Jonathan Glover, *Humanity. A moral history of the twentieth century* (New Haven and London: Yale University Press, 2012).

130 See Chapter 5.

131 ". . . empathy oils the wheels of social life." See: David Howe, *Empathy. What it is and why it matters* (London: Palgrave Macmillan, 2013), 187. Empathy is "the glue that binds us together in functioning and beneficial families, communities and countries." See: Peter Bazalgette, *The empathic instinct. How to create a more civil society* (London: John Murray, 2017), 2. According to Rifkin, empathy is "the soul of democracy." The ability to recognize oneself in the other and the other in oneself lies at the heart of decency and democracy. See Jeremy Rifkin, *The empathic civilization. The race to global consciousness in a world in crisis* (Cambridge: Polity Press, 2018), 161.

132 Frans de Waal, *The age of empathy. Nature's lessons for a kinder society* (London: Souvenir Press, 2019), 209.

133 Christakis, *Blueprint*, 237–239, 240 ff.

134 Avishai Margalit, *The decent society* (Cambridge and London: Harvard University Press, 1996).

135 Axel Honneth: *Disrespect. The normative foundations of critical theory* (Cambridge: Polity Press, 2007).

136 Dignity is a "form of conduct and interaction between people, a way of being with others and with herself." See: Sayer, *Why things matter to people*, 193.

137 J. LeBron McBride, "The relational soul of family medicine," *Family Practice Management* 20, no. 2 (2013): 40; Charles R. Perakis, "What about the soul?" *Academic Medicine* 88, no. 10 (2013): 1521.

138 Mark G. Kuczewski, "The soul of medicine," *Perspectives in Biology and Medicine* 50, no. 3 (2007): 410–420.

139 Terrence C. Wright, "Phenomenology and the moral imagination," *Logos: A Journal of Catholic Thought and Culture* 6 (2003): 104–121.

140 Edvin Schei, Abraham Fuks, and J. Donald Boudreau, "Reflection in medical education: Intellectual humility, discovery, and know-how," *Medicine Health Care and Philosophy* 22, no. 2 (2019): 167–178.

141 Seyedeh Z. Nahardani, Fazlollah Ahmadi, Shoaleh Bigdeli, and Soltani Arabshahi, "Spirituality in medical education: A concept analysis," *Medicine Health Care and Philosophy* 22, no. 2 (2019): 179–189.

142 Henk ten Have, "The fundamental role of education," in *Equal beginnings, but then? A global responsibility*, eds. Vincenzo Paglia and Renzo Pegoraro (Rome: Pontifical Academy for Life, 2019), 63–80.

# Bibliography


Accad, Michel. "How Western medicine lost its soul." *The Linacre Quarterly* 83, no. 2 (2016): 144–146.

Adams, S., P. Blokker, N. Doyle, J. Krummel, and J. Smith, "Social imaginaries in debate." *Social Imaginaries* 1 (2015): 15–52.

Adams, Samantha, and Antoinette de Bont. "Information Rx: Prescribing good consumerism and responsible citizenship." *Health Care Analysis* 15 (2007): 273–290.

Adams, Tony E. "A review of narrative ethics." *Qualitative Inquiry* 14, no. 2 (2008): 175–194.

Adorno, Theodore, Else Frenkel-Brunswik, Daniel J. Levinson, and R. Newitt Sanford. *The authoritarian personality*. New York: Harper, 1950.

Agich, George, J. "Education and the improvement of clinical ethics services." *BMC Medical Education* 13 (2013): 41; doi:10.1186/1472-6920-13-41.

Akhavan, Payam. *In search of a better world. A human rights Odyssey*. Toronto, Canada: Anansi, 2017.

Aldred, Jonathan. *Licence to be bad. How economics corrupted us*. London: Allen Lane/ Penguin Random House, 2019.

Alexander, Eben. *Proof of heaven. A neurosurgeon's journey into the afterlife*. New York: Simon & Schuster, 2012.

Allison, Dale C. *The Sermon on the mount: Inspiring the moral imagination*. New York: Crossroad Publications, 1999.

American Board of Internal Medicine (ABIM) Foundation. *Medical Professionalism in the New Millennium: A Physician Charter*, 2002; https://abimfoundation.org/wp-content/uploads/2015/12/Medical-Professionalism-in-the-New-Millenium-A-Physician-Charter.pdf.

American Board of Medical Specialties. *ABMS Definition of Medical Professionalism*. Long Form. Adopted by the ABMS Board of Directors (18 January 2012); www.abms.org/media/84742/abms-definition-of-medical-professionalism.pdf.

Ancelovici, Marcos, Pascale Dufour and Héloïse Nez, eds. *Street politics in the age of austerity. From the Indignados to Occupy*. Amsterdam: Amsterdam University Press, 2016.

Anderson, Elizabeth. *Value in ethics and economics*. Cambridge and London: Harvard University Press, 1993.

Andone, Dakin, and Artemis Moshtaghian. "A doctor in California appeared via video link to tell a patient he was going to die. The man's family is upset." *CNN* (11 March 2019); www.cnn.com/2019/03/10/health/patient-dies-robot-doctor/index.html.

Andrade, Chittaranjan, and Pajiv Radhakrihnan. "Prayer and healing: A medical and scientific perspective on randomized controlled trials." *Indian Journal of Psychiatry* 51, no. 4 (2009): 247–253.

Andrews, Lori B. "My body, my property." *Hastings Center Report* 16, no. 5 (1986): 28–38.

Angus, Ian H. "Disenchantment and modernity: The mirror of technique." *Human Studies* 6, no. 2 (1983): 141–166.

Antoniou, Stavros A., George A. Antoniou, Robert Learney, Frank A. Granderath, and Athanasios I. Antoniou. "The rod and the serpent: History's ultimate healing symbol." *World Journal of Surgery* 35 (2011): 217–221.

Archard, David. "Selling yourself: Titmuss's argument against a market in blood." *The Journal of Ethics* 6, no. 1 (2002): 87–103.

Ashby, Michael A., and Bronwen Morrell. "To the barricades or the blackboard: Bioethics activism and the "stance of neutrality." *Journal of Bioethical Inquiry* 15 (2018): 479.

Astrow, Alan, S. "On the disenchantment of medicine: Abraham Joshua Heschel's 1964 address to the American Medical Association." *Theoretical Medicine and Bioethics* 39 (2018): 483–497.

Atran, Scott, and Robert Axelrod. "Reframing sacred values." *Negotiation Journal* 24, no. 3 (2008): 221–246.

Bachelard, Gaston. *L'eau et les rêves. Essai sur l'imagination de la matière*. Paris: Librairie José Corti, 1942; http://classiques.uqac.ca/classiques/bachelard_gaston/eau_et_les_reves/eau_et_les_reves.pdf.

Bachelard, Gaston. *L'Air et les Songes. Essai sur l'imagination du movement*. Paris: Librairie José Corti, 1943; http://classiques.uqac.ca/classiques/bachelard_gaston/air_et_les_songes/air_et_les_songes.pdf.

Bachelard, Gaston. *The poetics of space*. New York: Penguin Books, 2014; original: *La Poétique de l'Espace*. Paris: Les Presses Universitaires de France, 1957; https://gaston-bachelard.org/wp-content/uploads/2015/07/BACHELARD-Gaston-La-poetique-de-l-espace.pdf.

Bachelard, Gaston. *Le nouvel esprit scientifique*. Paris: Presses Universitaires de France, 1968; original 1934.

Bachelard, Gaston. *On Poetic Imagination and Reverie*. New York: Spring Publications, 2014.

Baehr, Peter. "The 'Iron cage' and the 'Shell as hard as steel': Parsons, Weber, and the Stahlhartes Gehäuse in the Protestant Ethics and the Spirit of Capitalism." *History and Theory* 40, no. 2 (2001): 153–169.

Bailey, Anthony. *A view of Delft. Vermeer then and now*. London: Chatto & Windus, 2001.

Baker, Gordon, and Katherine J. Morris. *Descartes' dualism*. London and New York: Routledge, 1996.

Baker, Lynne Rudder. *Naturalism and the first-person perspective*. Oxford: Oxford University Press, 2013.

Balboni, Michael J., and Tracy A. Balboni. "Reintegrating care for the dying, body and soul." *The Harvard Theological Review* 103 (2010): 351–364.

Baron, Jonathan, and Sarah Leshner. "How serious are expressions of protected values?" *Journal of Experimental Psychology* 6, no. 3 (2000): 183–194.

Barrena, Sara. "Reason and imagination in Charles S. Peirce." *European Journal of Pragmatism and American Philosophy* 5, no. 1 (2013): 1–15.

Barrett, William. *Death of the soul. From Descartes to the computer*. New York: Anchor Books, Doubleday, 1986.

Bastian, Brock, Thomas F. Denson, and Nick Haslam. "The roles of dehumanization and moral outrage in retributive justice." *PLoS One* 8, no. 4 (2013): e61841; doi:10.1371/journal.pone.0061842.

Batson, C. Daniel, Christopher L. Kennedy, Lesly-Anne Nord et al. "Anger at unfairness: Is it moral outrage?" *European Journal of Social Psychology* 37 (2007): 1272–1285.

Baudelaire, Charles. "La Reine de Facultés." In *Charles Baudelaire. Curiosités esthétiques et l'art romantique*, edited by H. Lemaitre. Paris: Garnier, 1962.

Bauman, Zygmunt. *Wasted lives: Moderity and its outcasts*. Cambridge, UK: Polity Press, 2004.

Baumgaertner, Bert, Juliet E. Carlisle, and Florian Justwan. "The influence of political ideology and trust on willingness to vaccinate." *PLoS One* 13, no. 1 (2018): e0191728; doi.org/10.1371/journal.pone.0191728.

Bazalgette, Peter. *The empathic instinct. How to create a more civil society*. London: John Murray, 2017.

Beall, Jeffrey. "Dangerous predatory publishers threaten medical research." *Journal of Korean Medical Science* 31 (2016): 1511–1513.

Beall, Jeffrey. "Predatory journals threaten the quality of published medical research." *Journal of Orthopaedic & Sports Physical Therapy* 47, no. 1 (2017): 3–5.

Bekker, Balthasar. *De betoverde wereld*. Amsterdam: Daniel van den Dalen, 1691; www.dbnl.org/tekst/bekk001beto01_01/.

Benatar, Solomon. "Moral imagination: The missing component in global health." *PLoS Medicine* 2, no. 12 (2005): e400; doi.org/10.1371/journal.pmed.0020400.

Benatar, Solomon, Abdallah Daar, and Peter Singer. "Global health challenges: The need for an expanded discourse on bioethics." *PLoS Medicine* 2, no. 7 (2005): e143; doi:10.1371/journal.pmed.0020143.

Bennett, Jane. *The enchantment of modern life. Attachments, crossings, and ethics*. Princeton and Oxford: Princeton University Press, 2001.

Bensing, Jozien, Myrian Deveugele, Francesca Moretti, Ian Fletcher, Liesbeth van Vliet, Marjolein Van Bogaert, and Michela Rimondini. "How to make the medical consultation more successful from a patient's perspective? Tips for doctors and patients from lay people in the United Kingdom, Italy, Belgium and the Netherlands." *Patient Education and Counseling* 84 (2011): 287–293.

Bensing, Jozien, Michela Rimondini, and Adriaan Visser. "What patients want." *Patient Education and Counseling* 90 (2013): 287–290.

Bensing, Jozien, Debra L. Roter, and Robert L. Hulsman. "Communication patterns of primary care physicians in the United States and The Netherlands." *Journal of General Internal Medicine* 18 (2003): 335–342.

Berlin, Isaiah. *The hedgehog and the fox. An essay on Tolstoy's view of history*. London: Weidenfeld & Nicolson, 1953; www.blogs.hss.ed.ac.uk/crag/files/2016/06/the_hedgehog_and_the_fox-berlin.pdf.

Berlin, Leonard. "Accuracy of diagnostic procedures: Has it improved over the past five decades?" *American Journal of Roentgenology* 188 (2007): 1173–1178.

Bernstein, Richard J. "Dewey's naturalism." *The Review of Metaphysics* 13, no. 2 (1959): 340–353.

Bishop, Jeffrey P. *The anticipatory corpse. Medicine, power, and the care of the dying*. Notre Dame: University of Notre Dame Press, 2011.

Bishop, John D. "Adam Smith's invisible hand argument." *Journal of Business Ethics* 14, no. 3 (1995): 165–180.

Blendon, Robert J., and John M. Benson. American's view on health policy: A fifty-year historical perspective." *Health Affairs* 20, no. 2 (2001): 33–46.

Blum, Lawrence A. *Moral perception and particularity*. New York: Cambridge University Press, 1994.

Blumhagen, Dan W. "The doctor's white coat. The image of the physician in modern America." *Annals of Internal Medicine* 91 (1979): 111–116.

Blythe, Jacob, A., and Farr A. Curlin, "'Just do your job': Technology, bureaucracy, and the eclipse of conscience in contemporary medicine." *Theoretical Medicine and Bioethics* 39 (2018): 431–452.

Boff, Leonardo, and Virgilio Elizondo. "Ecology and poverty: Cry of the earth, cry of the poor." *Concilium: International Journal of Theology* 5 (1995): ix–x.

Bollnow, Otto Friedrich. "Marcel's concept of availability." In *The philosophy of Gabriel Marcel*, edited by Paul A. Schilpp and Lewis E. Hahn, 177–199. Open Court: La Salle, 1984.

Borrell-Carrió, Francesc, Anthony L. Suchman, and Ronald M. Epstein. "The biopsychosocial model 25 years later: Principles, practice, and scientific inquiry." *Annals of Family Medicine* 2, no. 6 (2004): 576–582.

Borry, Pascal, Paul Schotsmans, and Kris Dierickx. "The birth of the empirical turn in bioethics." *Bioethics* 19, no. 1 (2005): 49–71.

Botha, Danie. "Are we at risk of losing the soul of medicine?" *Canadian Journal of Anaesthesia* 64 (2017): 122–127.

Bowden, Brett. *The empire of civilization: The evolution of an imperial idea*. Chicago and London: The University of Chicago Press, 2009.

Bowden, Brett. "The thin ice of civilization." *Alternatives: Global, Local, Political* 36, no. 2 (2011): 118–135.

Bowen, Anthony, and Arturo Casadevall. "Increasing disparities between resource inputs and outcomes, as measured by certain health deliverables, in biomedical research." *Proceedings of the National Academy of Sciences* 112, no. 36 (2015): 11335–11340.

Bowles, Samuel. *The moral economy. Why good incentives are no substitute for good citizens*. New Haven and London: Yale University Press, 2016.

Bowles, Samuel, and Herbert Gintis. "Homo reciprocans." *Nature* 415, no. 6868 (2002): 125–128.

Bowles, Samuel, and Herbert Gintis. "Social preferences, homo economicus and zoon politicon." In *The Oxford Handbook of Contextual Political Analysis*, edited by Robert E. Goodin and Charles Tilly, 172–186. Oxford: Oxford University Press, 2006.

Breeur, Roland. "Individualism and personalism." *Ethical Perspectives* 6, no. 1 (1999): 67–81.

Brennan, Jason. *Against democracy*. Princeton and Oxford: Princeton University Press, 2016.

Briggs, Charles L., and Daniel C. Hallin. "Biocommunicability. The neoliberal subject and its contradictions in news coverage of health issues." *Social Text* 25, no. 4 (2007): 43–66.

British Educational Research Association. "Most teenagers believe they have a soul." *Press Release* (14 September 2016); www.bera.ac.uk/bera-in-the-news/press-release-most-teenagers-believe-they-have-a-soul.

Brown, Candy Gunther. *Testing prayer. Science and healing*. Boston: Harvard University Press, 2012.

Brown, Kate. "Child's play. The global quest for a Green New Deal." *Times Literary Supplement* (7 June 2019).

Brown, Warren S., Nancy Murphy, and H. Newton Malony, eds. *Whatever happened to the soul? Scientific and theological portraits of human nature*. Minneapolis: Fortress Press, 1998.

Brueggemann, Walter. *The prophetic imagination*. Minneapolis: Fortress Press, 2018 (originally 1978).

Bruni, Luigino. *Reciprocity, altruism and the civil society. In praise of heterogeneity*. London and New York: Routledge, 2008.

Bruni, Luigino. *The wound and the blessing. Economics, relationships, and happiness*. Hyde Park and New York: New City Press, 2012.

Bruno, Luigino, and Stefano Zamagni. *Civil economy. Another idea of the market*. Newcastle upon Tyne: Agenda Publishing, 2016.

Butalid, Ligaya, Jozien M. Bensing, and Peter F. M. Verhaak. "Talking about psychosocial problems: An observational study on changes in doctor-patient communication in general practice between 1977 and 2008." *Patient Education and Counseling* 94 (2014): 314–321.

Butler, Stuart M., Davna Bowen Matthew, and Marcela Cabello. *Re-balancing medical and social spending to promote health: Increasing state flexibility to improve health through housing*. Washington: Brookings Institute, 15 February 2017; www.brookings.edu/blog/usc-brookings-schaeffer-on-health-policy/2017/02/15/re-balancing-medical-and-social-spending-to-promote-health-increasing-state-flexibility-to-improve-health-through-housing/.

Buytendijk, Frederik J. J. "De relatie arts-patiënt." *Nederlands Tijdschrift voor Geneeskunde* 103 (1959): 2504–2508.

Caenazzo, Luciana, Lucia Mariani, and Renzo Pegoraro, eds. *Medical Humanities. Italian Perspectives*. Padova: Cooperativa Libraria Editrice Universita di Padova, 2015.

Cahn, Steven M. ed. *New studies in the philosophy of John Dewey*. Hanover: The University Press of New England, 1977.

Calcagno, Antonio. *The philosophy of Edith Stein*. Pittsburgh: Duquesne University Press, 2007.

Callahan, Daniel. "Individual good and common good: A communitarian approach to bioethics." *Perspectives in Biology and Medicine* 46, no. 4 (2003): 496–507.

Callero, Peter. *The myth of individualism. How social forces shape our lives*. Lanham, Boulder, New York and London: Rowman & Littlefield, 2018 (3rd edition).

Campbell, Alastair V. *The body in bioethics*. London and New York: Routledge, 2009.

Campbell, Courtney S. "Body, self, and the property paradigm." *Hastings Center Report* 22, no. 5 (1992): 34–42.

Campelia, Georgina, and Tyler Tate. "Empathic practice. The struggle and virtue of empathizing with a patient's suffering." *Hastings Center Report* 49, no. 2 (2019): 17–24.

Caplan, Arthur. "He Jankui's moral mess." *PLOS Biologue* (3 December 2018); https://blogs.plos.org/biologue/2018/12/03/he-jiankuis-moral-mess/.

Carel, Havi. "Phenomenology as a resource for patients." *Journal of Medicine and Philosophy* 37 (2012): 96–113.

Carel, Havi. *Phenomenology of illness*. Oxford: Oxford University Press, 2016.

Carroll, Chandler W. "Spotting the wolf in sheep's clothing: Predatory open access publications." *Journal of Graduate Medical Education* 8, no. 5 (2016): 662–664.

Casey, Edward S. *Imagining. A phenomenological study*. Bloomington and Indianapolis: Indiana University Press, 2000.

Cha, In-Suk. *The mundalization of home in the age of globalization: Towards a transcultural ethics*. Münster: LIT Verlag, 2012.

Cha, In-Suk. *Essais sur la mondialisation de notre demeure: vers une éthique transculturelle*. Paris: L'Harmattan, 2013.

Chalcraft, David. "Bringing the text back in: On ways of reading the iron cage metaphor in the two editions of *The Protestant Ethic*." In *Organizing modernity. New Weberian perspectives on work, organization and society*, edited by Larry J. Ray and Michael Reed, 16–45. London: Routledge, 1994.

Chambers, Tod S. "The bioethicist as author: The medical ethics case a rhetorical device." *Literature and Medicine* 13, no. 1 (1994): 60–78.

Chambliss, J. J. "John Dewey's idea of imagination in philosophy and education." *The Journal of Aesthetic Education* 25 (1991): 43–49.

Charon, Rita. "Narrative medicine. A model for empathy, reflection, profession, and trust." *JAMA* 286 (2001): 1897–1902.

Charon, Rita. *Narrative medicine. Honoring the stories of illness*. New York: Oxford University Press, 2006.

Charon, Rita, and Martha Montello, eds. *Stories matter. The role of narrative in medical ethics*. New York and London: Routledge, 2002.

Cherry, Mark J. "The scandal of secular bioethics: What happens when the culture acts as if there is no God?" *Christian Bioethics* 23, no. 2 (2017): 85–99.

Chida, Yoichi, Andrew Steptoe, and Lynda H. Powell. "Religiosity/spirituality and mortality." *Psychotherapy and Psychosomatics* 78 (2009): 81–90.

Chilton, Paul, and Mikhail Ilyin. "Metaphors of political discourse: The case of the 'common European house'." *Discourse & Society* 4, no. 1 (1993): 7–31.

Chokshi, Niraj. "Americans are among the most stressed people in the world, poll finds." *The New York Times* (25 April 2019); www.nytimes.com/2019/04/25/us/americans-stressful.html.

Christakis, Nicholas A. *Blueprint. The evolutionary origins of a good society*. New York, Boston and London: Little, Brown Spark, 2019.

Chuwa, Leonard Tumaini. *African indigenous ethics in global bioethics*. Interpreting Ubuntu. New York: Springer, 2014.

Claassen, Jan, Kevin Doyle, Adu Matory, Caroline Couch, et al. "Detection of brain activation in unresponsive patients with acute brain injury." *New England Journal of Medicine* 380, no. 26 (2019): 2497–2505.

Cocking, J. M. *Imagination. A study in the history of ideas*. London and New York: Routledge, 1991.

Cohen, Alain, Michel André Maréchal, David Tannenbaum, and Christian Lukas Zünd. "Civic honesty around the globe." *Science* 365 (2019): 70–73.

Cohen, Daniel. *Homo economicus, prophète (égaré) des temps nouveaux*. Paris: Albin Michel, 2012.

Collier, Paul. "Greed is dead. The recognition that we need to rely on each other rather than ourselves." *Times Literary Supplement* (6 December 2019): 4–6.

Collingwood, R. G. *The new Leviathan. Or man, society, civilization and barbarism*. Oxford: Clarendon Press, 1992 (revised edition); original 1942.

Coluci, Massimiliano, and Renzo Pegoraro. "Towards a Medicine of the Invisible: Bioethics and Relationship in *The Little Prince*." *Medical Humanities* 43 (2017): 9–14.

Constas, Nicholas. "Icons and the imagination." *Logos: A Journal of Catholic Thought and Culture* 1, no. 1 (1997): 114–127.

Cook, Chad. "Predatory journals: The worst thing in publishing, ever." *Journal of Orthopaedic & Sports Physical Therapy* 47, no. 1 (2017): 1–2.

Coriat, Benjamin, ed. *Le retour des communs. La crise de l'idéologie propriétaire*. Paris: Éditions Les Liens qui Libèrent, 2015.

Cosgrove, Denis. "Contested global visions: One-world, whole-earth, and the Apollo space photographs." *Annals of the Association of American Geographers* 84 (1994): 270–294.

Coulehan, Jack, ed. *Chekhov's Doctors. A collection of Chekhov's medical tales*. Kent and London: The Kent State University Press, 2003.

Cousineau, Phil, ed. *Soul. An archaeology*. New York: HarperCollins Publishers, 1995.

Crick, Francis. *The astonishing hypothesis. The scientific search for the soul*. New York: Simon & Schuster, 1994.

Crockett, M. J. "Moral outrage in the digital age." *Nature Human Behavior* 1 (2017): 769–771.

Curlin, Farr A., John D. Lantos, Chad J. Roach, Sarah A. Sellergren, and Marshal H. Chin. "Religious characteristics of U. S. Physicians. A national survey." *Journal of General Internal Medicine* 20 (2005): 629–634.

Dadkhah, Mehdi, and Giorgio Bianciardi. "Ranking predatory journals: Solve the problem instead of removing it!" *Advanced Pharmaceutical Bulletin* 6, no. 1 (2016): 1–4.

Dallmayr, Fred. "The return of philosophical anthropology." In *Philosophy and anthropology: Border crossing and transformations*, edited by Ananta Kumar Giri and John Clammer, 357–364. London: Anthem Press, 2013.

Dancer, Marie. "Le climat en tête des préoccupations des Européens," *La Croix* (25 November 2019); www.la-croix.com/Monde/Europe/DAthenes-Stockholm-climat-tete-preoccupations-Europeens-2019-11-25-1201062503.

Danevska, Lenche, Mirko Spiroski, Doncho Donev, Nada Pop-Jordanova, and Momir Polenakovic. "How to recognize and avoid potential, possible, or probable predatory open-access publishers, standalone, and hijacked journals." *Contributions, Section of Medical Sciences* 37, no. 2–3 (2016): 5–13.

Dardot, Pierre, and Christian Laval. *The new way of the world. On neo-liberal society*. London and New York: Verso, 2017.

Daston, Lorraine. "On scientific observation." *Isis* 99, no. 1 (2008): 97–110.

Daston, Lorraine, and Peter Galison, *Objectivity*. New York: Zone Books, 2010.

Davenport, Beverly Ann. "Witnessing and the medical gaze: How medical students learn to see at a free clinic for the homeless." *Medical Anthropology Quarterly* 14, no. 3 (2000): 310–327.

Davies, Brian. *The thought of Thomas Aquinas*. Oxford: Clarendon Press, 1992.

Davies, Sara E., Adam Kamradt-Scott, and Simon Rushton, *Disease diplomacy. International norms and global health security*. Baltimore: Johns Hopkins University Press, 2015.

Dawson, Angus, Christopher F. C. Jordens, Paul Macneill, and Deborah Zion. "Bioethics and the myth of neutrality." *Journal of Bioethical Inquiry* 15 (2018): 483–486.

De Vries, Raymond. "Good without God: Bioethics and the sacred." *Society* 52 (2015): 438–447.

De Vries, Rob, and Bert Gordijn. "Empirical ethics and its alleged meta-ethical fallacies." *Bioethics* 23, no. 4 (2009): 193–201.

De Waal, Frans. *The age of empathy. Nature's lessons for a kinder society*. London: Souvenir Press, 2019.

De Witte, Joke, and Henk ten Have. "Ownership of genetic material and information." *Social Science & Medicine* 45, no. 1 (1997): 51–60.

Deese, Richard. "The artefact of nature: 'Spaceship Earth' and the dawn of global environmentalism." *Endeavour* 33, no. 2 (2009): 70–75.

Dekkers, Wim. "Dwelling, house and home: Towards a home-led perspective on dementia care." *Medicine Health Care and Philosophy* 14 (2011): 291–300.

Delgado, Janet. "Re-thinking relational autonomy: Challenging the triumph of autonomy through vulnerability." *Bioethics Update* 5 (2019): 50–65.

Dell'Oro, Roberto. "On the ultimate that is first: Thinking beyond bioethics." *Gregorianum* 100, no. 3 (2019): 621–647.

Deneen, Patrick J. *Why liberalism failed*. New Haven and London: Yale University Press, 2019.

Descartes, René. *Oeuvres de Descartes*, edited by Charles Adam and Paul Tannery. Paris: Vrin, 1897–1913.

Dewey, John. *Human nature and conduct. An introduction to social psychology*. New York: Henry Holt & Company, 1922.

Dewey, John. "Half-hearted naturalism." *The Journal of Philosophy* 24, no. 3 (1927): 57–64.

Dewey, John. *A common faith*. New Haven: Yale University Press, 1934.

Diallo, Rokhaya. "Why are the 'yellow vests' protesting in France?" *Al Jazeera* (10 December 2018).

Dijksterhuis, Eduard, J. *De mechanisering van het wereldbeeld*. Amsterdam: Meulenhoff, 1950 (English translation: *The mechanization of the world picture*. New York: Oxford University Press, 1961).

Disivestro, Russell. "The ghost in the machine is the elephant in the room: Souls, death, and harm at the end of life." *Journal of Medicine and Philosophy* 57 (2012): 480–502.

Do Ceu Patrão Neves, Maria. "On scientific integrity: Conceptual clarification." *Medicine, Health Care and Philosophy* 21, no. 2 (2018): 181–187.

Domagala, Alicja, Malgorzata M. Bala, Juan Nicolas-Sanchez, Dawid Storman, Mateusz J. Schwierz, Mateusz Kaczmarczyk, and Monika Storman. "Satisfaction of physicians working in hospitals within the European Union: State of the evidence based on systematic review." *European Journal of Public Health* 29, no. 2 (2018): 232–241.

Dove, Edward S., Susan E. Kelly, Federica Lucivero, Mavis Machirori, Sandi Dheensa, and Barbara Prainsack. "Beyond individualism: Is there a place for relational autonomy in clinical practice and research? *Clinical Ethics* 12, no. 3 (2017): 150–165.

Downie, Robin. "Patient and consumers." *Journal of the Royal College of Physicians of Edinburgh* 47 (2017): 261–265.

Duhigg, Charles. "Why are we so angry? The untold story of how all got so mad at one another." *The Atlantic* (January–February 2019): 63–75.

Dumont, Louis. *Essays on individualism. Modern ideology in anthropological perspective*. Chicago and London: The University of Chicago Press, 1992.

Duncan, Grant. "Mind-body dualism and the biopsychosocial model of pain: What did Descartes really say?" *Journal of Medicine and Philosophy* 25, no. 4 (2000): 485–513.

Durkheim, Émile. *The elementary forms of religious life*. Oxford: Oxford University Press, 2001; original in French 1912.

Dworkin, Ronald, *Life's dominion. An argument about abortion and euthanasia*. London: Harper & Collings Publishers, 1993.

The Earth Charter, 2000; https://earthcharter.org/invent/images/uploads/echarter_english.pdf.

Editorial. "Coping with peer rejection." *Nature* 425 (2003): 645.

Editorial. "Physician burnout: A global crisis." *The Lancet* 394, no. 10193 (2019): 93.

Ehrenreich, Barbara. *Natural causes. An epidemic of wellness, the certainty of dying, and killing ourselves to live longer*. New York and Boston: Twelve/Hachette Book Group, 2018.

Elias, Norbert. *The civilizing process. Sociogenetic and psychogenetic investigations*. Malden: Blackwell Publishing, 2017 (revised edition); original 1939.

Ells, Carolyn, Matthew Hunt, and Jane Chambers-Evans. "Relational autonomy as an essential component of patient-centered care." *International Journal of Feminist Approaches to Bioethics* 4, no. 2 (2011): 79–101.

Encyclopedia Brittanica. "Naturalism" (2019); www.britannica.com/topic/naturalism-philosophy.

Engel, George L. "The need for a new medical model: A challenge for biomedicine." *Science* 196, no. 4286 (1977): 129–136.

English, Andrea. "John Dewey and the role of the teacher in a globalized world: Imagination, empathy, and 'third voice'." *Educational Philosophy and Theory* 48 (2016): 1046–1064.

Eriksson, Stefan, and Gert Helgesson. "The false academy: Predatory publishing in science and bioethics." *Medicine Health Care and Philosophy* 20, no. 2 (2017): 163–170.

Evans, Tony. *The politics of human rights. A global perspective*. London and Ann Arbor: Pluto Press, 2005 (2nd edition).

Farmer, Paul, and Nicole Gastineau Campos. "Rethinking medical ethics: A view from below." *Developing World Bioethics* 4 (2004): 17–14.

Federman, Adam. "Revealed: US listed climate activist group as 'extremists' alongside mass killers." *The Guardian* (13 January 2020); www.theguardian.com/environment/2020/jan/13/us-listed-climate-activist-group-extremists.

Feigl, Herbert. *The 'mental' and the 'physical'. The essay and a postscript*. Minneapolis: University of Minneapolis Press, 1967.

Fesmire, Steven. *John Dewey and moral imagination. Pragmatism in ethics*. Bloomington and Indianapolis: Indiana University Press, 2003.

Fevre, Ralph. *Individualism and inequality. The future of work and politics*. Cheltenham and Northampton: Edward Elgar Publishing, 2017.

Figley, Charles R. "The empathic response in clinical practice: Antecedents and consequences." In *Empathy. From bench to bedside*, edited by Jean Decety, 263–273. Cambridge and London: The MIT Press, 2014.

Fins, Joseph J., and James L. Bernat. "Ethical, palliative, and policy considerations in disorders of consciousness." *Neurology* 91, no. 10 (2018): 471–475.

Flew, Annis. "Images, supposing, and imagining." *Philosophy* 28, no. 106 (1953): 246–254.

Ford, Richard Thompson. *Universal rights down to earth*. New York and London: W. W. Norton & Company, 2011.

Foucault, Michel. *The birth of the clinic. An archaeology of medical perception*. New York: Pantheon Books, 1973).

Fox, Maggy. "Fewer Americans believe in God – Yet they still believe in afterlife." *NBC News*, 21 March 2016; www.nbcnews.com/better/wellness/fewer-americans-believe-god-yet-they-still-believe-afterlife-n542966.

Fox, Renée C. *The sociology of medicine: A participant observer's view*. Englewood Cliffs: Prentice Hall, 1989.

Frank, Arthur W. "Why study people's stories? The dialogical ethics of narrative analysis." *International Journal of Qualitative Methods* 1, no. 1 (2002): 109–117.

Frank, Jason R., Linda Snell, and Jonathan Sherbino, eds. *CanMEDS 2015 Physician Competency Framework*. Ottawa: Royal College of Physicians and Surgeons of Canada, 2015; file:///C:/Users/Henk%20ten%20Have/Downloads/canmeds-full-framework-e.pdf.

Franklin, Sarah. "Ethical research – the long and bumpy road from shirked to shared." *Nature* 574, no. 7780 (2019): 627–630.

Freedberg, David. *The power of images. Studies in the history and theory of response*. Chicago and London: The University of Chicago Press, 1989.

Friedman, Milton. "The social responsibility of business is to increase its profits." The *New York Times Magazine* (13 September 1970); http://umich.edu/~thecore/doc/Friedman.pdf.

Friedman, Thomas. "Finding the 'common good' in a pandemic." *New York Times*, 24 March 2020.

Gauchet, Marcel. *The disenchantment of the world. A political history of religion*. Princeton: Princeton University Press, 1997.

Gaudin, Colette. "Preface." In *On Poetic Imagination and Reverie*, Gaston Bachelard. New York: Spring Publications, 2014.

Gawande, Atul. *Being Mortal. Medicine and what matters in the end*. New York: Metropolitan Book/ Henry Holt and Company, 2014.

Gehlen, Arnold. *Man. His nature and place in the world*. New York: Columbia University Press, 1988; original German edition 1974.

Gelhaus, Petra. "The desired moral attitude of the physician: (I) empathy." *Medicine Health Care and Philosophy* 15 (2012): 103–113.

Gelhaus, Petra. "The desired moral attitude of the physician: (II) compassion." *Medicine Health Care and Philosophy* 15 (2012): 397–410.

General Medical Council. *Medical professionalism matters. Report and recommendations*, 2016; www.gmc-uk.org/-/media/documents/mpm-report_pdf-68646225.pdf.

Geppert, Cynthia M. A., and Wayne N. Shelton. "A comparison of general medical and clinical ethics consultations: What can we learn from each other?" *Mayo Clinic Proceedings* 87, no. 4 (2012): 381–398.

Gerhard, E. S. "Schiller's 'Die Götter Griechenlands'." *The German Quarterly* 15, no. 2 (1942): 86–92.

Gerring, John. "Ideology: A definitional analysis." *Political Research Quarterly* 50, no. 4 (1997): 957–994.

Giacino, Joseph T., Douglas I. Katz, Nicholas D. Schiff, John Whyte, et al. "Practice guideline update recommendations summary: Disorders of consciousness." *Neurology* 91, no. 10 (2018): 450–460.

Gintis, Herbert. "Strong reciprocity and human sociality." *Journal of Theoretical Biology* 206 (2000): 169–179.

Gintis, Herbert. *Individuality and entanglement: The moral and material bases of social life*. Princeton and Oxford: Princeton University Press, 2017.

Glannon, Walter. "Tracing the soul: Medical decisions at the margins of life." *Christian Bioethics* 6, no. 1 (2000): 49–69.

Glover, Jonathan. *Humanity. A moral history of the twentieth century*. New Haven and London: Yale University Press, 2012 (2nd edition; 1st edition 1999).

Goddard, Maria. "Competition in healthcare: Good, bad or ugly?" *International Journal of Health Policy and Management* 4, no. 9 (2015): 567–569.

Goetz, Stewart, and Charles Taliaferro, *Naturalism*. Grand Rapids and Cambridge: William B. Eerdmans Publishing Company, 2008.

Gottschalk, Andrew, and Susan A. Flocke. "Time spent in face-to-face patient care and work outside the examination room." *Annals of Family Medicine* 3 (2005): 488–493.

Gowing, Lawrence. *Vermeer*. London: Giles de la Mare Publishers Limited, 1997 (1st edition 1952).

Granovetter, Mark. *Society and economy. Framework and principles*. Cambridge and London: The Belknap Press of Harvard University Press, 2017.

Greaves, David. *Mystery in Western medicine*. Aldershot: Avebury, 1996.

Greene, Jeremy A., and Joseph Loscalzo. "Putting the patient back together – Social medicine, network medicine, and the limits of reductionism." *New England Journal of Medicine* 377 (2017): 2493–2499.

Greisman, H. C. "Disenchantment of the world: Romanticism, aesthetics and sociological theory." *The British Journal of Sociology* 27, no. 4 (1976): 495–507.

Grierson, Jamie, Vikram Dodd, and Peter Walker. "Putting Extinction Rebellion on extremist list 'completely wrong,' says Keir Starmer." *The Guardian* (13 January 2020); www.theguardian.com/environment/2020/jan/13/priti-patel-defends-inclusion-of-extinction-rebellion-on-terror-list.

Grimley, Naomi. "Identity 2016: 'Global citizenship' rising, poll suggests." *BBC News* (28 April 2016); www.bbc.com/news/world-36139904.

Groopman, Jeremy. *How doctors think*. Boston: Houghton Mifflin: Boston, 2007.

Grosby, Steven. "Max Weber, religion, and the disenchantment of the world." *Sociology* 50 (2013): 301–310.

Habermas, Jürgen. "Technology and science as 'ideology'." In *Toward a rational society*, edited by Jürgen Habermas, 81–122. Boston: Beacon, 1970.

Haldar, Antara. "Intrinsic goodness," *Times Literary Supplement* (2 November 2018): 10–11.

Halpern, Jodi. *From detached concern to empathy. Humanizing medical practice*. Oxford and New York: Oxford University Press, 2010.

Halpern, Jodi. "From idealized clinical empathy to empathic communication in medical care." *Medicine Health Care and Philosophy* 17 (2014): 301–311.

Hammond-Browning, Natasha. "When doctors and parents don't agree: The story of Charlie Gard." *Bioethical Inquiry* 14 (2017): 461–468.

Han, Sam. "Disenchantment revisited: Formations of the 'secular' and 'religious' in the technological discourse of modernity." *Social Compass* 62, no. 1 (2015): 76–88.

Hanegraaf, Wouter J. "How magic survived the disenchantment of the world." *Religion* 33 (2003): 357–380.

Hanson, Mark G. "Imaginative ethics – bringing ethical practice into sharper relief." *Medicine, Health Care and Philosophy* 5 (2002): 33–42.

Harding, Jeremy. "Among the gilets jaunes." *London Review of Books* 21 March 2019, 3–11.

Harris, James C. "Towards a restorative medicine – The science of care." JAMA 301, no. 16 (2009): 1710–1712.

Harvey, H. B., and D. F. Weinstein. "Predatory publishing: An emerging threat to the medical literature." *Academic Medicine* 92 (2017): 150–151.

Hauser, David J., and Norbert Schwarz. "Medical metaphors matter: Experiments can determine the impact of metaphors on bioethical issues." *The American Journal of Bioethics* 16, no. 10 (2016): 18–19.

Hayek, Friedrich. *The road to serfdom*. Chicago and New York: University of Chicago Press, 2005.

Heaton, Janet. "The gaze and visibility of the carer: A Foucauldian analysis of the discourse of informal care." *Sociology of Health & Illness* 21, no. 6 (1999): 759–777.

Henderson, Saras, and Alan Petersen, eds. *Consuming health. The commodification of health care*. London and New York: Routledge, 2002.

Henrich, Joseph, Robert Boyd, Samuel Bowles, Colin Camerer, Ernst Fehr, Herbert Gintis, and Richard McElreath. "In search of homo economicus: Behavioral experiments in 15 small-scale societies." *American Economic Review* 91, no. 2 (2001): 73–84.

Hewa, Soma, and Robert W. Hetherington. "Specialists with spirit: Crisis in the nursing profession." *Journal of Medical Ethics* 16 (1990): 179–284.

Hobbs, Jennifer Lynn. "A dimensional analysis of patient-centered care." *Nursing Research* 58, no. 1 (2009): 52–62.

Hojat, Mohammadreza, Salvatore Mangione, Thomas J. Nasca, Susan Rattner, James B. Erdmann, Joseph S. Gonnella, and Mike Magee. "An empirical study of decline in empathy in medical school." *Medical Education* 38 (2004): 934–941.

Holmas, Tor Helge, Egil Kjerstad, Hilde Luras, and Odd Rune Straume. "Does monetary punishment crowd out pro-social motivation? A natural experiment on hospital length of stay." *Journal of Economic Behavior & Organization* 75 (2010): 261–267.

Honenberger, Philip. *Naturalism and philosophical anthropology. Nature, life, and the human between transcendental and empirical perspectives*. Houndmills: Palgrave Macmillan, 2016.

Honneth, Axel. *Disrespect. The normative foundations of critical theory*. Cambridge: Polity Press, 2007.

Hopgood, Stephen. *The endtimes of human rights*. Ithaca: Cornell University Press, 2013.

Horton, Richard. "Rediscovering human dignity." *The Lancet* 364 (2004): 1081–1085.

Howe, David. *Empathy. What it is and why it matters.* London: Palgrave Macmillan, 2013.

Howe, Lauren C., J. Parker Goyer, and Alia J. Crum. "Harnessing the placebo effect: Exploring the influence of physician characteristics on placebo response." *Health Psychology* 36, no. 11 (2017): 1074–1082.

Huang, Sui. "When peers are not peers and don't know it: The Dunning-Kruger effect and self-fulfilling prophecy in peer-review." *Bioessays* 35 (2013): 414–416.

Hunt, Lynn. *Inventing human rights. A history*. New York and London: W. W. Norton & Company, 2007.

Hunter, David J. "The case against choice and competition." *Health Economics, Policy and Law* 4 (2009): 489–501.

Hurwitz, Brian, and Victoria Bates. "The roots and ramifications of narrative in modern medicine." In *The Edinburgh Companion to the Critical Medical Humanities*, edited by Anne Whitehead, Angela Woods, Sarah Atkinson, Jane Macnaughton, and Jennifer Richards, 559–576. Edinburgh: Edinburgh University Press, 2016.

Husserl, Edmund. *Die Krisis der europäische Wissenschaften und die transzendentale Phänomenologie. Eine Einleitung in die phänomenologische Philosophie*. Hamburg: Felix Meiner Verlag, 1977.

Hvistendahl, Mara. "China's publication bazaar." *Science* 342 (2013): 1035–1039.

Ignatieff, Michael. "Human rights as politics and idolatry." In *Human rights as politics and idolatry*, edited by Amy Gutmann, 3–98. Princeton and Oxford: Princeton University Press, 2001.

Ignatieff, Michael. *The ordinary virtues. Moral order in a divided world*. Cambridge: Harvard University Press, 2017.

Illouz, Eva. *Cold intimacies: The making of emotional capitalism*. Cambridge: Polity Press, 2007.

Illouz, Eva. *Saving the modern soul. Therapy, emotions, and the culture of self-help*. Berkeley, Los Angeles and London: University of California Press, 2008.

Ingold, Tom. "Globes and spheres. The topology of environmentalism." In *The perception of the environment. Essays on livelihood, dwelling and skill*, edited by Tom Ingold, 209–218. London and New York: Routledge, 2000.

Intergovernmental Panel on Climate Change, *Global warming of 1.5°C*. Switzerland: IPCC, 2018; https://report.ipcc.ch/sr15/pdf/sr15_spm_final.pdf.

Ironson, Gail, Rick Stuetzle, Dale Ironson, Elizabeth Balbin, Heidemarie Kremer, Annie George, Neil Schneiderman, and Mary Ann Fletcher. "View of God as benevolent and forgiving or punishing and judgmental predicts HIV disease progression." *Journal of Behavioral Medicine* 34 (2011): 414–425.

Irving, Greg, Ana Luisa Neves, Hajira Dambha-Miller, Ai Oishi, Hiroko Tagashira, Anistasiya Verho, and John Holden. "International variations in primary care physician consultation time: A systematic review of 67 countries." *BMJ Open* 7 (2017): e017902; doi:10.1136/bmjopen-2017-017902.

Jackson, Stanley W. "The imagination and psychological healing." *Journal of the History of the Behavioral Sciences* 26 (1990): 345–358.

Jacobson, Kirsten. "A developed nature: A phenomenological account of the experience of home." *Continental Philosophy Review* 42 (2009): 355–373.

Jacobson, N. P. "The problem of civilization." *Ethics* 63, no. 1 (1952): 14–32.

Jacoby, Russell. *The end of utopia. Politics and culture in an age of apathy*. New York: Basic Books, 1999.

Jacoby, Russell. *Picture imperfect. Utopian thought for an anti-utopian age*. New York: Columbia University Press, 2005.

James, William. *Principles of Psychology*. Chicago: University of Chicago: Encyclopaedia Britannica, Inc, 1990; original 1890.

Jantos, Marek, and Hosen Kiat. "Prayer as medicine: How much have we learned?" *Medical Journal of Australia* 186, no. 10 (2007): S51; doi:10.5694/j.1326-5377.2007.tb01041.x.

Jasanoff, Sheila. *Can science make sense of life?* Cambridge: Polity Press, 2019.

Jefferson, T., M. Rudin, F. S. Brodney, and F. Davidoff. "Editorial peer review for improving the quality of reports of biomedical studies." *Cochrane Database of Systematic Reviews* 18, no. 2 (2007): MR000016.

Jelley, Jane. *Traces of Vermeer*. Oxford: Oxford University Press, 2017.

Jenkins, Richard. "Disenchantment, enchantment and re-enchantment: Max Weber at the Millennium." *Max Weber Studies* 1 (2000): 11–32.

Jennings, Bruce. "Reconceptualizing autonomy: A relational turn in bioethics." *Hastings Center Report* 46, no. 3 (2016): 11–16.

Jennings, Bruce, and Angus Dawson. "Solidarity in the moral imagination of bioethics." *Hastings Center Report* 45 (2015): 31–38.

Jewson, Nicholas D. "The disappearance of the sick-man from medical cosmology, 1770–1870." *Sociology* 10, no. 2 (1976): 225–244.

Jha, Kirti Nath. "How to write articles that get published." *Journal of Clinical and Diagnostic Research* 8, no. 9 (2014): XG01–XG03.

Joas, Hans. *The genesis of values*. Cambridge: Polity Press, 2000.

Joas, Hans. *The sacredness of the person. A new genealogy of human rights*. Washington: Georgetown University Press, 2013.

Joas, Hans. *Sind die Menschenrechte westlich?* München: Kösel Verlag, 2015.

Joas, Hans. *Die Macht des Heiligen. Eine Alternative zur Geschichte der Entzaubering*. Berlin: Suhrkamp Verlag, 2017.

Johnson, Mark. *Moral imagination. Implication of cognitive science for ethics*. Chicago and London: The University of Chicago Press, 1993.

Jones, Anne Hudson. "Narrative in medical ethics." *British Medical Journal* 318 (1999): 253–256.

Jors, Karin, Arndt Büssing, Niels Christian Hyidt, and Klaus Baumann, "Personal prayer in patients dealing with chronic illness: A review of the research literature," *Evidence-Based Complementary and Alternative Medicine* 2015; doi:10.1155/2015/927973.

Josephson-Storm, Jason, Ā. *The myth of disenchantment. Magic, modernity, and the death of the human sciences*. Chicago and London: The University of Chicago Press, 2017.

Jung, Carl Gustav. *Modern man in search of a soul*. New York: Harcourt, Brace and Company, 1933.

Kahn, Abraham, and Sarab Sodhi. "Professionalism sans humanism: A body without a soul." *Academic Medicine* 91, no. 10 (2016): 1331–1332.

Kalberg, Stephen. "Max Weber's types of rationality: Cornerstones for the analysis of rationalization processes in history." *American Journal of Sociology* 85, no. 5 (1980): 1145–1179.

Kalberg, Stephen. "Max Weber's sociology of civilizations: The five major themes." *Max Weber Studies* 14, no. 2 (2014): 205–232.

Kaplan, Edward J. "Gaston Bachelard's philosophy of imagination: An introduction." *Philosophy and Phenomenological Research* 33, no. 1 (1972): 1–24.

Kaplan, Robert M. *More than medicine. The broken promise of American health*. Cambridge and London: Harvard University Press, 2019.

Kaplan, Robert M., and Veronica L. Irvin. "Likelihood of null effects of large NHLBI clinical trials has increased over time." *PLoS One* 10, no. 8 (2015): e0132382; https://doi.org/10.1371/journal.pone.0132382.

Kaplan, Robert M., Suzanne Bennett Johnson, and Patricia Clem Kobor. "NIH Behavioral and Social Sciences Research Support: 1980–2016." *American Psychologist* 72, no. 8 (2017): 808–821.

Kaptchuk, Ted J., John M. Kelley, Lisa A. Conboy, Roger B. Davis, et al. "Components of placebo effect: Randomized controlled trial in patients with irritable bowel syndrome." *British Medical Journal* 336 (2008): 999–1003.

Käsler, Dirk. *Max Weber. An introduction to his life and work*. Chicago: The University of Chicago Press, 1988.

Kass, Leon R. "Thinking about the body." *Hastings Center Report* 15, no. 1 (1985): 20–30.

Keane, Webb. *Ethical life. Its natural and social histories*. Princeton and Oxford: Princeton University Press, 2016.

Kearney, Richard. *The wake of imagination. Toward a postmodern culture*. London: Routledge, 2001.

Kearney, Richard. *On stories*. London and New York: Routledge, 2002.

Kearney, Richard, and James Williams. "Narrative and ethics." *Proceedings of the Aristotelian Society, Supplementary Volumes* 70 (1996): 29–61.

Kearns, Robert A., and J. Ross Barnett. "Consumerist ideology and the symbolic landscapes of private medicine." *Health & Place* 3, no. 3 (1997): 171–180.

Kekes, John. "Disgust and moral taboos." *Philosophy* 67 (1992): 431–447.

Kekes, John. *The enlargement of life. Moral imagination at work*. Ithaca and London: Cornell University Press, 2006.

Kelly, Edward F., Adam Crabtree, and Paul Marshall, eds. *Beyond physicalism. Toward reconciliation of science and spirituality*. Lanham, Boulder, New York and London: Rowman & Littlefield, 2015.

Kennedy, Jonathan. "Populist politics and vaccine hesitancy in Western Europe: An analysis of national-level data." *European Journal of Public Health* 29, no. 3 (2019): 512–516.

Keysers, Christian. "Mirror Neurons." *Current Biology* 19, no. 21 (2010): R971–973.

Keyvanara, Mahmoud, Saeed Karimi, Elahe Khorasani, and Marzie Jarfarina Jazi. "Experts' perceptions of the concept of induced demand in healthcare: A qualitative study in Isfahan, Iran." *Journal of Education & Health Promotion* 3, no. 27 (2014); doi:10.4103/2277-9531.131890.

Khullar, Dhruv. "Do you trust the medical profession? A growing distrust could be dangerous to public health and safety." *The New York Times* (23 January 2018); www.nytimes.com/2018/01/23/upshot/do-you-trust-the-medical-profession.html.

Kinkeldey, Otto. "The music of the spheres." *Bulletin of the American Musicological Society* 11/12/13 (1948): 30–32.

Kirschner, Kristin L. "Rethinking and advocacy in bioethics." *American Journal of Bioethics* 1 (2002): 60–62.

Kleinman, Arthur. "Moral experience and ethical reflection: Can ethnography reconcile them? A quandary for 'The new bioethics'." *Daedalus* 128, no. 4 (1999): 69–97.

Kornfield, Donald, S. "What is the role of a clinical ethics consultant?" *The American Journal of Bioethics* 16, no. 3 (2016): 40–42.

Kotsis, Sandra V., and Kevin C. Chung. "Manuscript rejection: How to submit a revision and tips on being a good peer reviewer." *Plastic and Reconstructive Surgery* 133 (2014): 958–963.

Kraft-Todd, Gordon T., Diego A. Reinero, John M. Kelley, Andrea S. Heberlein, Lee Baer, and Helen Riess. "Empathic nonverbal behavior increases ratings of both warmth and competence in a medical context." *PLoS One* 12, no. 5 (2017): e0177758; doi.org/10.1371/journal.pone.0177758.

Kravitz, Richard, L., Peter Franks, Mitchel D. Feldman, Martha Gerrity, Cindy Byrne, and William M. Tierney. "Editorial peer reviewers' recommendations at a general medical journal: Are they reliable and do editors care?" *PLoS One* 5, no. 4 (2010): e10072; doi:10.1371/journal.pone.0010072.

Krupinski, Elizabeth A. "Editorial: Medical image perception: Understanding how radiologists understand images." *Journal of Medical Imaging* 3, no. 1 (2016): 01101; doi:10.1117/1.JMI.3.1.011001.

Kuczewski, Mark G. "The soul of medicine." *Perspectives in Biology and Medicine* 50, no. 3 (2007): 410–420.

Kumar, Pradeep, and Deepak Saxena. "Pandemic of publications and predatory journals: Another nail in the coffin of academics." *Indian Journal of Community Medicine* 41, no. 3 (2016): 169–171.

Lachman, Peter. "Redefining the clinical gaze." *BMJ Quality and Safety* (2013): 1–3; doi:10.1136/bmjqs-2013-002322.

Lakoff, George, and Mark Johnson. *Metaphors we live by*. Chicago and London: The University of Chicago Press, 2003 (1st edition 1980).

Lalonde, Marc. *A new perspective on the health of Canadians. A working document*. Ottawa, 1974; www.phac-aspc.gc.ca/ph-sp/pdf/perspect-eng.pdf.

Landy, Joshua, and Michael Saler, eds. *The re-enchantment of the world. Secular magic in a rational age*. Stanford: Stanford University Press, 2009.

Lanzerath, Dirk, and Minou Friele, eds. *Concepts and values in biodiversity*. London and New York: Routledge, 2014.

Latour, Bruno. "Visualisation and cognition: Drawing things together." In *Knowledge and Society. Studies in the Sociology of Culture Past and Present*, edited by Elizabeth Long and Henrika Kuklick, 1–40. Greenwich: Jai Press, 1986.

Lavely, John H. "What is personalism." *The Personalist Forum* 7, no. 2 (1991): 1–33.

Lederach, John Paul. *The moral imagination. The art and soul of building peace*. New York: Oxford University Press, 2005.

Lee, Eric Austin, and Samuel Kimbriel, eds. *The resounding soul. Reflections on the metaphysics and vivacity of the human person*. Eugene: Cascade Books, 2015.

Lee, Nancy S. "Framing choice: The origins and impact of consumer rhetoric in US health care debates." *Social Science & Medicine* 138 (2015): 136–143.

Lei, Ruipeng, and Renzong Qiu. "Chinese bioethicists: He Jiankui's crime is more than illegal medical practice." *The Hastings Center*, 4 January 2020; www.thehastingscenter.org/chinese-bioethicists-he-jiankuis-crime-is-more-than-illegal-medical-practice/.

Leibowitz, Kari A., Emerson J. Hardebeck, J. Parker Goyer, and Alia J. Crum. "Physician assurance reduces patient symptoms in US adults: An experimental study." *Journal of General Internal Medicine* 33, no. 12 (2018): 2051–2052.

Levinas, Emmanuel. *Totality and Infinity: An essay on exteriority*. Dordrecht: Kluwer Academic Publishers, 1991.

Levitas, Ruth. *Utopia as method. The imaginary reconstruction of society*. Houndmills: Palgrave Macmillan, 2013.

Lindau, Richard L. ". . . And the least of these is empathy." In *Empathy and the practice of medicine. Beyond pills and the scalpel*, edited by Howard M. Spiro, Mary G. McCrea

Curnen, Enid Peschel, and Deborah St. James, 103–109. New Haven and London: Yale University Press, 1993.

Lindeboom, Gerrit A. *Descartes and medicine*. Amsterdam: Rodopi, 1979.

Little, Paul, Hazel Everitt, Ian Williamson, Greg Warner, Michael Moore, Clare Gould, Kate Ferrier, and Sheila Payne. "Observational study of the effect of patient centredness and positive approach on outcomes of general practice consultations." *British Medical Journal* 323, no. 7318 (2001): 908–911.

Livesey, Finbarr. *From global to local. The making of things and the end of globalization*. New York: Pantheon Books, 2017.

Lloyd, G. E. R. *In the grip of disease. Studies in the Greek imagination*. Oxford: Oxford University Press, 2003.

Lorey, Isabell. *Die Regierung der Prekären*. Berlin: Turia + Kant, 2012.

Lortie, Christopher J., Stefano Allesina, Lonnie Aarssen, Olyana Grod, and Amber E. Budden. "With great power comes great responsibility: The importance of rejection, power, and editors in the practice of scientific publishers." *PLoS One* 8, no. 12 (2013): e85382; doi:10.1371/journal.pone.0085382.

Lutz, Mattew, and James Lenman. "Moral naturalism." In *The Stanford Encyclopedia of Philosophy*, edited by Edward N. Zalta (Fall 2018 edition); https://plato.stanford.edu/archives/fall2018/entries/naturalism-moral.

Lynch, Michael. "Discipline and the material form of images: An analysis of scientific visibility." *Social Studies of Science* 15, no. 1 (1985): 37–66.

Lyons, William. *Gilbert Ryle. An introduction to his philosophy*. Brighton: The Harvester Press, 1980.

Lysaught, M. Therese, and Michael McCarthy, eds. *Catholic bioethics and social justice. The praxis of US health care in a globalized world*. Collegeville: Liturgical Press Academic, 2018.

Määttä, Sylvia M. "Closeness and distance in the nurse-patient relation. The relevance of Edith Stein's concept of empathy." *Nursing Philosophy* 7 (2006): 3–10.

Machamer, Peter, Lindley Darden, and Carl F. Craver. "Thinking about mechanisms." *Philosophy of Science* 67, no. 1 (2000): 1–25.

MacIntyre, Alasdair. *After virtue. As study in moral theory*. Notre Dame: University of Notre Dame Press, 1984.

MacIntyre, Alasdair. *Dependent rational animals. Why human beings need the virtues*. London: Duckworth, 1999.

MacIntyre, Alasdair. *Edith Stein. A philosophical prologue, 1931–1922*. Lanham: Rowman & Littlefield Publishers, 2007.

Mackenzie, Catriona, and Natalie Stoljar, eds. *Relational autonomy. Feminist perspectives on autonomy, agency, and the social self*. New York and Oxford: Oxford University Press, 2000.

Major-Kincade, Terri, L., Jon E. Tyson, and Kathleen A. Kennedy. "Training pediatric house staff in evidence-based ethics: An exploratory controlled trial." *Journal of Perinatology* 21 (2001): 161–166.

Mallet, Shelley. "Understanding home: A critical review of the literature." *Sociological Review* 52, no. 1 (2004): 62–89.

Marcel, Gabriel. *Homo viator. Introduction to a metaphysic of hope*. New York: Harper & Row, 1962.

Marcel, Gabriel. "Reply to John E. Smith." In *The philosophy of Gabriel Marcel*, edited by Paul A. Schilpp and Lewis E. Hahn, 350–351. Open Court: La Salle, 1984.

Marcel, Gabriel. *Man against mass society*. South Bend: St. Augustine's Press, 2008; original 1952.

Marchant, Jo. *Cure. A journey into the science of mind over body*. New York: Broadway Books, 2016.

Marcum, James A. "Reflections on humanizing biomedicine." *Perspectives in Biology and Medicine* 51, no. 3 (2008): 392–405.

Margalit, Avishai. *The decent society*. Cambridge and London: Harvard University Press, 1996.

Maritain, Jacques, and John T. FitzGerald. "The person and the common good." *The Review of Politics* 8, no. 4 (1946): 419–455.

Maskulak, Marian. "Edith Stein: A proponent of human community and a voice for social change." *Logos: A Journal of Catholic Thought and Culture* 15, no. 2 (2012): 64–83.

Mauron, Alex. "Is the genome the secular equivalent of the soul?" *Science* 291 (2001): 831–832.

Mauron, Alex. "Renovating the house of being. Genomes, souls, and selves." *Annuals of the New York Academy of Sciences* 1001 (2003): 240–252.

May, Todd. *A decent life. Morality for the rest of us*. Chicago and London: The University of Chicago Press, 2019.

Mazzi, Maria Angela, Michela Rimondini, Wienke G. W. Boerma, Christa Zimmerman, and Jozien M. Bensing. "How patient would like to improve medical consultations: Insights from a multicenter European study." *Patient Education and Counseling* 99 (2016): 51–60.

McBride, L. LeBron. "The relational soul of family medicine." *Family Practice Management* 20, no. 2 (2013): 40.

McCaffrey, Anne M., David M. Eisenberg, Anna T. Legedza, et al. "Prayer for health concerns: Results of a national survey on prevalence and patterns of use." *Archives of Internal Medicine* 164 (2004): 858–862.

McCann, Peter. "Suffering and empathy in the stories of Anton Chekhov and their relevance to healthcare today." *Hektoen International. A Journal of Medical Humanities* 6, no. 1 (2014); https://hekint.org/2017/01/27/suffering-and-empathy-in-the-stories-of-anton-chekhov-and-their-relevance-to-healthcare-today/.

McCullough, Thomas E. *The moral imagination and public life. Raising the ethical question*. Chatham: Chatham House Publishers, 1991.

McElwain, Gregory S. *Mary Midgley. An introduction*. London: Bloomsbury Academic, 2020.

McGuire, Meredith B. "Religion and healing the mind/body/self." *Social Compass* 43 (1996): 101–116; doi:10.1177/003776896043001008.

McKibben, Bill. *Falter. Has the human game begun to play itself out?* London: Wildfire, 2019.

Mead, Margaret. "Towards more vivid utopias." *Science* 126, no. 3280 (1957): 957–961.

Mechanic, David. "Physician discontent. Challenges and opportunities." JAMA 290, no. 7 (2003): 941–946.

Meilaender, Gilbert C. *Body, soul, and bioethics*. Notre Dame: University of Notre Dame Press, 2009; original 1995.

Mickey, Sam. *On the verge of a planetary civilization. A philosophy of integral ecology*. London and New York: Rowman & Littlefield, 2014.

Midgley, Mary. *The ethical primate: Humans, freedom and morality*. London and New York: Taylor & Francis Group, 1994.

Midgley, Mary. "Souls, minds, bodies, and planets." In *The resounding soul. Reflections on the metaphysics and vivacity of the human person*, edited by Eric Austin Lee and Samuel Kimbriel, 175–195. Eugene: Cascade Books, 2015.

Midgley, Mary. *What is philosophy for?* London: Bloomsbury Academic, 2018.

Milanovic, Branko. *Capitalism alone. The future of the system that rules the world*. Cambridge and London: The Belknap Press of Harvard University Press, 2019.

Milbank, John, and Adrian Pabst. *The politics of virtue. Post-liberalism and the human future*. London and New York: Rowman & Littlefield, 2016.

Miles, Andrew, and Juan E. Mezzich. "The care of the patient and the soul of the clinic: Person-centered medicine as an emergent model of modern clinical practice." *The International Journal of Person Centered Medicine* 1, no. 2 (2011): 207–222.

Miles, Nancy O. "The individual in the individualism/communitarianism debate: In defense of personism." *Legon Journal of the Humanities* 29, no. 2 (2018): 241–263.

Miller, Hugh. "DNA blueprints, personhood, and genetic privacy." *Health Matrix. The journal of Law-Medicine* 8, no. 2 (1998): 179–221.

Mills, C. Wright. *The sociological imagination*. Oxford and New York: Oxford University Press, 2000; original 1959.

Mitchell, W. J. T. *What do pictures want? The lives and loves of images*. Chicago and London: The University of Chicago Press, 2005.

Mitzman, Arthur. *The iron cage. An historical interpretation of Max Weber*. New Brunswick and Oxford: Transaction Books, 2005; original 1969.

Moffitt, Benjamin. *The global rise of populism. Performance, political style, and representation*. Stanford: Stanford University Press, 2016.

Mold, Alex. "Repositioning the patient: Patient organizations, consumerism, and autonomy in Britain during the 1960s and 1970s." *Bulleting of the History of Medicine* 87 (2013): 225–249.

Montez, Jennifer Karas, and Mark D. Hayward. "Cumulative childhood adversity, educational attainment, and active life expectancy among U.S. adults." *Demography* 51, no. 2 (2014); 413–435; doi:10.1007/s13524-013-0261-x.

Montgomery, Jeremy. "Bioethics as a governance practice." *Health Care Analysis* 24 (2016): 3–23.

Moore, Jeanne. "Placing *home* in context." *Journal of Environmental Psychology* 20 (2000): 207–217.

Moore, Thomas. *Care of the soul. A guide for cultivating depth and sacredness in everyday life*. New York: HarperCollins Publishers, 1992.

Moore, Thomas. "Does America have a soul?" *Mother Jones* (September–October 1996): 26–32.

Moran, Dermot. "Husserl's transcendental philosophy and the critique of naturalism." *Continental Philosophy Review* 41 (2008): 401–425.

Moreland, James P., and Scott B. Rae. *Body & Soul. Human nature & the crisis in ethics*. Downers Grove: InterVarsity Press, 2000.

Morris, David B. "Narrative medicines: Challenge and resistance." *The Permanente Journal* 12, no. 10 (2008): 88–96.

Morrisey, Clair, and Rebecca L. Walker. "Funding and forums for ELSI research: Who (or What) is setting the agenda?" *AJOB Primary Research* 3, no. 3 (2012): 51–60; doi:10.1080/21507716.2012.678550.

Mortensen, Jonas Norgaard. *The common good. An introduction to personalism*. Wilmington: Vernon Press, 2017.

Mounier, Emmanuel. *Le personalisme*. Paris: Presses Universitaires de France, 1949.

Moustafa, Khaled. "The disaster of the impact factor." *Science and Engineering Ethics* 21 (2015): 139–142.

Moyn, Samuel. *The last utopia. Human rights in history*. Cambridge and London: The Belknap Press of Harvard University Press, 2010.

Moyn, Samuel. *Not enough. Human rights in an unequal world*. Cambridge and London: The Belknap Press of Harvard University Press, 2018.

Mudde, Cas, and Cristobal Rovira Kaltwasser. *Populism. A very short introduction*. Oxford: Oxford University Press, 2017.
Muir, Star A. "The web and the spaceship: Metaphors of the environment." *ETC: A Review of General Semantics* 51, no. 2 (1994): 145–152.
Müller, Jan-Werner. *What is populism?* London: Penguin Books, 2017.
Müller, Jan-Werner. "Populism and the People." *London Review of Books* (23 May 2019): 35–37.
Murdoch, Iris. "Ethics and the imagination." *Irish Theological Quarterly* 52, no. 1–2 (1986): 81–95.
Nagel, Thomas. *Mind and cosmos: Why the materialist Neo-Darwinian conception of nature is almost certainly false*. Oxford: Oxford University Press, 2012.
Nahardani, Seyedah A., Fazlollah Ahmadi, Shoaleh Bigdeli, and Soltani Arabshahi. "Spirituality in medical education: A concept analysis." *Medicine Health Care and Philosophy* 22, no. 2 (2019): 179–189.
Neier, Aryeh. *The international human rights movement. A history*. Princeton and Oxford: Princeton University Press, 2012.
Nelkin, Dorothy. "Molecular metaphors: The gene in popular discourse." *Nature Reviews: Genetics* 2, no. 7 (2001): 555–559.
Nelkin, Dorothy, and Lori Andrews. "Homo economicus. Commercialization of body tissue in the age of biotechnology." *Hastings Center Report* 28, no. 5 (1998): 30–39.
Nelkin, Dorothy, and M. Susan Lindee. *The DNA mystique: The gene as a cultural icon*. New York: W. H. Freeman and Company, 1995.
Neumann, Melanie, Friedrich Edelhäuser, Diethard Tauschel, Martin R. Fischer, Markus Wirtz, Christiane Woopen, Aviad Haramati, and Christian Scheffer. "Empathy decline and its reasons: A systematic review of studies with medical students and residents." *Academic Medicine* 86 (2011): 996–1009.
Newman, John Henry. *Essays and Sketches*, 2. New York, London and Toronto: Longmans, Green and Co, 1948.
Newton, Bruce W., Laurie Barber, James Clardy, Elton Cleveland, and Patricia O'Sullivan. "Is there a hardening of the heart during medical school?" *Academic Medicine* 83, no. 3 (2008): 244–249.
Nie, Jing-Bao, Adam Gilbertson, Malcolm de Roubaix, Ciara Staunton, Anton van Niekerk, Joseph D. Tucker, and Stuart Rennie. "Healing without waging war: Beyond military metaphors in medicine and HIV cure research." *The American Journal of Bioethics* 16, no. 10 (2016): 3–11.
Nitzke, Solvejg, and Nicholas Pethes, eds. *Imagining Earth. Concepts of wholeness in cultural constructions of our home planet*. Bielefeld: Transcript Verlag, 2017; file:///C:/Users/Henk%20ten%20Have/Downloads/1004718.pdf.
NIVEL. *Nederlanders hebben nog steeds veel vertrouwen in de gezondheidszorg*. Utrecht, 27 October 2016; www.nivel.nl/nl/nieuws/nederlanders-hebben-nog-steeds-veel-vertrouwen-de-gezondheidszorg.
Nordgren, Anders. "Ethics and imagination. Implications of cognitive semantics for medical ethics." *Theoretical Medicine and Bioethics* 19 (1998): 117–141.
Nordgren, Lars. "Mostly empty words – what the discourse of 'choice' in health care does." *Journal of Health Organization and Management* 24, no. 2 (2010): 109–126.
Nortjé, Nico, Willem A. Hoffmann, and Jo-Celene De Jongh, eds. *African perspectives on ethics for healthcare professionals*. New York: Springer, 2018.
Nortvedt, Per. "Empathy." In *Encyclopedia of Global Bioethics*, edited by Henk ten Have, 1105–1112, Vol. 2. Switzerland: Springer International Publishing, 2016.

Nuland, Sherwin B. *The soul of medicine. Tales from the bedside*. New York: Kaplan Publishing, 2010.

Nye, Linda S. "The minds' eye. Biomedical visualization: The most powerful tool in science." *Biochemistry and Molecular Biology Education* 32, no. 2 (2004): 123–131.

O'Connell, David. *Louis-Ferdinand Céline*. Boston: Twayne Publishers, 1976.

O'Connell, Paul. "On reconciling irreconcilables: Neo-liberal globalization and human rights." *Human Rights Law Review* 7, no. 3 (2007): 483–509.

Olafson, Frederick A. *Naturalism and the human condition. Against scientism*. London and New York: Routledge, 2001.

O'Leary, Diane. "Why bioethics should be concerned with medically unexplained symptoms." *The American Journal of Bioethics* 18, no. 5 (2018): 6–15.

Papanicolas, Irene, et al. "Health care spending in the United States and other high-income countries." *JAMA* 318 (13 March 2018): 1024–1039.

Papineau, David. "Naturalism." In *The Stanford Encyclopedia of Philosophy*, edited by Edward N. Zalta (Winter 2016 edition); https://plato.stanford.edu/archives/win2016/entries/naturalism.

Parnia, Sam, and Peter Fenwick. "Near death experiences in cardiac arrest: Visions of a dying brain or visions of a new science of consciousness." *Resuscitation* 52 (2002): 5–11.

Peabody, Francis W. "The care of the patient." *JAMA* 88 (1927): 877–882.

Peabody, Francis W. "The soul of the clinic," *JAMA* 90, no. 15 (1928): 1193–1197.

Pedersen, Reidar. "Empathy: A world in sheep's clothing?" *Medicine Health Care and Philosophy* 11 (2008): 325–335.

Pejic, Rade Nicholas. "The symbol of medicine: Aesculapius or Caduceus? *JAMA* 275, no. 16 (1996): 1232.

Pellegrino, Edmund D., and David C. Thomasma, *A philosophical basis of medical practice*. New York: Oxford University Press, 1989.

Perakis, Charles R. "What about the soul?" *Academic Medicine* 88, no. 10 (2013): 1521.

Petsko, Gregory A. "'The blue marble'." *Genome Biology* 12 (2011): 112.

Pew Research Center. "Religious and/or spiritual people say they have a soul" (23 May 2018); www.pewforum.org/2018/05/29/attitudes-toward-spirituality-and-religion/pf_05-29-18_religion-western-europe-05-05/.

Philippon, Thomas. *The great reversal. How America gave up on free markets*. Cambridge and London: The Belknap Press of Harvard University Press, 2019.

The Physicians Foundation, *2018 Survey of America's Physicians. Practice Patterns & Perspectives*. Merritt Hawkins, September 2018; https://physiciansfoundation.org/wp-content/uploads/2018/09/physicians-survey-results-final-2018.pdf.

Pierce, Anne R. *A Perilous Path: The Misguided Foreign Policy of Barack Obama, Hillary Clinton & John Kerry*. New York: Post Hill Press, 2016.

Plato, *Charmides*, 156e–157a; http://classics.mit.edu/Plato/charmides.html.

Plattel, Martin. *Utopie en kritisch denken*. Bilthoven: Amboboeken, 1970.

Plessner, Helmuth. *Levels of organic life and the human. An introduction into philosophical anthropology*. New York: Fordham University Press, 2019; original 1928.

Plotkin, Bill. *Nature and the human soul. Cultivating wholeness and community on a fragmented world*. Novato, CA: New World Library, 2008.

Poirier, Agnès. *Notre-Dame. The soul of France*. London: Oneworld Publications, 2020.

Pope Francis. *Encyclical letter Laudato Si' – On care for our common home*. Rome: Vatican, 2005.

Pope Francis. *Humana Communitas, Letter to the President of the Pontifical Academy for Life*. Vatican City: Libreri Editrice Vaticana, 2019.

Porter, Dorothy. *Health, civilization and the state: A history of public health from ancient to modern times*. London and New York: Routledge, 1999.

Posner, Eric A. *The twilight of human rights law*. Oxford: Oxford University Press, 2014.

Post, Stephen G. "A moral case for nonreductive physicalism." In *Whatever happened to the soul?* edited by Warren S. Brown, Nancy Murphy, and H. Newton Malony, 195–212. Minneapolis: Fortress Press, 1998.

Potter, Van Rensselaer. *Bioethics: Bridge to the future*. Englewood Cliffs: Prentice-Hall, 1971.

Potter, Van Rensselaer. *Global bioethics. Building on the Leopold legacy*. East Lansing: Michigan State University Press, 1988.

Potter, Van Rensselaer. "Moving the culture toward more vivid utopias with survival as the goal." *Global Bioethics* 14, no. 4 (2001): 19–30.

Prescott, Susan L., and Alan C. Logan. "Narrative medicine meets planetary health: Mindsets matter in the Anthropocene." *Challenges* 10, no. 17 (2019); doi:10.3390/challe10010017.

Preston, Jesse Lee, Ryan S. Ritter, and Justin Hepler. "Neuroscience and the soul: Competing explanations for the human experience." *Cognition* 127 (2013): 31–37.

Quinn, Tom. "The death of compassion in Louis-Ferdinand Céline's *Voyage au bout de la nuit*." *Irish Journal of French Studies* 1 (2001): 67–74.

Rabin, Paulinc L. "Francis Peabody's 'The care of the patient'." *JAMA* 252 (1984): 819–820.

Radin, Margaret Jane. *Contested commodities*. Cambridge and London: Harvard University Press, 2001.

Rand, Ayn. *The virtue of selfishness: A new concept of egoism*. New York: Signet/Penguin, 2014.

Ratcliffe, Matthew. "The phenomenology of depression and the nature of empathy." *Medicine Health Care and Philosophy* 17 (2014): 269–280.

Remen, Rachel N. "Recapturing the soul of medicine." *Western Journal of Medicine* 174 (2001): 4–5.

Rich, Nathaniel. *Losing earth. The decade we could have stopped climate change*. London: Picador, 2019.

Richardson, Mary Ann, Tina Sanders, J. Lynn Palmer, Anthony Greisinger, and S. Eva Rosendal, Marianne, Tim C. Olde Hartman, Aase Aamland, Henriette van der Horst, Peter Lucassen, Anna Budtz-Lilly, and Christopher Burton. "'Medically unexplained' symptoms and symptom disorders in primary care: Prognosis-based recognition and classification." *BMC Family Practice* 18, no. 18 (2017); doi:10.1186/s12875-017-0592-6.

Richmond, Caroline. "Dame Cicely Saunders. Founder of the modern hospice movement." *British Medical Journal* 331 (2005): 238.

Ricoeur, Paul. "Imagination in discourse and in action." In *Rethinking imagination. Culture and creativity*, edited by Gillian Robinson and John Rundell, 119–135. London and New York: Routledge, 1994.

Ricoeur, Paul. "Approaching the human person." *Ethical Perspectives* 6, no. 1 (1999): 45–54.

Rifkin, Jeremy. *The empathic civilization. The race to global consciousness in a world in crisis*. Cambridge: Polity Press, 2009.

Rio Declaration on Environment and Development, 1992; www.unesco.org/education/pdf/RIO_E.PDF.

Roberts, Leanne, Irshad Ahmed, and Andrew Davidson. "Intercessory prayer for the alleviation of ill health." *Cochrane Database of Systematic Reviews*, no. 2 (2009). Art. No.: CD000368; doi:10.1002/14651858.CD000368.pub3.

Rogers-Vaughn, Bruce. *Caring for souls in a neoliberal age*. New York: Palgrave Macmillan, 2019.

Rosanvallon, Pierre. *Counter-democracy. Politics in an age of distrust*. Cambridge: Cambridge University Press, 2008.

Rosanvallon, Pierre. *De democratie denken. Werk in uitvoering*. Nijmegen: Uitgeverij Vantilt, 2019.

Rose, Nikolas. *Governing the soul. The shaping of the private self*. London and New York: Free Association Books, 1999 (2nd edition); original 1989.

Roth, Alvin E. "Repugnance as a constraint on markets." *The Journal of Economic Perspectives* 21, no. 3 (2007): 37–58.

Rovisco, Maria. "The indignados social movement and the image of the occupied square: The making of a global icon." *Visual Communication* 16, no. 3 (2017): 337–359.

Royal Dutch Medical Association (KNMG). *Medical Professionalism*. Utrecht: KNMG, 2007.

Rozzi, Ricardo. "Biocultural ethics: Recovering the vital links between the inhabitants, their habits, and habitats." *Environmental Ethics* 34 (2012): 27–50.

Runciman, David. *How democracy ends*. London: Profile Books, 2019.

Rundell, John. "Creativity and judgement: Kant on reason and imagination." In *Rethinking imagination. Culture and creativity*, edited by Gillian Robinson and John Rundell, 88–117. London and New York: Routledge, 1994.

Ryle, Gilbert. *The concept of mind*. Harmondsworth: Penguin Books, 1949.

Sachs, Wolfgang. *Planet dialectics. Explorations in environment and development*. London: Zed Books, 2015.

Sandel, Michael J. *Liberalism and the limits of justice*. Cambridge: Cambridge University Press, 1982.

Sandel, Michael J. *Public philosophy. Essays on morality in politics*. Cambridge, MA and London: Harvard University Press, 2005.

Sandel, Michael J. *What money can't buy. The moral limits of markets*. London: Allen Lane, 2012.

Sandler, Ronald, and Phaedra C. Pezzullo, eds. *Environmental justice and environmentalism. The social justice challenge to the environmental movement*. Cambridge and London: The MIT Press, 2007.

Sarewitz, Daniel. "Saving science." *The New Atlantis* 49 (Spring–Summer 2016): 5–40.

Sayer, Andrew. *Why things matter to people. Social science, values and ethical life*. Cambridge: Cambridge University Press, 2011.

Scaff, Lawrence, A. *Fleeing the iron cage. Culture, politics, and modernity in the thought of Max Weber*. Berkeley, Los Angeles and London: University of California Press, 1989.

Schama, Simon. *Kunstzaken. Over Rembrandt, Rubens, Vermeer en vele andere schilders*. Amsterdam and Antwerpen: Uitgeverij Contact, 1997.

Schei, Edvin, Abraham Fuks, and J. Donald Boudreau. "Reflection in medical education: Intellectual humility, discovery, and know-how." *Medicine Health Care and Philosophy* 22, no. 2 (2019): 167–178.

Schiller, Friedrich. *Die Götter Griechenlands* (1788); www.uni-due.de/lyriktheorie/texte/1788_schiller.html.

Schmidt, Elke Elisabeth. "The dilemma of moral naturalism in Nagel's Mind and Cosmos." *Ethical Perspectives* 25, no. 2 (2018): 203–231.

Schneider, Carl E., and Mark A. Hall. "The patient life: Can consumers direct health care?" *American Journal of Law & Medicine* 35, no. 1 (2009): 7–65.

Schotsmans, Paul. "Personalism in medical ethics." *Ethical Perspectives* 6, no. 1 (1999): 10–20.

Schouten, Jan. *The rod and serpent of Aesculapius: Symbol of medicine*. London: Elsevier Publishing, 1967.

Schram, Sanford F. *The return of ordinary capitalism. Neoliberalism, precarity, occupy*. Oxford: Oxford University Press, 2015.

Schroeder, Ralph. "'Personality' and 'inner distance': The conception of the individual in Max Weber's sociology." *History of the Human Sciences* 4, no. 1 (1991): 61–78.

Schroeder, Ralph. "Disenchantment and its discontents: Weberian perspectives on science and technology." *The Sociological Review* 43, no. 2 (1995): 227–250.

Schwartz, Michael A., and Osborne P. Wiggins. "Psychosomatic medicine and the philosophy of life." *Philosophy, Ethics, and Humanities in Medicine* 5, no. 2 (2010); doi:10.1186/1747-5341-5-2.

Schweitzer, Albert. *The Philosophy of Civilization. Part II. Civilization and ethics*. New York: The Macmillan Company, 1959.

Scruton, Roger. *On human nature*. Princeton and Oxford: Princeton University Press, 2017.

Selâl Şengör, A. M. "Our home, the planet earth." *Diogenes* 39, no. 155 (1991): 25–51.

Sen, Amartya K. "Rational fools: A critique of the behavioral foundations of economic theory." *Philosophy & Public Affairs* 6, no. 4 (1977): 317–344.

Shamseer, L., D. Moher, O. Maduekwe, L. Turner, V. Barbour, R. Burch, J. Clark, J. Galipeau, J. Roberts, and B. J. Shea. "Potential predatory and legitimate biomedical journals: Can you tell the difference? A cross-sectional comparison." *BMC Medicine* 15 (2017): 28; doi:10.1186/s12916-017-0785-9.

Shapiro, Johanna. "The use of narrative in the doctor-patient encounter." *Family Systems Medicine* 11, no. 1 (1993): 47–53.

Shapiro, Johanna. "(Re)examining the clinical gaze through the prism of literature." *Families, Systems and Health* 20, no. 2 (2002): 161–170.

Shapiro, Johanna. "The paradox of teaching empathy in medical education." In *Empathy. From bench to bedside*, edited by Jean Decety. Cambridge and London: The MIT Press, 2014, 275–290.

Sheikh, Anees A. ed. *Imagination and healing*. Farmingdale, NY: Baywood Publishing Company, 1984.

Sheikh, Anees A. ed. *Healing images. The role of imagination in health*. Amityville, NY: Baywood Publishing Company, 2003.

Sherry, Patrick. "Disenchantment, re-enchantment, and enchantment." *Modern Theology* 25 (2009): 369–386.

Shuman, Joel James. "Re-enchanting the body: Overcoming the melancholy of anatomy." *Theoretical Medicine and Bioethics* 39 (2018): 473–481.

Siedentop, Larry. *Inventing the individual. The origins of Western liberalism*. Cambridge: The Belknap Press of Harvard University Press, 2014.

Sikkink, Kathryn. *Evidence for hope. Making human rights work in the 21st century*. Princeton and Oxford: Princeton University Press, 2017.

Silver, Lee M. "Biotechnology and conceptualizations of the soul." *Cambridge Quarterly of Healthcare Ethics* 12 (2003): 335–341.

Silvers, Stuart. "Nonreductive naturalism." *Theoria: An International Journal for Theory, History and Foundations of Science* 12, no. 1 (1997): 163–184.

Sinsky, Christine, Lacey Colligan, Ling Li, Mirela Prgomet, San Reynolds, Lindsey Goders, Johanna Westbrook, Michael Tutti, and George Blike. "Allocation of physician time in ambulatory practice: A time and motion study in 4 specialties." *Annals of Internal Medicine* 165 (2016): 753–760.

Slaby, Jan. "Empathy's blind spot." *Medicine Health Care and Philosophy* 17 (2014): 249–258.

Smajdor, Anna, Andrea Stöckl, and Charlotte Salter, "The limits of empathy: Problems in medical education and practice." *Journal of Medical Ethics* 37, no. 6 (2011): 380–383.

Smith, Adam. *An Inquiry into the Nature and Causes of the Wealth of Nations*. Edited by S. M. Soares. Amsterdam: Meta Libri Digital Library, 2007; original 1776, II.ii.2; www.ibiblio.org/ml/libri/s/SmithA_WealthNations_p.pdf.

Smith, Roch C. *Gaston Bachelard. Philosopher of science and imagination*. Albany: SUNY Press, 2016 (1st edition 1982).

Smith, Sandy G. "The essential qualities of a home." *Journal of Environmental Psychology* 14 (1994): 31–46.

Soares, Conceição. "The philosophy of individualism: A critical perspective." *International Journal of Philosophy & Social Values* 1, no. 1 (2018): 11–34.

Song, Fujian, Yoon Loke, and Lee Hooper. "Why are medical and health-related studies not being published? A systematic review of reasons given by investigators." *PLoS One* 9, no. 10 (2014): e110418; doi:10.1371/journal.pone.0110418.

Sontag, Susan. *Illness as metaphor & Aids and its metaphors*. London: Penguin Books, 1991.

Sowell, Thomas. *Basic economics. A common sense guide to the economy*. New York: Basic Books, 2015 (5th edition).

Spencer, John. "Decline in empathy in medical education: How can we stop the rot?" *Medical Education* 38, no. 9 (2004): 916–918.

Sperling, Daniel. "(Re)disclosing physician financial interests: Rebuilding trust or making unreasonable burdens on physicians?" *Medicine Health Care and Philosophy* 20, no. 2 (2017): 179–186.

Spiro, Howard M., Mary G. McCrea Curnen, Enid Peschel, and Deborah St. James, eds. *Empathy and the practice of medicine. Beyond pills and the scalpel*. New Haven and London: Yale University Press, 1993.

Sposato, Luciano A., Bruce Ovbiagle, S. Claiborne Johnston, Marc Fisher, and Gustavo Saposnik. "A peek behind the curtain: Peer review and editorial decision making at *Stroke*." *Annals of Neurology* 76 (2014): 151–158.

Sridhar, Devi. "Health policy: From the clinical to the economic gaze." *The Lancet* 378 (2011): 1909.

Stahl, Devan. "Patient reflections on the disenchantment of techno-medicine." *Theoretical Medicine and Bioethics* 39 (2018): 499–513.

Stegenga, Jacob. *Medical nihilism*. Oxford: Oxford University Press, 2018.

Stein, Edith. *On the problem of empathy*. Washington: ICS Publications, 1989 (3rd edition); original 1917.

Steinhauser, Karen E., Nicholas A. Christakis, Elizabeth C. Clipp, Maya McNeilly, Lauren McIntyre, and James A. Tulsky. "Factors considered important at the end of life by patient, family, physicians, and other care providers." *JAMA* 284, no. 19 (2000): 2476–2482.

Stent, Gunther. "That was the molecular biology that was." *Science* 160, no. 3826 (1968): 390–395.

Stewart, Moira. "Towards a global definition of patient centred care: The patient should be the judge of patient centred care." *British Medical Journal* 322, no. 7284 (2001): 444–445.

Stoljar, Daniel. *Physicalism*. London and New York: Routledge, 2010.

Stoljar, Daniel. "Physicalism." In *The Stanford Encyclopedia of Philosophy*, edited by Edward N. Zalta (Winter 2016 edition); https://plato.stanford.edu/archives/win2017/entries/physicalism.

Stone, Neil J. "Critical confidence and the three C's: Caring, communicating, and competence." *The American Journal of Medicine* 119 (2006): 1–2.

Straus, Erwin W., and Michael A. Machado. "Gabriel Marcel's notion of incarnate being." In *The philosophy of Gabriel Marcel*, edited by Paul A. Schilpp and Lewis E. Hahn, 123–155. Open Court: La Salle, 1984.

Strech, Daniel, Matthis Synofzik, and Georg Marckmann. "Systematic review of empirical bioethics." *Journal of Medical Ethics* 34 (2008): 471–477.

Strong, Kimberley A., Wendy Lipworth, and Ian Kerridge. "The strengths and limitations of empirical bioethics." *Journal of Law and Medicine* 18, no. 2 (2010: 316–319.

Stroud, Joanne H. *Gaston Bachelard. An elemental reverie on the world's stuff*. Dallas: The Dallas Institute of Humanities and Culture, 2015.

Stuurman, Siep. *The invention of humanity. Equality and cultural difference in world history*. Cambridge and London: Harvard University Press, 2017.

Sulmasy, Daniel P. *The rebirth of the clinic. An introduction to spirituality in health care*. Washington: Georgetown University Press, 2006.

Svenaeus, Fredrik. *Phenomenological bioethics. Medical technologies, human suffering, and the meaning of being alive*. London and New York: Routledge, 2018.

Swinburne, Richard. *The evolution of the soul*. Oxford: Clarendon Press, 1997 (revised edition; 1st edition 1986).

Swinburne, Richard. *Are we bodies or souls?* Oxford: Oxford University Press, 2019.

Tai-Seale, Ming, Cliff W. Olson, Jinnan Li, Albert S. Chan, Criss Morikawa, Meg Durbin, Wei Wang, and Harold S. Luft. "Electronic health record logs indicate that physicians split time evenly between seeing patients and desktop medicine." *Health Affairs* 36, no. 4 (2017): 655–662.

Taliaferro, Charles. "The virtues of embodiment." *Philosophy* 76, no. 295 (2001): 111–125.

Tarzian, Anita, Lucia D. Wocial, and the ASBH Clinical Ethics Consultation Affairs Committee. "A code of ethics for health care ethics consultants: Journey to the present and implications for the field." *American Journal of Bioethics* 15, no. 5 (2015): 38–51.

Taylor, Charles. *Modern social imaginaries*. Durham and London: Duke University Press, 2004.

Teding van Berkhout, Emily, and John M. Malouff. "The efficacy of empathy training: A meta-analysis of randomized controlled trials." *Journal of Counseling Psychology* 63, no. 1 (2016): 32–41.

The Telegraph. "Most people believe in life after death, study finds" (13 April 2009); www.telegraph.co.uk/news/religion/5144766/Most-people-believe-in-life-after-death-study-finds.html.

Ten Have, Henk. "Medicine and the Cartesian image of man." *Theoretical Medicine* 8 (1987): 235–246.

Ten Have, Henk. "The anthropological tradition in philosophy of medicine." *Theoretical Medicine* 16 (1995): 3–14.

Ten Have, Henk. "The need and desirability of an (Hippocratic) Oath or Pledge for scientists." In *New perspectives in academia*, edited by Jüri Engelbrecht and Johannes J. F. Schroots, 19–30. Amsterdam: KNAW; ALLEA Biennial Yearbook 2006, 2007.

Ten Have, Henk. *Global bioethics. An introduction*. London and New York: Routledge, 2016.

Ten Have, Henk. *Vulnerability. Challenging bioethics*. London and New York: Routledge, 2016.

Ten Have, Henk. "The fundamental role of education." In *Equal beginnings, but then? A global responsibility*, edited by Vincenzo Paglia and Renzo Pegoraro, 63–80. Rome: Pontifical Academy for Life, 2019.

Ten Have, Henk. *Wounded planet. How declining biodiversity endangers health and how bioethics can help*. Baltimore: Johns Hopkins University Press, 2019.

Tessman, Lisa. *Moral failure. On the impossible demands of morality*. New York: Oxford University Press, 2015.

Tessman, Lisa. *When doing the right thing is impossible*. New York: Oxford University Press, 2017.

Tetlock, Philip E. "Thinking the unthinkable: Sacred values and taboo cognitions." *Trends in Cognitive Sciences* 7, no. 7 (2003): 320–324.

Thatcher, Margaret. Interview for the Sunday Times (7 May 1988); www.margaretthatcher.org/document/104475.

Thibodeau, Paul H., Cynthia McPherson Frantz, and Matias Berretta. "The earth is our home: Systemic metaphors to redefine our relationship with nature." *Climatic Change* 142, no. 1 (2017): 287–300.

Titmuss, Richard M. *The gift relationship: From human blood to social policy*. London: Allen and Unwin, 1970.

Tivnan, Edward. *The moral imagination. Confronting the ethical issues of our day*. New York: Simon & Schuster, 1995.

Tolstoy, Leo. *The death of Ivan Ilyich*, chapter IV; www.classicallibrary.org/tolstoy/ivan/index.htm.

Tomes, Nancy. *Remaking the American patient. How Madison Avenue and modern medicine turned patients into consumers*. Chapel Hill: The University of North Carolina Press, 2016.

Tooze, Adam. "Democracy and its discontents." *The New York Review of Books* (6 June 2019): 52–57.

Trappenburg, Margo J. "Active solidarity and its discontents." *Health Care Analysis* 23 (2015): 207–220.

Trotter, Gregory A. "Toward a non-reductive naturalism: Combining the insights of Husserl and Dewey." *William James Studies* 12, no. 1 (2016): 19–35.

Turner, Denys. *Thomas Aquinas. A Portrait*. New Haven and London: Yale University Press, 2013.

UK Human Rights Blog. "UK not doing enough to combat human trafficking and domestic slavery" (28 November 2012); https://ukhumanrightsblog.com/2012/11/28/uk-not-doing-enough-to-combat-human-trafficking-and-domestic-slavery/.

UNESCO. *Recommendation on science and scientific researchers*, 2017; https://unesdoc.unesco.org/ark:/48223/pf0000263618.

United Nations, General Assembly, Seventieth session. Extreme poverty and human rights (4 August 2015); https://documents-dds-ny.un.org/doc/UNDOC/GEN/G16/088/20/PDF/G1608820.pdf?OpenElement.

Van der Schee, Evelien. *Public trust in health care. Exploring the mechanisms*. Utrecht: NIVEL, 2016.

Van Lommel, Pim. *Consciousness beyond life. The science of the near-death experience*. New York: HarperCollins, 2010.

Van Lommel, Pim, Ruud van Wees, Vincent Meyers, and Ingrid Elfferich. "Near-death experience in survivors of cardiac arrest: A prospective study in the Netherlands." *The Lancet* 358 (2001): 2039–2045.

Van Nuland, Sonya, and Kem A. Rogers. "Academic Nightmares: Predatory publishing." *Anatomical Sciences Education* (December 2016); doi:10.1002/ase.1671.

Van Oudenhove, Lukas, and Stefan Cuypers, "The philosophical 'mind-body problem: And its relevance for the relationship between psychiatry and the neurosciences." *Perspectives in Biology and Medicine* 53, no. 4 (2010): 545–557.

Van Oudenhove, Lukas, and Stefan Cuypers. "The relevance of the philosophical 'mind-body problem' for the status of psychosomatic medicine: A conceptual analysis of the biopsychosocial model." *Medicine Health Care and Philosophy* 17 (2014): 201–213.

Van Peursen, Cees A. *Feiten, waarden, gebeurtenissen. Een deiktische ontologie*. Kampen: J. H. Kok N.V, 1972.

Van Peursen, Cornelis A. *Lichaam – ziel – geest. Inleiding tot een fenomenologische antropologie*. Utrecht: Erven J. Bijleveld, 1970 (4th edition).

Van Ruler, Han. "Minds, forms, and spirits: The nature of Cartesian disenchantment." *Journal of the History of Ideas* 61, no. 3 (2000): 381–395.

Van Tellingen, C. "About hearsay – or reappraisal of the role of the anamnesis as an instrument of meaningful communication." *Netherlands Heart Journal* 15, no. 10 (2007): 359–362.

Vellenga, Sipco J. "Longing for health. A practice of religious healing and biomedicine compared." *Journal of Religion and Health* 47, no. 3 (2008): 326–337.

Vest, Matthew Vest, and Ashley Moyse. "Understanding modern, technological medicine: Enchanted, disenchanted, or other?" *Theoretical Medicine and Bioethics* 39 (2018): 407–417.

Vidal, Fernando. *The sciences of the soul: The early modern origins of psychology*. Chicago and London: Chicago University Press, 2011.

Villegas, Robert. *Individualism*. Self-published, USA, 2015.

Vintzileos, A. M., C. V. Ananth, A. O. Odibo, S. P. Chauban, J. C. Smulian, and Y. Oyelese. "The relationship between a reviewer's recommendation and editorial decision of manuscripts submitted for publication in obstetrics." *American Journal of Obstetrics & Gynecology* 211 (2014): 703.e1–5.

Von Mises, Ludwig. *Human action: A treatise on economics*. Auburn: Ludwig von Mises Institute, 1998; original 1949; https://mises.org/sites/default/files/Human%20Action_3.pdf.

Von Weizsäcker, Viktor. "Medizin, Klinik und Psychoanalyse." In *Zwischen Medizin und Philosophie*, edited by Viktor von Weizsäcker and Dieter Wyss. Göttingen: Vandenhoeck & Ruprecht, 1957; original 1928.

Von Weizsäcker, Viktor. "Psychosomatische Medizin." In *Zwischen Medizin und Philosophie*, edited by Viktor von Weizsäcker and Dieter Wyss. Göttingen: Vandenhoeck & Ruprecht, 1957; original 1949.

Wagner, Steven J., and Richard Wagner, eds. *Naturalism. A critical appraisal*. Notre Dame: University of Notre Dame, 1993.

Wallace-Wells, David. *The uninhabitable earth. A story of the future*. London: Penguin Books, 2019.

Walsham, Alexandra. "The reformation and 'the disenchantment of the world' reassessed." *The Historical Journal* 51, no. 2 (2008): 497–528.

Walt, Vivienne. "France's yellow vests straitjacket Macron." *Time* (17 December 2018): 8.

Walter, Jennifer K., and Lainie Friedman Ross. "Relational autonomy: Moving beyond the limits of isolated individualism." *Pediatrics* 133 (2014): S16–S23.

Wangmo, Tenzin, and Veerle Provoost. "The use of empirical research in bioethics: A survey of researchers in twelve European countries." *BMC Medical Ethics* 18 (2017): 79; doi 10.1186/s12910-017-0239-0.

Warnock, Mary. *Imagination*. Berkeley and Los Angeles: University of California Press, 1978.

Watson, James. *DNA. The secret of life*. New York: Alfred A. Knopf, 2003.

Weber, Max. "Science as a vocation." *Daedalus* 87, no. 1 (1958): 111–134.

Weber, Max. *Gesammelte Afsätze zur Wissenschaftlehre*. Edited by J. Winckelmann. Tübingen: J. C. B. Mohr (Paul Siebeck), 1968 (3rd edition).

Weber, Max. *Gesamtausgabe*. Tübingen: J. C. B. Mohr (Paul Siebeck), 1984, I/15.

Weber, Max. *The Protestant ethics and the 'spirit' of capitalism and other writings*. New York: Penguins Books, 2002.

Wellcome Global Monitor 2018. *How does the world feel about science and health?* London: Wellcome, 2019; https://wellcome.ac.uk/sites/default/files/wellcome-global-monitor-2018.pdf.

Whatley, Shawn D. "Borrowed philosophy: Bedside physicalism and the need for a *sui generis* metaphysic of medicine." *Journal of Evaluation of Clinical Practice* 20 (2014): 961–964.

Widdershoven, Guy, Tineke Abma, and Bert Molewijk. "Empirical ethics as dialogical practice." *Bioethics* 23, no. 4 (2009): 236–248.

Wiley, Lindsay F. "The struggle for the soul of public health." *Journal of Health Politics, Policy and Law* 41, no. 6 (2016): 1083–1096.

Williams, Oliver F., ed. *The moral imagination. How literature and films can stimulate ethical reflection in the business world*. Notre Dame: The University of Notre Dame Press, 1997.

Williams, Thomas D., and Jan Olof Bengtsson, "Personalism." In *The Stanford Encyclopedia of Philosophy*, edited by Edward N. Zalta (Winter 2018); https://plato.stanford.edu/archives/win2018/entries/personalism.

Wilson, David, and William Dixon. *A history of Homo Economicus. The nature of the moral in economic theory*. London and New York: Routledge, 2012.

Wispé, Lauren. "The distinction between sympathy and empathy: To call forth a concept, a word is needed." *Journal of Personality and Social Psychology* 50, no. 2 (1986): 314–321.

Wolf, Gunter. "Portrayal of negative qualities in a doctor as a potential teaching tool in medical ethics and humanism: *Journey to the End of Night* by Louis-Ferdinand Céline." *Postgraduate Medical Journal* 82 (2006): 154–156.

Woods, Philip, A. "Rationalisation, disenchantement and re-enchantement. Engaging with Weber's sociology of modernity." In *The Routledge International Handbook of the Sociology of Education*, edited by Michael W. Apple, Stephen J. Ball, and Luis Amando Gandin, 121–131. London and New York: Routledge, 2010.

Wootton, David. *Bad medicine. Doctors doing harm since Hippocrates*. Oxford: Oxford University Press, 2007.

World Health Organization. "Ten threats to global health in 2019"; www.who.int/emergencies/ten-threats-to-global-health-in-2019.

World Medical Association. *Declaration of Helsinki* (2013); www.wma.net/policies-post/wma-declaration-of-helsinki-ethical-principles-for-medical-research-involving-human-subjects/.

Wright, Terrence C. "Phenomenology and the moral imagination." *Logos: A Journal of Catholic Thought and Culture* 6 (2003): 104–121.

Yang, Wei. "Research integrity in China." *Science* 342 (2013): 1019.

Yarmolinsky, Rachel. "Ethics for ethicists? The professionalization of clinical ethics consultation." *AMA Journal of Ethics* 18, no. 5 (2016): 506–513.

Young, Richard A., Sandra K. Burge, Kaparaboyna A. Kumar, Jocelyn M. Wilson, and Daniela F. Ortiz. "A time-motion study of primary care physicians' work in the electronic record era." *Family Medicine* 50, no. 2 (2018): 91–99.

Zahavi, Dan. *Subjectivity and selfhood. Investigating the first-person perspective*. Cambridge and London: The MIT Press, 2005.

Zahavi, Dan, and Søren Overgaard. "Empathy without isomorphism: A phenomenological account." In *Empathy. From bench to bedside*, edited by Jean Decety, 3–20. Cambridge and London: The MIT Press, 2014.

Zahurek, Rothlyn P. "Intentionality: The matrix of healing creates caring, healing presence." *Beginnings (American Holistic Nurses' Association)* (April 2014): 6–9.

Zhang, Joy Y. *The cosmopolitanization of science. Stem cell governance in China*. Houndmills: Palgrave Macmillan, 2012.

Zuger, Abigal. "Dissatisfaction with medical practice." *The New England Journal of Medicine* 350 (2004): 69–75.

Zukier, Henri. "The soul in medicine: Rabbinic and scientific controversies." *Journal of Religion and Health* 55 (2016): 2174–2188.

Zweig, Stefan. *Die Welt von Gestern. Erinnerungen eines Europäers*. London and Stockholm: Hamish-Hamilton and Bermann-Fischer Verlag AB, 1942.

# Index